MANAGING YOUR HEALTH

MANAGING YOUR HEALTH

STRATEGIES FOR LIFELONG GOOD HEALTH

Peter A. Gross, M.D.; Jonathan L. Halperin, M.D.;
Mack Lipkin, Jr., M.D.; Joan H. Marks, M.S.;
Richard S. Rivlin, M.D.; Thomas N. Wise, M.D.;
Constance Grzelka; and the Editors of
Consumer Reports Books

Consumer Reports Books
A Division of Consumers Union
Yonkers, New York

The ideas, procedures, and suggestions contained in this book are not intended to replace the services of a physician. All matters regarding your health require medical supervision, and you should consult a physician before adopting any procedures in this book. Any application of the treatments set forth herein are at the reader's discretion, and neither the authors nor the publisher assume any responsibility or liability therefor.

Library of Congress Cataloging-in-Publication Data
Managing your health : strategies for lifelong good health / Peter A. Gross . . . [et al.].
p.   cm.
Includes bibliographical references and index.
ISBN 0–89043–438–7 (HC)
1. Health.   I. Gross, Peter A.
RA776.M255 1991
613—dc20   90–23293
CIP
Rev.

Design by GDS / Jeffrey L. Ward
First printing, April 1991
Manufactured in the United States of America

Figure 1 on page 108 reprinted courtesy of American Cancer Society, Inc., from the brochure "Personal Touch," copyright 1987.

The sections "Warning Signs of a Heart Attack" and "Warning Signs of a Stroke" (pages 67 and 73) are taken from *1990 Heart and Stroke Facts* by the American Heart Association. Copyright © 1989 by the American Heart Association. Reproduced with permission.

Guidelines on page 41 are taken from Position Stand, "The Recommended Quantity and Quality of Exercise for Developing and Maintaining Cardiorespiratory and Muscular Fitness in Healthy Adults," *Medicine and Science in Sports Exercise* 22:2 (1990), pp. 265–274. Copyright © 1990 by the American College of Sports Medicine.

Chart on page 8 by Benedict Carey. Excerpted from *In Health* magazine. Copyright © 1990.

Managing Your Health is a Consumer Reports Book published by Consumers Union, the nonprofit organization that publishes *Consumer Reports,* the monthly magazine of test reports, product Ratings, and buying guidance. Established in 1936, Consumers Union is chartered under the Not-for-Profit Corporation Law of the State of New York.

The purposes of Consumers Union, as stated in its charter, are to provide consumers with information and counsel on consumer goods and services, to give information on all matters relating to the expenditure of the family income, and to initiate and to cooperate with individual and group efforts seeking to create and maintain decent living standards.

Consumers Union derives its income solely from the sale of *Consumer Reports* and other publications. In addition, expenses of occasional public service efforts may be met, in part, by nonrestrictive, noncommercial contributions, grants, and fees. Consumers Union accepts no advertising or product samples and is not beholden in any way to any commercial interest. Its Ratings and reports are solely for the use of the readers of its publications. Neither the Ratings nor the reports nor any Consumers Union publications, including this book, may be used in advertising or for any commercial purpose. Consumers Union will take all steps open to it to prevent such uses of its materials, its name, or the name of *Consumer Reports.*

Contents

Acknowledgments

Special thanks to Diane Goetz and Faith Hamlin for helping to launch this project; to Linda Piccirilli, R.N., for serving as a discerning test audience and offering constructive criticism; to Nellie Grzelka, for her unfailing support; and to the editors of Consumer Reports Books, especially Julie Henderson and Sarah Uman.

MANAGING YOUR HEALTH

Introduction

For the last few decades, Americans have hopped on and off the health bandwagon. After hearing so many mixed messages about what to eat, how many miles to run, and how to achieve peace of mind, many have thrown up their hands, thoroughly confused and frustrated.

Not surprisingly, the old idea of moderation, balance, and responsibility still seems the most realistic and sound approach to good health and to a good life. *Managing Your Health* stresses those health habits and practices that are known to work, and helps *you* choose what is best for your individual needs. The health care marketplace is overloaded with products, services, and fraudulent claims. It's up to you to take the responsibility to sort through the conflicting wealth of information and make your choices—always in conjunction with your doctor's advice, of course.

A Working Partnership

Each of us has an individual health profile that's influenced by our genes, personal risk factors, environment, age, habits, and luck. Of all these factors, your heredity and your life-style habits are the most important. There's not much we can do about our genes, but we can modify our diet and exercise habits, and avoid those practices that are known

1

to be potentially dangerous, such as smoking, drinking alcohol, taking drugs, and not wearing seat belts when we drive.

The belief that we must take personal responsibility for our health is increasingly gaining recognition. A 1981 report from the surgeon general of the United States clearly stated: "You, the individual, can do more for your own health and well-being than any doctor, any hospital, any drugs, any exotic medical devices." In 1989 a panel of medical experts, known collectively as the U.S. Preventive Services Task Force, released its recommendations on the appropriate use of preventive medicine in a clinical setting. The group's final report cited all the personal health practices that lead to overall good health and compared them to yearly batteries of screening tests for early disease detection. It is the contention of the Task Force that good personal health habits are a more likely route to a long, healthy life, and that education and counseling by physicians is more valuable in the long run to patients than performing blood cell counts or chest X rays.

What does this mean to the average medical consumer? Simply that if doctors are cast as educators, patients will be expected to take an active role in maintaining their own health. In a sense, you will form a partnership with your physician and work on ways to improve your day-to-day health maintenance. You will be expected to ask questions, read up on your particular problem, and take the responsibility to inquire about possible courses of treatment. As an official at the U.S. Office of Disease Prevention and Health Promotion remarked, "The days of the doctor just lecturing to the patient are gone. One of the important messages that emerges from the Task Force recommendations is that of a new attitude—a shifting of control from the doctor to the patient."

The Task Force recommendations on how to do this are stated throughout *Managing Your Health*.

How to Use This Book

Managing Your Health contains eight chapters, each divided into sections dealing with basic issues of interest to a wide range of health care consumers. Each chapter has been written under the supervision and guidance of a leading physician or expert, and all the material has received a peer review for accuracy and currency.

Chapter 1 looks at the growing interest in preventive medicine and explains how the recently released Task Force recommendations can affect your future medical care. A chart is included for you to use in planning your periodic health checkups based on your own personal risk factors.

Chapter 2 covers diet, nutrition, and exercise. Special attention is given to food labeling, health claims, and weight control.

Chapter 3 gives you the latest information on taking care of your heart. *Chapter 4* covers the important issue of sex and sexuality, including the role of contraceptives, fertility, and sexually transmitted diseases.

The mind and the brain are the focus of *Chapter 5*. You'll learn how to recognize and deal with stress, depression, and anxiety. *Chapter 6* is about growing older—something we would all like to do well. This chapter gives a look at what to expect, what to be concerned about, and how you can continue to look and feel well through the years ahead of you.

Chapter 7 is a major section of the book and deals with the most common health complaints—causes, symptoms, diagnosis, treatment, and prevention. Some of these problems subside on their own with self-care; others require medical attention. This chapter will help you decide when professional care is needed.

To use all this information effectively, you have to know how to use the health care system wisely. *Chapter 8* offers practical advice on choosing a health care plan and a doctor, advises you on what questions to ask, and suggests how best to communicate with health personnel for optimum results.

Managing Your Health is as reliable and accurate as we can make it. We hope it helps you to understand and recognize the vital importance of your participation in your own health care. Your life may depend on it.

1

A Dose of Preventive Medicine

Mack Lipkin, Jr., M.D.

Americans are a reasonably healthy and hardy population and most of us want to stay that way. Occasionally, we hear about medical scientists who would like to extend the human life span, but for the most part, the majority of us are focused on our own present health and hopeful that we'll be able to maintain it as we grow older. Now, we have more to go on than hope.

Each year in this country billions of dollars are spent treating a myriad of diseases and debilitating conditions. But only about 3 percent of this total is used to teach people *prevention*—how to avoid all these diseases and conditions. Well aware of this, the Department of Health and Human Services created the U.S. Preventive Services Task Force in 1984 to come up with recommendations on what doctors can do to promote the idea of prevention in medical care.

After a four-year evaluation of more than 169 medical interventions and procedures to prevent 60 different illnesses and conditions, the Task Force published its findings in 1989 as the *Guide to Clinical Preventive Services*. The recommendations take a different tack from what most doctors are used to providing, yet sound a lot like what most patients want.

Task Force chairman Robert S. Lawrence, M.D., director of the Division of Primary Care at Harvard Medical School, calls the guide an "operational blueprint" for doctors.

The guide urges doctors to see themselves as special consultants who can motivate their patients to change patterns of personal behavior— smoking, substance abuse, or a sedentary life-style—that are destructive to good health. The hope is that doctors can help patients acquire the attitudes and skills to make important life-style changes, thus leaving patients in control of their own health decisions.

Simple talk aimed at patient education is one of the most effective health-maintenance services a doctor can offer. But this aspect of prevention requires more than just talk. It also involves recognizing obstacles to change and helping the patient overcome them, getting the patient to make a commitment to the needed change, and then designing a behavior modification plan for the patient.

The publication of these guidelines for doctors marks the first attempt to develop standards for the practice of preventive medicine. Persuading doctors to use the guidelines and strategies would help lower the demand for those costly tests and treatment regimens that do not promise some health benefit. In the end, however, the doctor who works in a free-market economy will respond most directly to the demands of his or her own patients. Just as your doctor has a responsibility to educate you about things he or she knows will improve your prospects for remaining healthy, you have a responsibility to educate your doctor about the fact that you expect him or her to provide such information.

Unfortunately, preventive care isn't often covered by insurance or by government agencies that deliver health services. Because patients are forced to pay for this kind of health benefit out of their own pockets, and doctors don't get reimbursed by insurers, it's a seriously underutilized health strategy.

The unwillingness of most third-party payers to cover preventive health-care services stems from the argument that there have never been enough solid data demonstrating the effectiveness of prevention. But the Task Force report now presents more than enough proof, especially in regard to cardiovascular disease and cancer.

Periodic Examinations

The traditional rationale for the annual physical checkup may be faltering, but it's not completely out. Nor should it be. The only part of the periodic physical that should be counted out is the performance of a set battery of head-to-toe tests every year.

Even if you're well, it's important to see your doctor for a periodic checkup. The visit should include a review of your general health, your present life-style, and your risk factors. Based on these findings, your doctor may then prescribe certain specific tests.

A good way to view health examinations is to see them as part of a long-term plan for your personal preventive health care. This plan entails your getting checked at the appropriate intervals for the problems for which you are at risk.

The intervals vary with each individual. It's reasonable, for example, to have your blood pressure checked at least every two years. If you're a woman over 40, an annual clinical breast examination is recommended. If you're a sexually active woman, then it's advisable to have a Pap smear every one to three years. (If two consecutive tests have been normal, Pap smears can be done every three years.) A woman 50 or over should receive mammography testing every one or two years and more frequently if there is a family history of breast cancer. And blood cholesterol levels should be monitored every five years. You don't need any other routine tests unless you're in a risk group for a particular health problem.

Once you're aware of your individual risk profile, you ought to create a lifetime (or at least a long-term) health screening plan based on the appropriate guidelines. (See chart on page 8.)

Having a family history of certain problems might affect both the frequency of your checkups and the kind of tests you receive at these times. Some of these family problems might be genetic diseases, such as sickle cell disease, thalassemia, hemophilia, cancer, or polyps of the colon.

Certain other risk factors increase your need for regular checkups, such as: acute or chronic illness, exposure to an infectious agent, occupational exposure to toxins, personal stresses, environmental hazards, or life-style factors.

To benefit the most from these recommendations, it's important to develop a strong relationship with your doctor. Now that a physician's role is changing to include patient education and counseling on health behavior, you and your doctor should be able to get to know each other well.

Basic Checkup Plan

Instead of going for a traditional annual physical examination and receiving a battery of broad-scale disease detection tests, the emphasis now is on your *personal risk profile*. The tests in the following chart are important for everyone—whether you have symptoms or not. Your doctor should obtain a detailed and complete health history to determine whether you are at increased risk for conditions that require additional tests or more frequent monitoring.

The age level suitability and timing of some of these tests remains controversial. The following recommendations are based on the findings of the U.S. Preventive Services Task Force and are not meant to set a standard for individual care.

When to Check Up on Yourself

For most healthy adults, the classic head-to-toe annual physical is a thing of the past. But there are certain tests you should have routinely, even if you have no symptoms. Your doctor will know if there are any special tests that you need in addition to these.

TEST	AGE			
	20 to 29	30 to 39	40 to 49	50 and over
Blood Pressure	Every 2 years*	Every 2 years*	Every 2 years*	Every 2 years*
Cholesterol	—	Once between 35 and 39	Every 4 to 5 years*	Every 4 to 5 years to age 65*
Pap Smear	Every 1 to 3 years**	Every 1 to 3 years**	Every 1 to 3 years**	Every 1 to 3 years to age 70**
Breast Exam	Every 2 to 3 years***	Every 2 to 3 years***	Annually	Annually
Mammography	—	—	Once around 40***	Every 1 to 2 years
Fecal Occult Blood	—	—	—	Every 1 to 2 years

*More often if person is overweight, a smoker, or has a family history of heart disease.

**More often if woman takes the pill, has been exposed to DES, has multiple sex partners, or has a family history of cervical cancer.

***More often if woman has a family history of breast cancer.

Self-Awareness

The technological advances of the last few decades have resulted in scores of tests capable of checking out all the nooks and crannies of the human body. But they can't replace the intuitive wisdom of the body. Learn how to listen for messages that come to you in the form of a lingering pain, a sense of discomfort, or a sudden change in any of your body's routines that cannot be attributed to outside causes. Unfortunately, many disorders produce no signs or symptoms. High blood pressure and osteoporosis are two of these "silent" but dangerous or debilitating diseases. But many other serious diseases and disorders have early warning signs that are specific for that illness. Symptoms that we all should be aware of include

- weight loss of more than 10 pounds for no explicable reason over a period of two to three months
- a thickening or lump that appears under the skin
- a sore in the mouth or on the skin that doesn't heal after a few weeks
- any change in the color, shape, or size of a mole or skin blemish. Such changes also include bleeding and a change in texture
- a recurrent headache accompanied by vomiting, but without any feeling of nausea
- brief loss of consciousness—fainting—for no apparent reason. Or fainting followed by numbness and tingling in parts of the body, confusion, blurred vision, and difficulty speaking
- sudden changes in vision, including new sensitivity to bright light, blurry vision, the appearance of flashing lights or black dots, or the sudden loss of part or all of the field of vision
- a growing difficulty in swallowing that may or may not have rapid weight loss as a companion symptom
- a persistent cough, hoarseness, or loss of voice
- shortness of breath that is severe and progressive
- swollen ankles accompanied by gradually increasing shortness of breath
- coughing up blood or blood in the phlegm or sputum
- vomiting red blood or dark clumps of blood that look like coffee grounds
- recurrent pain in the upper abdomen with appetite loss and weight loss. Recurring pain in the lower abdomen with a change in bowel habits
- a change in bowel habits—especially going from a state of regularity to constipation or diarrhea
- a change in the appearance of bowel movements. Black and tarry bowel movements may indicate blood in the stool. Pale-colored bowel movements could point to other disorders

- passing urine that is pink, red, cola-colored, or brownish
- bleeding from the rectum (other than hemorrhoidal bleeding)
- painful urination
- abnormal discharge from the penis or vagina
- swelling of one testicle without any accompanying pain
- irregular vaginal bleeding that may occur between normal menstrual cycles or following the cessation of periods during menopause

Many subtle changes reflect gradual declines in function that are a normal part of the aging process (see Chapter 6). There are also times when minor symptoms can respond to rest or over-the-counter remedies. When to take symptoms seriously enough to seek medical advice is a decision each of us must make on our own, taking into account the type, intensity, frequency, and onset of symptoms, and our own personalities. If you tend to be generally cautious about things, trust your body. If you tend to let things go, listen to your body, but then add an extra measure of caution, so that if you err it will be on the safe rather than the sorry side.

Whenever the changes are not subtle but pronounced, it is sensible to consult your doctor before attempting to treat yourself.

Talking to Your Doctor

When you consult a physician for your symptoms, don't let fear, pride, shame, or embarrassment get in the way. Your feelings, concerns, and any facts that relate to the problem are important and may help in the diagnosis and treatment.

A large part of the solution to your problem may depend on your close observation of the symptoms. A concrete, down-to-earth description of what you feel will be much more helpful than a few well-chosen technical words.

When you describe your problem to the doctor, be sure to include

- when the symptoms first began to bother you
- the order in which your symptoms appeared. Which symptom occurred first?
- the area of the body in which the pain or changes have occurred
- exactly how the symptoms felt when they began. Was it a stabbing pain? A squeezing pain? A scorching sensation? A jolt—as if you were struck on the head from behind? A tingling? Did any other symptoms occur?
- how intense the symptoms were when they first appeared

- how often the symptoms occur. Are they constant or just occasionally troublesome?
- what seems to trigger the symptoms and how long each episode lasts. Mention any treatments you have received for these or similar symptoms in the past.
- what actions seem to make a symptom better or worse
- a brief description of any changes in your life-style that may have occurred around the time the problem first began to bother you.

What You Can Do on Your Own

It's trite but true that those who have good health take it for granted. Yet the body suffers abuse every day, whether from inhaling pollutants, living with nonstop stress, or eating fatty foods. Although the body has its own repair system for many kinds of damage, the system has its limits. Subjected to enough abuse, even the hardiest constitution finally gives in to sickness. A little kindness toward your body—such as eating nutritious food, exercising regularly, getting adequate rest, and maintaining a positive attitude—can go a long way in holding off disease.

You can't eliminate or neutralize external agents such as disease-causing microbes or invisible toxic materials that may enter your body, disrupt normal cell growth, and cause cancerous changes. But you can eliminate those bad habits of your own that promote disease and shorten your life expectancy. Smoking is one of the most lethal. And lack of exercise is next.

Smoking

One telephone survey of 13,013 adult smokers found that people who quit smoking on their own are twice as successful as those who participate in organized smoking cessation programs. Most of the people who quit on their own used the "cold turkey" method. The cold-turkey quitters were considered less likely to relapse than smokers who gradually decreased their daily total of cigarettes or switched to a lower-tar or lower-nicotine cigarette.

This is not to say that organized smoking cessation programs aren't useful. They serve a real need among heavier smokers (those who smoke more than 25 cigarettes a day), many of whom are unable to quit on their own.

Relapse is a common problem. The odds of succeeding on your first try are somewhere around one in five. But you can expect to do better when you try again. It often takes six or seven tries before you learn some helpful behavioral technique, boost your motivation, benefit from how you went astray last time, and eventually become sick and tired of not quitting. The good news is: you can quit. The bad news remains the same: it is not easy and you have to be persistent.

Many smokers who make the decision to stop set a specific quit date. When that date arrives, so do nicotine withdrawal symptoms. Some smokers have minimal symptoms while others experience irritability, headaches, insomnia, sudden shifts of mood, anxiety, and difficulty concentrating. These symptoms usually last about a week or so. Cravings for nicotine continue for a longer time—in some cases, for years. First- and second-time quitters especially are likely to experience cravings at parties or social occasions where they were used to lighting up.

Quitting with Assistance

Getting formal help to quit smoking may include learning behavior modification techniques at a stop-smoking clinic or getting a prescription for nicotine gum or a medication.

How effective are these methods? Every form of therapy and every program claims its own success rate. Because these success rates may reflect the anecdotal experience of participants, rather than data developed in a scientifically based followup study, don't be unduly impressed or swayed by them.

Organized programs.   These programs can range from a free lecture at a hospital or community center to an eight-week program that either requires a nominal fee or costs a few hundred dollars. These programs emphasize behavior modification techniques, using a buddy or support system to help you when you feel an urge to smoke, and aversion therapy. They are usually sponsored by such organizations as the American Lung Association, the American Cancer Society, the American Heart Association, Smokers Anonymous, the General Council of Seventh-Day Adventists, local Y's, community centers, and some commercial services.

The programs usually attract heavy smokers, who seem to gain the most help from aggressive quitting techniques. (If you find that these organized programs are beyond your financial means, ask these organizations for any free self-help materials.)

Nicotine gum.   This gum contains enough nicotine to raise your blood level to the amount you'd get from smoking half a cigarette. As you chew the gum, it's absorbed into your bloodstream through the mucus lining of your mouth. When nicotine gum is used in combination with other stop-smoking methods, it may help you quit without undergoing nicotine withdrawal symptoms or at least diminish them.

Nicotine gum is usually reserved for heavy smokers and is not meant to be used longer than three to six months. The gum's cost and taste keep most users within the recommended usage time. However, a small percentage of users do manage to get hooked on the gum.

Medications.   Certain drugs are under investigation for their potential to assist heavy smokers in quitting. One such drug is clonidine (Catapres), an antihypertensive drug that has been used to treat alcohol and opiate withdrawal symptoms.

In a 1988 report published in *The Journal of the American Medical Association*, a team of investigators who analyzed 39 controlled studies determined which characteristics of smoking cessation programs are associated with higher success rates. They found that there is no single cessation technique or method that can make the difference. Instead, *reinforcement* of the value of nonsmoking is what counts—in a clear, consistent, and repeated message. Similarly, it appears that withholding or withdrawing reinforcement contributes to relapse.

One discouraging factor for some people is that weight gain is common in those who stop smoking. The increase is related to a nervous tendency to eat more after quitting, as well as to a slowdown in the body's metabolic rate that follows the removal of nicotine.

So if you're planning to quit and don't want to gain weight, devise a strategy in advance of your quit date. It will be necessary to consume fewer calories and to exercise more after quitting. Choose fresh fruit and raw vegetable snacks over high-fat, high-calorie foods. Regular physical activity of any type, such as a brisk walk every day, can help keep off the pounds.

It's a struggle, but a few weeks after you stop using nicotine, you will be able to tell the difference in terms of easier breathing and an improved sense of taste and smell. Most important, your risk of heart disease from smoking begins to decline, and after a few years, your heart and lungs should return to their presmoking state of health.

Passive Smoking

When a cigarette, cigar, or pipe is lit, the smoke it produces releases more than 4,000 chemicals into the air. About 200 of these substances are poisons, such as carbon monoxide, arsenic, DDT, and formaldehyde.

The burning tobacco is the source of two kinds of smoke: mainstream and sidestream. Mainstream smoke is that smoke inhaled or puffed by the smoker. When it is exhaled, nearby nonsmokers are exposed to the mainstream smoke. Sidestream smoke rises directly from the burning end of the cigarette, cigar, or pipe. Sidestream smoke is thought to be more of a health hazard for the nonsmoker than mainstream smoke because it has higher concentrations of irritating compounds, gases, and carcinogens.

Involuntary or passive smoking—being in breathing range of a lit cigarette in an enclosed area—has long been thought to be a serious health risk, but the data were not sufficient to prove it. Now, after years of studies and epidemiologic reviews, researchers see a clear association between the inhalation of secondhand smoke and diseases of the heart, blood vessels, and lungs.

Healthy nonsmokers who live with smokers have a 30 percent higher risk of dying from heart disease than other nonsmokers. The risk increases with the number of cigarettes smoked in the environment in which the nonsmoker lives.

Passive smoking can decrease heart function because the secondhand smoke reduces the amount of oxygen going to the heart. Biochemical changes that result from involuntarily inhaling smoke also are believed to adversely affect the stickiness of blood platelets and thus promote heart attacks.

Children of parents who smoke have a higher incidence of upper and lower respiratory problems and middle ear infections than children whose parents are nonsmokers.

The risk of developing lung cancer from regular exposure to passive smoking also appears to exist. A draft report of the Environmental Protection Agency released in 1990 concluded that passive smoke causes more than 3,800 lung cancer deaths each year.

The clinical effects of passive smoking on the development of the fetus during pregnancy have not been studied widely enough to give us a complete picture of the damage done. However, a pregnant woman who smokes has an increased risk of such complications as a low-birthweight infant, miscarriage, stillbirth, retarded growth, infant respiratory distress syndrome, and sudden infant death syndrome.

Exercise

Subsidizing the Sedentary

Americans appreciate the role of physical activity in maintaining health, but only about 10 percent exercise regularly enough to collect any health dividends.

It seems to be part of the American credo that inactivity is a personal choice affecting only the person who opts for the sedentary route. But that's not the case. Researchers have tallied up how much the rest of society pays to subsidize one person's sedentary habits. They computed the additional costs of higher medical bills, increased premiums for health-insurance coverage, sick-leave pay, disability insurance, and lost productivity on the job. Their final determination: society—meaning all of us—pays a $1,900 yearly subsidy for each sedentary person. Scientists say that by encouraging exercise, we all can end up saving money as well as preserving our national health.

2

Diet, Nutrition, and Exercise

Richard S. Rivlin, M.D.

Eating—long considered one of the simpler pleasures of life—is getting more complicated and less pleasurable, as many Americans wonder whether the food they consume is beneficial or dangerous to their health. The truth is, although we're inundated with dietary advice in the marketplace, much of it is inaccurate.

Any one of us would be hard put to recognize a nutrient if we saw one, but we all know good food. The problem is making choices about which foods to eat to get the nutrients we need.

By knowing the kind and amount of food you need for basic health maintenance and how to control total fat, saturated fat, cholesterol, and sodium in your diet, you can write your own meal ticket for healthy—and enjoyable—eating.

One of the reasons we pay so little attention to our eating habits is that the results aren't usually apparent until many years later. Some of the leading causes of death in the United States are associated with diet, especially coronary artery disease, cancer, and stroke. More than 40 million Americans are obese—at least 20 percent above their ideal weight. Obesity is a risk factor for hypertension and diabetes mellitus as well as for other disorders, such as osteoarthritis and gallbladder disease. Osteoporosis, constipation, diverticulitis, and tooth decay are also linked with nutritional factors.

Sadly, Americans waste billions of dollars a year in their search for the elusive holy grail of "miracle" nutrition and weight control. Food faddists, vitamin pushers, and quick-weight-loss promoters rely on fear and questionable claims to sell their products and services. Quacks claim to have the answer while scientific investigators readily admit that many unanswered questions remain. Knowing this, it's a better bet to be familiar with accepted dietary guidelines and use them to make your choices. They don't come with a guarantee, but they offer the best advice that nutritional science has to offer at the present time.

How to Eat

The food you eat—or your diet—provides a steady flow of nutrients to your body. The science of nutrition is concerned with what happens to the food you eat and how your body processes those nutrients and uses them for cell maintenance and growth.

Because it's more practical—and more interesting—to plan a meal in terms of food instead of nutrients, you don't have to know the intricacies of nutritional science to eat well. But you do need to have a working knowledge of which nutrients are available in the foods you eat.

Despite the many kinds of food, there are only three main categories—protein, carbohydrates, and fats—which are called *macronutrients* because the human body requires sizable quantities of each group every day. Vitamins and minerals—or *micronutrients*—are needed in very small quantities to help your body process nutrients and to help regulate several body functions.

In 1989, the National Research Council, an arm of the National Academy of Sciences, published *Diet and Health,* a comprehensive review of the latest scientific evidence on nutrition and health. The report offers sound dietary advice with specific recommendations on which foods are best emphasized, decreased, or eliminated to help avoid chronic diseases.

The advice is as follows for healthy adults and children:

• *Fat.* Reduce total fat intake to 30 percent or less of your total calories. Cut *saturated* fats to less than 10 percent of calories.

• *Cholesterol.* Keep your intake to less than 300 milligrams daily. (To reduce your consumption of both fat and cholesterol, substitute fish, poultry without skin, lean meats, and low- or nonfat dairy products for fatty meats and whole milk dairy products. Limit most oils, fats, egg yolks, and fried and other fatty foods.)

• *Vegetables and fruits.* Eat five or more servings (half-cup each) of vegetables and fruits every day, especially green and yellow vegetables and citrus fruits.

• *Starches and complex carbohydrates.* Eat six or more half-cup servings of a combination of breads, cereals, and legumes every day.

• *Protein.* Maintain a moderate level of intake, no more than two three-ounce servings of lean meat a day. As a rule of thumb, protein intake should be no more than 1.6 grams (1 ounce = 28 grams) per day per kilogram (2.2 pounds) of an adult's body weight.

• *Weight.* Balance your food intake and physical activity to maintain appropriate body weight.

• *Alcohol.* Alcohol isn't recommended. But if you do drink, limit your consumption to less than one ounce of pure alcohol a day. This equals two cans of beer, two small glasses of wine, or two average-sized cocktails. Pregnant women should avoid alcohol altogether.

• *Salt.* Limit your total daily intake to 6,000 milligrams or less, with a goal of 4,500 milligrams a day. (Remember: Salt, or sodium chloride, is about 40 percent sodium. That works out to a range of 2,400 milligrams of sodium for the top figure and 1,800 milligrams for the low number.)

• *Calcium.* Consume low- or nonfat dairy products and dark-green vegetables.

• *Dietary supplements.* Avoid taking supplements in excess of the Recommended Dietary Allowance (see following) in any one day. To obtain the recommended level of nutrients, eat a variety of foods.

• *Fluoride.* Maintain an optimal intake (by drinking fluoridated water), especially during childhood when the teeth are forming and growing.

The RDAs: Nutritional Guidelines

To help guide the American population toward making the best possible choices, nutritional scientists designed a list of guidelines called *Recommended Dietary Allowances,* or RDAs. The first RDA report, prepared by the National Academy of Sciences, appeared in 1943, and has since been revised periodically to incorporate new scientific data. The RDAs are used primarily by nutritionists who plan menus for large groups of people and by manufacturers developing new food products.

It's important to note that the RDAs are simply guidelines, not requirements or minimums. These standards for individual nutrient intake are generous and are intentionally set higher than most people need on a daily basis. In setting each RDA, scientists estimate the range of normal human needs, select a number at the high end of the range, and add a safety factor for each nutrient. Nearly all healthy people can meet the RDA requirements by eating a varied and well-balanced diet.

The Food and Drug Administration uses a different set of RDAs to formulate the standards used for nutritional labeling on food products. These guidelines, known as the United States Recommended Daily Allowances, or USRDAs, give the percentages of protein and certain vitamins and minerals. The USRDAs are intended for use by four general groups: pregnant or lactating women, infants up to one year old, children under age four, and adults and children over age four.

The most recent RDA report (1989) recommended higher levels of calcium for adolescents and young adults up to age 25. The new level is 1,200 milligrams daily. The change is based on scientific evidence that bone mass continues to build in young adults until at least age 25. Those who build calcium-rich bones early in life may be less vulnerable to the damage of the bone-thinning disease osteoporosis in their later years.

A newly issued RDA was targeted to smokers. The panel increased the recommended intake of vitamin C to 100 milligrams daily for smokers, but left it at 60 milligrams for nonsmokers. This revision was based on data that shows that a person smoking half a pack of cigarettes a day or more depletes the supply of vitamin C 40 percent more than do nonsmokers. Taking vitamin C in extra amounts will not protect you from the cancer and heart disease caused by smoking.

Two nutrients gained RDA status: vitamin K and selenium. Vitamin K, found in leafy vegetables, assists in blood clotting. Selenium, an element present in seafood, meat, and grains, aids in inactivating dangerous chemical oxidants.

Some RDAs were reduced, including those for iron in adolescent and premenopausal women (from 18 milligrams to 15 milligrams), folate, vitamin B_6, and vitamin B_{12}.

There is now a minimum recommendation for sodium. The council specifies a minimum sodium requirement of 500 milligrams a day for adults 18 and older.

The Macronutrients

Proteins

Protein is the raw material your tissues need to build, maintain, and replace the cells in your body. The hormones and enzymes that regulate various body processes are also derived from protein. When you consume too much protein, the excess either gets burned up as part of your body's fuel supply or turns into body fat. The material from which protein is made isn't a single substance but a group of 22 amino acids, all of which play a part in your body's metabolism. Your body produces some of these amino acids, but it must get the others from the food you eat.

To refill your supply of essential amino acids, you can choose from complete proteins, such as eggs, milk, meat, fish, or cheese. If your diet emphasizes incomplete proteins, you can combine complementary foods to make a complete protein. Some examples include rice and beans, or combining a small amount of animal protein with a larger quantity of grains, beans, peas, or nuts and seeds.

A growing body of scientific evidence indicates that too much protein may pose some health risks. A diet high in meat can increase the risk of certain cancers and coronary heart disease. Excess protein intake is also thought to have a role in the accelerated aging of the kidneys. You don't have to stop eating meat, but keep your protein intake at moderate levels.

Carbohydrates

Carbohydrates are the body's main source of energy. There are two kinds of carbohydrates. The easily digested form—known as simple carbohydrates—is found in fruit, honey, and sugar and generally provides quick energy. The second type—the complex carbohydrates—takes longer to digest and thus delivers energy more slowly.

Foods containing complex carbohydrates have traditionally been considered the staples of life: grains, potatoes, pasta, rice, beans, barley, oats, and corn. These foods, commonly called the *starches,* are digestible. A second category of complex carbohydrates—the *fibers*—cannot be digested. Dietary fiber comes from the outer layer of cereal grains and from the fibrous parts of vegetables, fruits, and legumes. Fiber is considered essential for the healthy operation of your gastrointestinal system.

In countries and cultures where plant foods are the main source of meals, the risk of coronary artery disease is far lower than in the United States. Dietary fiber appears to play a protective role against cancer of the colon and rectum, as well as such disorders as diabetes, diverticulosis, and hypertension. Because scientific evidence on fiber remains inconclusive, the best advice is to increase your consumption of all types of complex carbohydrates with an eye on variety and moderation.

Fats

Fats are a group of various highly concentrated substances that don't mix with water. Dietary fats are carriers for fat-soluble vitamins. If there were no fat in the diet, it could eventually lead to a vitamin deficiency. Some fats are crucial for maintaining the structure of each cell in your body and producing hormones. While fats are essential to good nutrition, they are beneficial only when you consume certain types in limited amounts.

Several fats fall into a group of oily substances, some of which bear such familiar names as cholesterol, saturated and unsaturated fat, and triglycerides. There are three kinds of dietary fat, all of which affect your health differently:

Saturated fat raises your cholesterol level. Butter, lard, and meat drippings contain mostly saturated fats. Most of these saturated fats, which remain solid at room temperature, come from animal sources. The only exceptions are such tropical plant oils as coconut oil and palm kernel oil, which are liquid at room temperature.

Besides butter, some obvious sources of saturated fat are whole milk, cheese, and meat. Saturated fats also appear in hidden form as hydrogenated fats in many products—which means that hydrogen was added to harden the vegetable oils used in the food item to extend its shelf life. Other sources of saturated fats are fried foods, some commercial baked goods, and fat-laden spreads and dressings. Most health experts recommend that you limit your daily intake of saturated fats to less than 10 percent of your calories.

Monounsaturated fat gets its name from its molecular structure. It contains two fewer hydrogen atoms than saturated fat and, by virtue of being one step removed from saturated status, monounsaturated fat merits a place on the recommended list. Olive oil and canola oil are excellent sources of monounsaturated fat. Some studies have suggested that use of monounsaturated fat can help lower the level of so-called bad cholesterol.

Polyunsaturated fat has even less hydrogen than monounsaturated fat and helps lower cholesterol in the bloodstream. Polyunsaturated fat remains liquid at room temperature. Good sources include safflower oil, sunflower oil, corn oil, and soybean oil.

There are two types of polyunsaturated fats: *omega-6* oils, which are common in safflower, sunflower, corn, and soybean oil, and *omega-3* oils, found in cold-water seafish, such as mackerel and salmon.

When fat is added to food, it imparts flavor and a feeling of satisfaction after a meal. But excess fat in the diet can also lead to obesity, coronary artery disease, and an increased risk of certain cancers.

Your body needs only a small amount of fat to survive. Although it is recommended that you keep your fat intake to 30 percent or less of calories, evidence suggests that further reductions may be beneficial. One type of fat that your body requires is linoleic acid—an unsaturated fat that the body cannot produce itself. This essential fatty acid can be obtained from the omega-6 oils in your diet—corn, safflower, soybean, and sunflower oils.

Fat from food—whether it's of animal or plant origin, saturated or polyunsaturated—is absorbed by your body at the rate of 9 calories per gram. If you don't burn up the fat you take in, it goes into storage. Carbohydrate and protein when burned yield only 4 calories a gram and tend to burn off more rapidly. Alcohol is relatively caloric at 7 calories per gram and can be a significant source of calories in heavy drinkers.

Most food packaging labels tell you the breakdown of fat in grams. To estimate the number of calories derived from fat in any product, multiply the grams of fat listed on the product by 9. If you come up with a number that equals more than a third of the total calories listed, the food has a fairly high fat content and should be offset in your total daily diet by other low-fat meals or products.

The average American's fat intake is 40 to 45 percent a day, far higher than the recommended level of 30 percent.

Cholesterol

Cholesterol is a lipid—or insoluble fatty substance—that your body manufactures to build the outer membrane of each of your cells as well as certain hormones. Because it doesn't mix with water, cholesterol cannot travel alone. To gain passage through the bloodstream, cholesterol combines into little packages with high-density lipoproteins (HDL, or so-called good cholesterol), low-density lipoproteins (LDL, or bad cholesterol), or very-low-density lipoproteins (VLDL).

Animal foods contain cholesterol as a naturally occurring substance; you find some cholesterol in everything from beef, pork, lamb, veal, chicken, and fish to dairy products and eggs. A prudent diet contains no more than 300 milligrams of cholesterol a day.

The amount and the kind of cholesterol in your blood are a reflection of the fats you eat. But as always, there are exceptions to the rule. Some people can feast on high-fat foods and still have acceptable cholesterol levels, while others trim their fat intake to the bare minimum without achieving any significant decrease in blood cholesterol. And many premenopausal women with elevations in their cholesterol levels still remain relatively safe because their HDL ("good") cholesterol levels are at work protecting their arteries.

Research has provided much evidence about the association between diet, cholesterol, and heart disease. A very high level of blood cholesterol increases the risk of coronary artery disease in the group most studied—men between ages 25 and 55. The higher the cholesterol, the greater the risk. A very low cholesterol level does not carry any risk by itself.

Although some individuals feel that the cholesterol issue has been exaggerated, the consensus is that a high-cholesterol diet is unhealthy. While we await definitive answers in the cholesterol controversy, it's best to take a prudent course: be familiar with the cholesterol and saturated-fat content of foods and apply this knowledge to your food choices.

Triglycerides

Triglycerides are fatty substances that are found in food and in your body, especially in the bloodstream. Most body fat occurs in the form of triglycerides, which contain three fatty acids—saturated, monounsaturated, and polyunsaturated fat. Although unproven, elevated levels of triglycerides in the blood are believed to play a role in coronary artery disease. A diet that emphasizes cold-water seafish containing omega-3 polyunsaturated fatty acids can be somewhat effective in reducing blood triglyceride levels and may have other health benefits as well.

Controlling Cholesterol

To decrease saturated fats in your diet

- Read labels on food packages. Don't look only for cholesterol content. Look for saturated or hidden fats. This especially applies to commercially baked goods such as cakes, pies, cookies, doughnuts, crackers, and chips.
- Replace butter with vegetable oil. Use canola, corn, sunflower, safflower, soybean, and olive oil in food preparation. Avoid hydrogenated soybean or cottonseed oil.
- Use skim or low-fat (1 percent) milk.
- Shun products containing palm or coconut oil.
- Eat low-fat cheeses such as part-skim mozzarella.
- Instead of ice cream, choose ice milk, sherbet, or low-fat yogurt.
- Trim all visible fat from meat. Select lean cuts of beef, veal, or pork.
- Avoid high-fat meat products such as hot dogs, hamburgers, bacon, sausage, bologna, and salami.
- Eat more chicken and turkey (with the skin removed) and more fish.
- Choose turkey, lean roast beef, lean ham, and water-packed tuna fish for sandwiches.
- Prepare more meals that use meat sparingly. Soups, stews, stir-fry meals, and pasta dishes call for more vegetables and carbohydrates and less meat.
- Broil, bake, or steam foods instead of frying them.
- Make your own salad dressings, using less oil.

To decrease cholesterol in your diet

- Limit your consumption of egg yolks to one or two a week.
- Use egg whites in food preparation.
- Eat moderate portions of lean meat, fish, and poultry. Keep your daily consumption at 6 ounces.
- Avoid organ meats (liver, kidneys, brains).
- Eat fewer commercially baked products (cakes, pies, cookies, doughnuts, crackers, and chips).

- Regular physical exercise can help increase the level of HDL—or good—cholesterol. (See Chapter 3.)

The Micronutrients

Vitamins

Because your body generally cannot manufacture vitamins in adequate amounts, you must obtain these organic substances from external sources—preferably from the food you eat. Your body requires only tiny amounts of vitamins each day to serve as catalysts that trigger the biochemical conversion of protein, carbohydrates, and fats into energy. The vitamins themselves are not a source of energy.

Thirteen of the scientifically known vitamins are required by the human body. Four of these are fat-soluble—vitamins A, D, E, and K. The nine other vitamins are water-soluble and include vitamin C and the eight members of the B-complex family—thiamin, riboflavin, niacin, B_6, pantothenic acid, B_{12}, biotin, and folic acid. Each vitamin performs a specific job in your body.

Vitamins are essential to your cell and tissue maintenance and to your health—but only when taken in the recommended amounts for your age and sex. Anyone who eats a varied and well-balanced diet and meets the USRDAs for major nutrients is unlikely to develop a significant vitamin deficiency.

Since your diet is your best source of vitamins, evaluate your dietary patterns to ensure that you are eating a variety of foods from the Basic Four groups: (1) vegetables and fruits, (2) grains and cereals, (3) meats, fish, and poultry, and (4) milk and milk products. Or you can have a professional nutritionist or registered dietitian analyze your diet. If you consult with a professional, be sure to record what you eat at each meal and in between meals over a one-week period and take this list with you.

Minerals

Minerals are inorganic substances that occur in a variety of foods. Your body uses minerals to help control many metabolic processes, including the formation of bones, teeth, and blood cells. Minerals also play an important role in the regulation of body fluids.

Minerals generally remain intact when food is cooked and processed. The best way to obtain essential minerals is by eating a varied diet. The essential elements your body needs to maintain good health are divided into two groups:

The *macrominerals*—the seven major minerals that your body requires in relatively large amounts (more than 100 milligrams a day)—are calcium, magnesium, sodium, potassium, phosphorous, sulfur, and chlorine.

Of these, calcium has commanded the most attention because a deficiency of this mineral has been strongly associated with the brittle-bone disease osteoporosis. Both women and men should consume an adequate intake of dietary calcium as a preventive measure. For post-menopausal women concerned about osteoporosis, estrogen replacement therapy is considered far more effective than taking calcium supplements alone (see Chapter 6).

The *trace elements* are minerals that are required in smaller amounts. The 10 essential trace elements are iron, iodine, zinc, copper, manganese, chromium, cobalt, selenium, molybdenum, and fluoride.

In certain cases, the association between trace element deficiency and disease is clear: drinking fluoridated water protects against tooth decay; insufficient iodine can produce an enlarged thyroid gland, or goiter; a diet deficient in iron is a common cause of anemia.

Although trace elements have been implicated in the risk of certain chronic diseases—such as cancer and cardiovascular disease—the evidence remains weak.

Who Needs Supplements?

Vitamin enthusiasts—including some doctors and nutrition consultants—offer many reasons why people need vitamin supplements. Among the most commonly cited are stress, eating on the run, overprocessing of food, nutrition insurance, restoration of nutrients lost in dieting, food allergies, and combating a lowered immune resistance to disease.

Generally speaking, when water-soluble vitamins are taken in excess, they pass through your body without causing any harm. But megadoses of niacin, vitamin C, and vitamin B_6 each bring their own set of problems. Too much niacin can cause severe flushing, skin disorders, and liver damage. An excess of vitamin C—a popular remedy for colds—can cause kidney stones. When large doses of vitamin B_6 are taken for an extended period, they can produce permanent neurological damage.

The body doesn't dispose of excess fat-soluble vitamins as efficiently as it does the water-soluble types. Instead, these chemicals are stored for future use. If you keep stockpiling these vitamins in your tissues, eventually they can reach toxic levels. Vitamins A and D have the greatest potential to cause trouble because they accumulate in body fat. Excessive vitamin A can lead to headache, bone pain, and liver damage. Prolonged use of vitamin D can cause kidney stones and, eventually, kidney damage.

It is our recommendation that you not take anything above the RDA amounts unless your doctor prescribes a supplement.

Some cases may warrant the temporary use of a vitamin supplement. Women and teenage girls who are pregnant or breast feeding may require vitamin supplementation. People on very-low-calorie weight-loss programs need careful planning of their nutritional needs, as do elderly people who don't eat balanced diets. People with intestinal absorption disorders and alcoholics may need a full medical evaluation, not just a vitamin supplement. Children who have poor eating habits and people on strict vegetarian diets may also need supplementation of certain vitamins. These conditions often can be remedied by working with a qualified dietician who can offer guidance on food choices and changes in your personal eating habits.

Certain minerals are more likely than vitamins to be lacking in the diet. Of primary concern are fluoride for children and calcium and iron for women.

Beyond the Basic Four

In the 1950s, nutritionists developed an easy-to-understand food plan, called the *Basic Four Food Groups,* intended to meet everyone's nutritional needs. Just as with the RDAs, the Basic Four is designed to give you more than enough nutrients—as long as you eat a wide variety of foods. If you miss a few nutrients for a short period of time, it doesn't qualify you for deficiency status. But if you routinely omit certain foods, the lack will eventually take its toll on your body.

Because the Basic Four doesn't take fat, sodium, or sugar into account, you have to know what to look for and be able to set limits. An optimal diet emphasizes vegetables, fruits, grains, legumes, lean meat, fish, poultry, and low-fat dairy products. By eating these foods most of the time, you allow some room for occasional treats from the less-recommended categories, such as rich desserts or commercial fast-food meals.

Fats are ubiquitous in the American diet. Try to select unsaturated fats over saturated fats. Read the labels on processed and packaged food.

Sodium

Sodium is one of the most common ingredients found in the foods you buy. Sodium is essential in the diet, and the new RDAs set the estimated minimum requirement for sodium at 500 milligrams to cover a wide range of physical activities and climates.

Sodium occurs naturally in many foods. But in the commercial processing of food, more sodium is added. And many people still add more at the table. The estimated salt consumption in the United States ranges from 4,000 to 5,800 milligrams daily. The list of sodium-rich foods is long indeed:

- cured meats, including ham, bacon, sausage, hot dogs, and lunch meats
- cheeses, pickles, olives, condiments, sauces
- frozen and canned meat and fish entrées and dinners
- canned and dried soups
- commercial pasta, noodles, rice, and potato dishes
- commercial mixes for waffles, muffins, and cakes
- canned vegetables
- frozen vegetables with sauces
- salted snacks
- baking powder and baking soda
- certain food additives
- some regional drinking water supplies
- some antacids

The exact role of sodium in hypertension is not entirely clear. Some people can consume relatively large amounts of salt without registering any elevation in their blood pressure. Others are salt-sensitive and their blood pressure goes up or down depending on how much salt is consumed. Obesity, the presence of potassium, and many other factors also seem to affect blood pressure.

Researchers are investigating evidence that excessive consumption of salted, dried, and pickled foods may increase the risk of stomach cancer by breaking down the gastric lining and allowing invasion by a carcinogen. Salt-cured, smoked, and nitrite-cured foods are believed to increase the risk of stomach and esophageal cancer when eaten frequently.

Sugar

Each year, the average American consumes about 67 pounds of sugar. About half of this comes from sucrose, or table sugar, and much of the rest from corn syrup sweeteners found in many commercial foods and beverages.

Sugar often occurs in foods under several different names, including honey, corn syrup, molasses, fructose, and sucrose. We expect to find it in candy, cookies, cakes, pies, ice cream, soft drinks, cereals, and some milk drinks. However, it is also contained in soups, sauces, fruits, vegetables, and juices.

The human body needs the glucose in sugars in order to function.

You can get sugar in your diet in the form of simple sugars or complex carbohydrates. Since the glucose your cells need is readily supplied by complex carbohydrates contained in starchy and fiber-rich foods, it's wise to cut down on simple sugars.

There's a clear association between a high sugar intake and dental cavities. If your doctor has diagnosed you as having diabetes, or one of certain other endocrinological disorders, you may be put on a diet that severely restricts sugar intake. But other than in these situations, though eating sugar does your body little good, there's little evidence that sugar by itself causes any major health problem.

Diet and Disease Prevention

For decades, the federal government strictly forbade food manufacturers from making disease-prevention claims. Then in 1987, these rules were relaxed and a variety of health claims appeared on a diversity of food products. After growing concern that many manufacturers' claims were false and misleading, the Food and Drug Administration announced plans in 1990 to toughen the rules. Under the proposal, food manufacturers would be allowed to make disease prevention claims only in specific health areas where there is adequate scientific information to back up the claim.

Scientists are well aware that nutrition is powerful medicine. They have found that a steady diet of certain foods may increase the risk of disease while a variety of other foods may reduce it. Indeed, the prevalence of heart disease, cancer, kidney disease, and adult-onset diabetes in the United States has a strong association with diet.

Epidemiological studies and sophisticated laboratory technologies have led to the isolation of various components of foods that may have some protective effect against disease. However, eating foods that contain these components offers no assurance of future good health. In fact, exclusive reliance on these foods could very well prove hazardous or even toxic if certain of them are eaten to excess. So, though it's worthwhile to know about these foods and to make sure they are included in your diet, don't overdo your consumption of any one food in the cause of disease prevention. Eat moderate amounts of a wide variety of foods—in other words, a balanced diet. Among the food components now under study for their beneficial effects are:

Omega-3 Fatty Acids

There is some evidence—although preliminary—that eating three or more servings of fish each week may help lower the risk of coronary heart disease. The most commonly occurring omega-3 acids in fish oils are eicosapentaenoic acid and docosahexaenoic acid. These oils seem to reduce the tendency of blood platelets to stick together and form potentially dangerous blood clots.

The best sources of fish oil are the red- or dark-meat fish, especially mackerel, herring, sablefish, salmon, albacore tuna, and bluefish. White-meat fish and shellfish contain much less body oil, but still remain good sources of omega-3 acids. (Farm-raised fish are more likely to be fed grains and oats, such as soybean meal, which are rich in omega-6 polyunsaturated fats. These commercially grown fish may contain only about a third to half as much omega-3 fatty acids as marine fish that feed on natural food in their environment.)

Fiber

The indigestible part of vegetables, fruits, and grains is classified as either *soluble* or *insoluble* fiber. Each works in a different way. It appears that soluble fiber, which dissolves in water, may disrupt the body's metabolism of cholesterol and lower the level of blood cholesterol. Good sources of soluble fiber are the pectin in prunes, pears, oranges, apples, and the soluble gums and mucilages found in legumes, carrots, cabbage, cauliflower, barley, and oat and corn bran.

Insoluble fiber works like a sponge inside the intestines by absorbing several times its weight in water to help speed the passage of digested food through your body. The three types of insoluble fiber are cellulose, lignin, and hemicellulose. The best way to obtain insoluble fiber is by eating whole-grain cereals—especially of the wheat bran variety—and whole-grain breads.

The evidence that fiber performs a role in protecting against cancer or coronary heart disease is still inconclusive. Until researchers produce a definitive study on fiber, increase all types of fiber in your diet while using moderation and variety as your guide.

Carotenoids

Foods in the carotenoid family—a group of compounds that give yellow, red, and orange fruits and vegetables their characteristic color—are currently under investigation for their possible effects against cancer. A diet rich in beta-carotene, a form of vitamin A, appears to confer a lower risk of cancer of the larynx, esophagus, and lung. Good sources of beta-carotene are carrots, tomatoes, spinach, apricots, peaches, and cantaloupes.

Cruciferous Vegetables

A diet that regularly includes the cruciferous vegetables—so named because their flowers have four leaves in the shape of a cross—may be protective against gastrointestinal and respiratory cancers. These vegetables include broccoli, brussels sprouts, cabbage, cauliflower, and kohlrabi.

Deciphering Food Labels

According to an FDA survey in the mid-1980s, 68 percent of American food shoppers who read food labels expressly do so to glean information on fat, cholesterol, sodium, sugar, and additives. But this kind of information isn't required under the current rules. Instead, food labels offer vitamin, mineral, and protein data, which reflect the concern over nutrition-deficiency diseases in the first half of this century.

In early 1990, the FDA proposed sweeping changes in the nation's food labeling system, calling for mandatory nutritional labeling on practically all packaged foods. The proposed new labels would require food manufacturers to show not just total fat in a product, but also the amount that comes from saturated fat. Besides listing total calories per serving, the label would have to specify the number of calories from fat. It also would be mandatory to provide information about dietary fiber and cholesterol.

Until new labeling requirements become a reality, make the best of the package information that's currently available. *New York Times* nutrition reporter Marian Burros has likened reading food labels to reading a contract: "The fine print is the most important part, even though much of it is unintelligible."

To make an informed choice about the food you buy, you need a working knowledge of the language of labeling. It's important to read both the nutrition label and the list of ingredients.

Nutrition labeling is not mandatory unless a food product has been fortified with vitamins and minerals or is promoted with a specific health claim. Labeling for most food products is under the regulation of the FDA; meat, poultry, and eggs fall under the jurisdiction of the federal Department of Agriculture.

FDA-regulated food product labels must first list the serving size and the number of servings per container. Next comes the following information: calories, protein, carbohydrate, fat, and sodium. The labels must also list the percentage of the U.S. Recommended Daily Allowance provided in a serving for protein, vitamins A and C, the three B vitamins thiamine, riboflavin, and niacin, and the minerals calcium and iron.

When a label states the size of a serving, compare it with similar products. Because there is no agreed-upon serving size, this number may vary to make it appear that there are fewer calories.

When a label doesn't list the amount of each ingredient, the FDA requires that the manufacturer list the ingredients in descending order by weight. The first ingredient listed is the one that is predominantly used in the product. If sodium appears in the number-three position, it's the third most-used ingredient.

Meat and poultry product labeling is different from that required for other foods. Under Department of Agriculture rules, beef is labeled according to its grade. The select grade contains 2.5 to 7.6 percent fat per three-and-a-half-ounce serving. A choice grade contains 3.9 to 10.2 percent fat per serving. The highest grade, prime, is the most expensive and has the highest fat content—6.2 to 14 percent per serving.

Beef producers now can label a package of beef as "lean" if it has no more than 10 percent fat by weight, not by calories. To qualify as "extra lean," it must have no more than 5 percent fat by weight. So-called light or "lite" beef is defined as having 25 percent less fat than the standard for the industry.

How to Read a Label

Smart shoppers should know the following most commonly used terms on food packages:

Cholesterol-free.   Currently there are no established standards for cholesterol labeling. This term becomes misleading in a food item that itself contains no cholesterol but is laden with saturated fat—like palm or coconut oil—which causes a rise in blood cholesterol.

Dietetic.   This product is intended to meet special dietary purposes. One or more specific ingredients, such as sugar or salt, has been replaced or substituted. The term *dietetic* does not necessarily indicate low in calories.

Enriched.   Nutrients lost in the refining process have been put back into the product.

Fiber.   No regulations govern the way fiber must be listed. It may appear as dietary or crude fiber and as soluble or insoluble fiber.

Fortified.   Additional nutrients have been added to the product. For instance, milk containing vitamins A and D is fortified.

Hydrogenated or partially hydrogenated.   Hydrogen has been added to an unsaturated fat to make it saturated, or solid at room temperature. Partially hydrogenated fat is saturated, but less so.

Light or lite. There is no standard definition for this term. The product may be light in color, taste, texture, calories, weight, or alcoholic content. It's up to the buyer to figure out which of these applies.

Low-calorie. Under FDA requirements, this food can contain no more than 40 calories in a serving and no more than 0.4 calories per gram.

Natural. By law, the word *natural* can appear only on meat or poultry that contains no artificial ingredients. When applied to other types of food, this term has little meaning, although it appears on many products. Natural may be confused with *pure,* a term that means a product is made from only one ingredient—for instance, juice or honey.

Organic. The implication of *organic* is that no synthetic fertilizers or pesticides were used to grow, process, or package the food product. There is no national standard or definition of organic, and therefore no guarantee that an organic label is true to its claims.

Reduced-calorie. The product must be at least one-third lower in calories when compared with a similar product.

Sodium-free. Fewer than 5 milligrams of sodium are contained in a serving. *Very-low sodium* means there's no more than 35 milligrams per serving. *Reduced sodium* indicates that the level of sodium has been reduced by at least 75 percent.

Sugar-free or sugarless. This product contains no sucrose, or table sugar. However, another form of sweetener may be used, such as fructose or sorbitol—which contain about as many calories by volume or weight as sucrose. Aspartame and saccharin are sometimes used to sweeten sugar-free products.

Eating Out

A recent food-service industry survey indicated that one of every five meals is eaten away from home. As a growing number of patrons demand nutritious as well as tasty food, restaurateurs are becoming more responsive. It's possible to make special requests such as having a dish served with sauce on the side or without butter. Most kitchens are willing to accommodate these requests—within reason. Here are some suggestions you may wish to try:

• When you're selecting a restaurant, look for one that serves a varied menu and offers different methods of food preparation. Choose one that serves à la carte dishes as well as regular-course meals. If you want fast food, look for a place that offers a salad bar or packaged salads as well as burgers and fries.

• When scanning a menu, look for such low-fat cooking methods as broiled, stir-fried, rack-grilled, poached, steamed, or roasted. If the menu says a food item is battered, buttered, breaded, creamed, fried, au gratin, or rich, that's a signal that it's higher in fat.

• Some terms that should alert you to the possibility that you'll be getting a high amount of sodium in your meal include *smoked, pickled, marinated, in soy sauce, teriyaki, Parmesan,* and *in a tomato base.*

• If the menu gives an entrée's name, but no description, ask your waiter or waitress how the dish is prepared.

• If you'd like your sauce or gravy on the side, or minimal butter on your broiled food, request it when ordering.

• Most restaurants serve generous entrées that many people can't (or shouldn't) finish at one sitting. Ask for a doggie bag and take the rest of your entrée home.

Fast Foods

Every day one out of every five Americans eats at a fast-food restaurant. Most fast-food meals deliver between 40 and 55 percent of their calories from fat—a far cry from public health recommendations of no more than 30 percent fat intake.

Whether you order from a five-star restaurant or a fast-food drive-up window, it's easy to get a high-fat meal—it all depends on what you order. A recent report on fast food by the Massachusetts Medical Society's Committee on Nutrition points out that the potential for getting too many calories and too few vitamins and minerals can exist as easily in a hamburger meal prepared at home, in a school cafeteria, or in an expensive restaurant.

Most people consider an occasional fast-food meal of a burger and fries either a treat or a quick solution when hunger sets in. In 1987, when *Consumer Reports* surveyed its readers, three out of five said they patronize fast-food restaurants "more to get in and out quickly" than for the quality of the food. There's nothing wrong with grabbing a fast-food meal occasionally, but don't make it part of your steady diet. And when you do eat out—whether at an elegant restaurant or a fast-food shop—be selective about what you order.

This may not always be as easy as it sounds. The Massachusetts Medical Society's report notes that "Health-conscious consumers may choose chicken or fish as lower-fat alternatives, but may be unaware that chicken nuggets and chicken patty sandwiches often contain ground-up chicken skin." The chicken or fish entrée also may be deep-fried in beef tallow or vegetable oil that is high in saturated fat. If you're at a fast-food outlet that offers grilled chicken sandwiches, order one of these instead.

Consumer Reports recently offered a survival guide for defensive dining when eating at a fast-food establishment. Among the suggestions are:

- Choose roast beef over burgers, if possible. Roast beef is leaner and contains less fat.
- Order your burger plain, without the cheese, mayonnaise, and special sauce.
- Order milk or juice instead of a shake or carbonated beverage. Opt for low-fat milk if it's available.
- If you order a baked potato, it's a low-calorie item until you add high-calorie toppings. Skip the french fries, or else split an order with someone.
- Order a salad or cole slaw. If you're composing your own at a salad bar, go for the dark green vegetables, carrots, tomatoes, and cucumbers. Go light on croutons, taco chips, and dressings. Remember that the pasta and potato salads contain high-calorie mayonnaise.

How to Get Reliable Nutrition Advice

Ideally, your *primary care physician* should offer guidance on the kind of diet and exercise that can allow you to achieve and maintain a desirable weight. When this isn't possible, the physician should refer you to a competent *nutritionist* or *dietitian* for counseling.

A reputable practitioner uses a simple approach: a review and analysis of your eating patterns in the context of total energy intake and energy expenditure. The emphasis is on identifying the problem areas and prescribing scientifically based suggestions for improving your diet and increasing your exercise.

Legitimate nutritionists have an academic degree in nutritional science and have earned professional certification in such groups as the American Institute of Nutrition and the American Society for Clinical Nutrition. Registered dietitians, or RDs, have successfully completed college studies in nutrition or dietetics. In order to gain registered status, they must pass a written test and participate in regular continuing education courses approved by the American Dietetic Association.

Certified nutritionists usually are affiliated with hospitals or medical schools, and conduct clinical research and serve as consultants to primary care doctors. Registered dietitians also may do research, but they are more likely to counsel patients and conduct classes for people with special dietary needs, such as pregnant women, heart and kidney patients, and diabetics. Many RDs have private practices and work with patients who are referred by their doctors. RDs translate the technical side of nutrition into practical information for their patients. When selecting a nutrition counselor, be sure to examine his or her credentials.

Many large *health organizations* such as the American Heart Association, the American Cancer Society, and the American Diabetes Association offer nutrition materials to the public. State and local dietetic associations, state health departments, and home economists at county cooperative extension services operated by the USDA are other sources of information about nutrition.

Controlling Your Weight

After years of trying one fad diet after another, Americans haven't shed many pounds. In fact, an estimated 60 percent of the population perceives itself as overweight. Many are turning to various weight-loss programs, systems, or plans with an eye on achieving weight control rapidly and painlessly. Are these approaches just a euphemism for dieting or are weight-conscious Americans on to something? That all depends on the method chosen, your expectations, and whether you're willing to accept the simple truth about permanent weight control: there are no miracles.

Anyone who weighs at least 20 percent more than his or her desirable weight (based on height and weight tables) is considered *obese*. In contrast, an *overweight* person is defined as one who exceeds the desirable weight for gender, height, and frame size as listed in a standard table. Athletes often weigh more than such tables indicate they should because they have a high muscle-to-weight ratio and very little excess body fat. Otherwise, there's often just a shade of a difference between obesity and overweight. Regardless of what you call it, the central issue is whether you are carrying excess weight and if it puts you at an increased risk of health problems.

Scientists at the National Institute on Aging's Gerontology Research Center recently drew up new weight tables that are adjusted for age. These tables make allowances for normal weight gain during early adulthood in healthy people who are not overweight. Reubin Andres, who created the tables, found that many studies showed that increased risk of mortality was minimal at the weights that the Metropolitan Life Insurance Company formerly had deemed too high.

When Fat Is Life-threatening

In addition to your age, sex, frame size, and when you gained the weight (early adulthood versus gradually during middle age), another factor may be significant: where you carry your fat.

The fat from a potbelly may present more of a health risk than fat that has accumulated elsewhere on the body. Apparently, excess fat cells in the abdomen may affect the metabolism of the liver and cause more fat to enter the bloodstream. In addition, the fat cells may become resistant to insulin and eventually increase the risk of diabetes. Extra fat in the abdominal area may also indicate higher blood triglyceride levels and more heart disease. Those whose fatty padding resides in the buttocks and hips—the classic pear-shaped figure—may have less of a health risk associated with the extra fat.

There are other risks. Overweight has been associated with an increased risk of heart attacks in men in their 40s. Hypertension occurs three times more frequently in overweight people. Cancers of the colon, rectum, prostate, gallbladder, biliary tract, endometrium, ovary, cervix, and breast tend to occur more frequently in people who carry a lot of excess weight. The risk of developing gallstones appears to increase in women who are only slightly overweight. And obese children have a greater likelihood of becoming obese adults.

For years, research on obesity and heart disease was limited to its effect on a certain segment of the male population. But recently, a long-term study of young and middle-aged women produced findings that have been described as "shocking." In 1990, researchers from Harvard Medical School and Brigham and Women's Hospital in Boston reported that virtually any degree of overweight in women may increase the risk of coronary heart disease.

After following nearly 116,000 nurses between ages 30 and 55 for eight years, only the leanest group of women studied had a low rate of coronary disease. Women who were mildly to moderately overweight had an 80 percent higher risk than the thinnest women. Up to 70 percent of the coronary events that occurred among the heaviest women and 40 percent of those in the overall group could be attributed to overweight.

If you're overweight and have other risk factors, such as cigarette smoking, hypertension, diabetes, high cholesterol, and a family history of heart attack, start to act *now*. Make weight loss a priority in your life.

Why We're Fat

Science still can't say with certainty what makes many of us fat. For years, everyone assumed that it was simply a matter of eating too much food. Now we know that obesity or overweight is much more complex—probably a combination of genetic, social, psychological, hormonal, and environmental factors. With one of every five Americans weighing in at levels 20 percent or more above their "desirable" weights, the subject of weight loss is on a lot of people's minds. They all want to know: what really works?

Anyone who faces the prospect of losing weight may have to search hard for role models to give inspiration. Of the millions of men and women who go on diets a few times every year, the failure rate is estimated to be in the range of 70 to 90 percent. Losing weight isn't easy; maintaining weight loss is even harder.

It helps to understand some of the possible causes of obesity and how the body responds to dieting. Once you're clear on what doesn't work, you can concentrate on the effective methods that do work.

Several studies have shown that, ironically, some overweight people actually consume fewer calories than slimmer folks. In some instances, obese people apparently burn those calories more slowly than thinner individuals. Genetic factors are thought to be a strong component of a tendency toward obesity. Your metabolism, or the rate at which your body burns calories, is a part of your genetic makeup. Whether your metabolism is slower or faster is an important factor in determining how much fat you end up storing. Obese individuals as a group tend to have lower heat production after eating than thinner people.

People differ in the amount of fat they burn as opposed to the fat they store. Fat that is burned disappears, but stored fat doesn't get permanently shelved in your body. A fat cell stores triglycerides, constantly forming new fat and burning old fat in a continuous cycle of cell renewal.

In 1990, two obesity researchers confirmed the long-held suspicion that heredity plays a major role in whether you're fat or lean. The studies, published in *The New England Journal of Medicine,* followed pairs of identical and fraternal twins under different circumstances.

Researchers at Laval University in Quebec compared weight gain in 12 pairs of lean identical twins who agreed to live on campus for four months. During this period, they had limited physical activity and planned overeating at the rate of 1,000 extra calories a day. Within each pair of twins, the location and amount of weight gain was the same. While both members of one pair tended to deposit fat on the abdomen, another pair was more prone to accumulating fat on the thighs and buttocks.

The differences in weight gain were more dramatic when comparisons were made among the sets of twins: one pair gained only 9½ pounds while another set of siblings gained 29 pounds. Those who added the least weight showed more of a gain in muscle than fat. Those recording heavier weight gains stored the extra energy as fat tissue.

In another study, University of Pennsylvania researchers studied two groups of identical twins and two groups of fraternal twins. Within each group, one section had been reared together in the same household while the other section had been reared apart in different homes. Once again, the identical twins had the same weights—whether they grew up together in the same environment or apart.

Genetic factors may account for up to 70 percent of the differences in weight gain in adults, according to the research results. But the scientists emphasize that the question of destiny versus diet doesn't completely rule out the role of the food you eat or your environment, for that matter. Instead, it serves as more of a warning: knowing in advance that you have a disposition to excess weight offers the opportunity to control the kind and quantity of food you eat.

A number of theories to explain obesity have emerged.

• *The fat-cell theory.* This theory postulates that some people were born with a predisposition toward producing a greater number of fat cells. Apparently, once the fat cells appear, they never go away. Losing weight and exercising can help shrink fat cells, but because these cells have an insatiable appetite for more fat, they may tend to accumulate fat easily. Scientists studying obesity have been able to measure the size and number of fat cells in research studies of severely obese patients.

• *The set-point theory.* The concept behind the set-point theory is that each person's body has a set notion of what it should weigh. The theory holds that if you stray above or below this set point, your metabolism steers your body right back to its biologically preprogrammed weight.

Repeated weight loss and weight gain from dieting—a phenomenon popularly called the "yo-yo syndrome"—may lower the body's metabolic set point. This is why dieters who fall into this cycle of weight loss/weight gain find it harder to lose weight the next time they begin a new diet.

• *The dietary fat theory.* According to this theory, a person who develops a taste for fat-laden and high-fat foods tends to gravitate toward these food choices—even when lower-fat alternatives are available. Repeatedly choosing fat-rich foods, of course, assures that obesity will eventually occur. It has been shown that obese people may be attracted to high-fat foods as opposed to items with a high-sugar content.

Clearly, it's better to avoid falling into the weight gain trap than to face the prospect of having to lose excess pounds. But if you're already overweight, forget about fad or crash diets. The only tried and true way to lose weight and keep it off is to change your eating habits permanently and to increase your physical activity on a regular basis.

The cornerstone of a successful weight-loss program consists of behavior modification and exercise. You can begin a program on your own or in a group. Some established weight-loss programs include behavior modification techniques that offer the added benefit of group support. But many people who choose to learn behavior modification methods take an independent route.

Diet Programs

Behavior Modification

The principles of behavioral therapy can be successfully used for virtually any kind of dietary or exercise program. The idea is to recognize the many cues—other than hunger—that trigger eating and to learn how to stop responding to them.

Your talent for observation, reflection, and patience comes into play during behavior modification. You'll need to monitor your activities continuously and make choices about how to act when faced with those stimuli that tell you to eat. You'll have to substitute considered responses for automatic responses regarding the kind and amount of food you eat as well as the circumstances under which you're accustomed to taking food.

• Keep a diary of everything you eat. Don't just list the food. Note also the time of day, the amount of food, whether you were alone or with someone, and your feelings while eating. After several days of logging every morsel, you should be able to detect a pattern that you can work to correct. The very fact of keeping a food diary may help to change your behavior.

• Be aware of the external cues that influence your desire for food. Learn to control them by limiting all opportunities to eat that don't coincide with your regular mealtimes. This may mean eating in only a certain room, keeping high-calorie snack foods out of your house, shopping for food after eating a meal as opposed to before, and preparing just enough food for a meal without any leftovers to tempt you. It's also important to eat slowly and learn to focus more on the sensory aspect of food as opposed to the mechanical act of eating.

• Select foods that are low in fat or calories. Calorie counting isn't a part of behavior modification. But a balanced diet is essential for all of us and should be part of your new attitude toward eating. Follow the suggested guidelines for increasing your consumption of complex carbohydrates.

• Adjust your attitude. Instead of feeling frustrated or unattractive, accentuate the positive: you've decided to change your habits and you feel good about your choice.

Behavior modification techniques are often successful on their own in people who have 20 to 25 pounds to lose. The weight loss is gradual, but encouraging—especially when combined with a program of regular exercise.

Very-Low-Calorie Diets

Very-low-calorie (VLC) diets were originally created for a select group of people whose severe obesity put them at risk for a host of medical problems. These drastic diets rely on liquid formulas that provide 400 to 800 calories a day—either alone or in combination with small amounts of food—over a period of several weeks or months.

Because such a restricted caloric intake carries the risk of dangerous changes in vital organs, all VLC dieters require medical supervision. Thousands of these weight-loss programs have been established all around the country in hospitals or through a doctor's office. The VLC participants buy their weight-loss formulas through these programs and are required to undergo weekly medical evaluation, including electrocardiograms and blood and urine tests. The better programs also offer support groups and behavior modification.

People who enroll in these formula-diet programs and stick with them often report dramatic results in terms of pounds lost. The biggest problem has been keeping the weight off when the program is over. After losing a sizable amount of weight during their weight-loss programs, many VLC dieters reported gaining it all back—and more—within two years or less.

Millions of Americans are overweight to some degree, a condition that some doctors call "cosmetically obese." If you've got up to 20 to 25 pounds to lose, behavior modification and regular exercise are often the best choices. However, the smaller number of people who qualify as seriously obese may find some real medical benefits from a VLC program—provided they keep the weight off.

VLC diet programs are expensive and the dropout rate is high. Many participants experience a range of side effects from constipation and bad breath to dizziness and hair loss. Some people may not be allowed on liquid-diet programs, including those who have had a recent heart attack, liver or kidney disease, or bleeding stomach ulcers.

Before signing up for a program, ask what kind of medical supervision is provided. Hospital-based programs usually offer a team of doctors, nurses, and dietitians. Programs conducted from a doctor's office may not have as extensive a team. Find out if the price includes the cost of the required medical tests. If not, ask how much extra you can expect to pay for them.

When the supervised part of the program ends, the maintenance part is up to you. Only by making permanent life-style and dietary changes can you expect to keep your lower weight.

Exercise

Previous guidelines called for exercising three to five times a week at a level intense enough to raise one's heart rate to 60 to 90 percent of its maximum and keep it there for 15 to 60 minutes. Less than 10 percent of American adults currently engage in this kind of exercise program.

However, recent studies point to the value of moderate and even low levels of physical activity in reducing the risk of early death. In 1989, researchers at the Institute for Aerobics Research in Dallas released the results of an eight-year study. People who stand to gain the most from modest amounts of exercise are those who move from the sedentary category to moderate activity. For inactive people, that's the equivalent of taking a brisk half-hour-to-45-minute walk six or seven days a week.

About a third of the population can be classified as regularly active, engaging in at least three 20-minute sessions of moderately intensive activity each week. Many in this group do not during their exercise sessions achieve and maintain the heart rates previously recommended by public health officials, but they have been making some of the right moves in terms of physical activity. Just by virtue of the exercise they have undertaken, they may have collected more health benefits than they were promised.

So regardless of how you do it and the extent to which you're able to take it, get moving on getting fit. Whether you choose moderate or vigorous levels of physical activity, there are many well-established health benefits, including a stronger heart and lungs, weight loss and maintenance of an appropriate weight level, a lower blood cholesterol level, reduced stress, and stronger bones.

How Much Exercise Is Enough?

In the not-too-distant past, when you jumped around a gym doing calisthenics and aerobics, went for a run, or pedaled off on your bicycle, you were exercising. Do the same thing today, and it's called physical activity. Semantics aside, the broader term *physical activity* takes in anything that keeps your body in motion.

Many people have negative perceptions about "exercise"—it's inconvenient, it can hurt, and it's expensive. In contrast, "physical activity" is more likely to be viewed as something that brings pleasure. Physical activity encompasses the entire range of possible motion from such vigorous activities as bicycling, swimming, and football to more moderate modes of movement such as walking, gardening, playing pool, raking leaves, mowing a lawn, climbing stairs, and ballroom dancing.

In order to be physically fit, you must first be physically active. *Fitness* is a measure of four basic elements: cardiovascular-respiratory endurance, body composition, muscular strength and endurance, and flexibility.

In 1990, the American College of Sports Medicine (ACSM) issued the following revised guidelines:

- Engage in physical activity three to five days a week.
- Exercise at an intensity that raises your heart rate to 60 to 90 percent of its maximum, or 50 to 85 percent of the most oxygen you can take in and use during exercise.
- Keep at your aerobic activity continuously for 20 to 60 minutes. If the activity is of lower or moderate intensity, a longer period of duration is recommended for the nonathletic adult.
- Perform any activity that continuously uses large muscle groups in a rhythmic motion, such as walking-hiking, running-jogging, rope skipping, rowing, stair climbing, swimming, and skating.
- Add resistance and strength training that is moderate in intensity to exercise all the major muscle groups of the body. (This new addition to the guidelines points to the need for developing and maintaining fat-free body weight.) The recommended minimum is one set of 8 to 12 repetitions of 8 to 10 exercises that condition the major muscle groups at least two days a week.

The ACSM notes that the amount and the quality of exercise you need to attain health-related benefits may not be the same as what is recommended for attaining cardiovascular fitness. In other words, levels of physical activity lower than those recommended may reduce the risk of certain chronic degenerative diseases, yet may not be intensive enough to raise your capacity to take in more oxygen. Also, just how much physical fitness is necessary for optimum health is unknown.

Remember, fitness is for people in all age groups. In a broad sense, it's the ability to perform moderate to vigorous levels of physical activity without becoming fatigued and being able to maintain this capability all your life. Just as genetic variations may play a role in other aspects of your physical makeup, they also account for differences in adapting to physical activity. Few of us have the genes it takes to be Olympic athletes, but nearly all of us possess the ability to work our way to better health.

Making Your Program Work

Before you begin a program of physical activity, consider your age and how long it's been since you were last physically active. If you have been sedentary for a long time, or are over 45, get medical clearance from your doctor before taking up any kind of intense physical activity. *Exercise tolerance testing*—in which you're hooked up to a machine with electrocardiographic leads that track your heart's electrical activity during exercise—may be recommended for people with symptoms of heart disease who are undertaking a new activity regimen.

Typically, people choose one activity and do the same thing time after time. Sports medicine experts now recommend *cross training*—or alternating among a few different kinds of physical activity. Ideally, combine one activity that is aerobic (using oxygen) with another that builds muscle strength and endurance. Cross training is beneficial because it works different groups of muscles in the lower and upper body to achieve balance and also reduces the risk of injury from overuse of any one set of muscles.

There isn't one single cross-training package that fits everyone. Depending on whether you're working out for pure enjoyment or with a definite goal in mind—weight control, stronger muscles, improving your sense of well-being, or to improve your performance in a sport—there are several activities from which to choose.

Aerobic Exercise	*Resistance Training*
Jogging/running	Traditional free weights
Swimming	(including barbells and
Bicycling	dumbbells)
Fast walking	Weight machines
Cross-country skiing	
Skating (ice or roller)	
Canoeing/rowing	
Aerobic dance	
Aerobic stair climbing	

Pastimes and Chores	Sports
Gardening	Softball
Walking	Tennis
Golf (carrying your clubs)	Volleyball
Bowling	Racquetball
Billiards/pool	Squash
Table tennis	Basketball
Raking leaves	Downhill skiing
Lawn mowing (with a	Hockey
hand mower)	Soccer
Shoveling snow	Touch football
Climbing stairs	

If your goal is weight control, you can select a few activities from the aerobics column as the centerpiece of your program for your thrice-weekly workout. To gain strength in your muscles, mix in resistance training.

For weight loss, aerobic activity is the exercise of choice. Aerobic exercise must be performed at least four times a week for a minimum of 20 minutes per session in order to burn fat. The key to burning up great quantities of fat calories is to exercise at low to moderate levels for longer periods of time.

Aerobic activity is highly beneficial to your heart and lungs. As your body becomes accustomed to a regular aerobic workout, your heart pumps a greater volume of blood to your tissues. Your lungs increase their ability to take in and use a larger volume of oxygen during exercise—something called VO_2 *max*. With your heart pumping more blood and delivering more oxygen to your body, your muscles work more efficiently—something that is often called the *training effect*. The effect is the result of your body's adaptation to progressively greater demands.

Your training zone should be within your *maximum heart rate,* which is one of the key indicators used to determine how intense your aerobic activity should be.

To determine your maximum heart rate (MHR), subtract your age from 220. If you are 40, you compute your MHR as $220 - 40 = 180$. To get maximum benefit from physical activity, you need to get your exercising heart rate up to at least 60 percent of its maximum. To compute your training heart zone, multiply your MHR by 60 percent. A 40-year-old, with an MHR of 180, would get a figure of 108 beats per minute.

If you increase the intensity of your workout to 70 percent, you would multiply your MHR by 70 percent for a rate of 126 beats. Although the ACSM guidelines give a maximum range of 90 percent of MHR, it's not necessary or prudent to go beyond 85 percent of MHR, and such levels should be attempted only by those who are sure they have no underlying heart disease.

According to ACSM, someone with a low fitness level can achieve a significant training effect with a sustained training heart rate as low as 40 to 50 percent of *heart rate max reserve*. The approximate figures are 130 to 135 beats per minute in younger people and 105 to 115 beats per minute in older individuals. Anyone taking beta-blocker medications is likely to have a lower heart rate.

Figuring Your Heart Rate

The standard method for determining your maximum heart rate is the target zone method. This begins with learning how to take your pulse properly. The best site is the radial artery of the wrist. Once you find this point, use the tips of your three middle fingers to feel the pulsations of the artery. Use a stopwatch or a watch with a second hand to count the number of times your pulse beats in 15 seconds. Then multiply this number by four.

You should take your pulse immediately after you stop your aerobic activity because the heart rate drops within 15 seconds and you won't get an accurate reading if you delay. Your pulse should fall between the 60 percent and 85 percent figures calculated earlier.

This formula isn't meant to trigger anxiety or to distract you from exercising. It's only a guide. Another method of gauging the intensity of your workout is the *rate of perceived exertion,* or RPE. The RPE scale is based on your own perception of how hard you're working out and has been found to be as accurate as an actual pulse check for most people.

The scale goes from a baseline of zero to a peak of 20. Anything under 10 is considered very light. Workouts rated 10 or 11 merit a light RPE classification. Twelve to 13 is considered moderate, or somewhat hard. The 14 to 16 zone is heavy intensity. Activity over 16 falls into the very hard category.

In most cases, an exerciser who becomes familiar with the relationship between heart rate and RPE should be able to rely on RPE instead of heart rate. The exceptions would be competitive athletes who may want to keep close tabs on their heart rates and people with heart disease or hypertension who must carefully monitor their heart rates.

Building Strength

Working out with weights—or resistance training—helps increase the amount of lean tissue in your body. The American College of Sports Medicine's 1990 general exercise prescription recommended resistance/ strength training as "a well-rounded program that exercises all the major muscle groups of the body."

Body composition changes with time once you pass your mid-20s. Slowly, but surely, you lose an estimated 3 to 5 percent of muscle mass each decade. If you're 40, you may proudly say that you weigh the same as you did at age 25. But if you haven't been following a consistent program of physical activity, your weight is more likely to reflect a higher proportion of fat than lean muscle tissue.

To avoid a common case of slowly shrinking muscles, include strength training among your physical activities. Strength training is not a substitute for regular aerobic activity but an adjunct to your program.

Resistance training doesn't produce Herculean-size muscles. (Body builders who want to develop very strong muscles work out at much higher levels than those recommended for overall fitness.) Instead, as you subject specific groups of muscles to an increased work load, they gain strength, endurance, and tone. With each regular workout, flabby muscles become tighter. By utilizing a muscle vigorously, you coax small groups of muscle fibers into becoming thicker.

Resistance training reshapes your body, but it doesn't burn fat. After a few months of weight training, your muscles should feel firmer and look more toned. But the scale won't show you any lighter, because muscle tissue is much heavier than fat.

When strength training is done in moderation, it can increase the flexibility of your joints, improve your posture, and make your reflexes a little quicker. Overall, the strength and balance you gain can offer some protection against bone, joint, and muscle injuries. Older adults especially may find a strength training program beneficial. The risk of injury is very small as long as the training is done properly.

If you are new to this activity, it is advisable to join a class or a club that offers instruction to beginners. After you learn the proper way to use weights, the right amount of weight to work with, how to breathe, and the best way to do your repetitions, you'll create the foundation to use in working out on your own.

There are three basic types of muscle training.

Isometric exercise. This static form of exercise calls for contracting certain muscles without moving the body area with which you're working. If you tense the muscles of your arm without moving it, that's a form of isometric exercise. This type of exercise is not advised for middle-aged and older adults with high blood pressure because the repeated muscle contractions could cause a dangerous rise in blood pressure.

Isotonic exercise.   This dynamic form of exercise involves moving against a resistance (weight lifting or calisthenics such as push-ups or sit-ups) while maintaining constant tension in a particular set of muscles. Isotonics are done in sets of repetitions. Newcomers to isotonic strength training should start off easily. Begin with low weights and work your way up. Start with one set of repetitions per exercise session, then progress to two sets, and move up gradually. Otherwise, you're likely to develop sore muscles that may discourage future training.

The ACSM advises caution on training that emphasizes an isotonic variation called *eccentric* contractions. Eccentric training emphasizes lengthening the muscle as it contracts and has greater potential for producing sore muscles.

Isokinetic exercise.   This training variation combines isometric and isotonic techniques. The special equipment required for this kind of exercise provides resistance to muscles as well as range of motion. This advanced equipment may be available in some gyms.

The Benefits of Exercise

A primary care physician should be your first resource for advice about physical activity. Your doctor can explain the health benefits of exercise, your individual risk of developing illnesses linked to inactivity, and the need for starting your activity at a level safe for you. This discussion with your doctor should give you a better idea of what kind and level of physical activity is best for you.

Regular physical activity clearly has many positive side effects and is a simple, not to mention inexpensive, means of preventing certain diseases. For these reasons, when a doctor can recommend physical activity instead of medication, this is just the kind of prescription you should be eager to follow.

Physical activity is effective in preventing several diseases. The conditions that have undergone the most study are coronary artery disease, hypertension, non-insulin-dependent diabetes mellitus, osteoporosis, obesity, and depression.

Coronary artery disease.   People who are physically inactive are twice as likely to develop coronary heart disease as those who perform regular physical activity. Regular aerobic activity boosts the power of the heart and blood vessels, so that your heart pumps more blood with less effort. However, the protective effect of exercise is good only as long as you continue your physical activity.

Hypertension.   A heart that pumps blood more efficiently as a result of regular physical activity appears to be at reduced risk of developing high blood pressure. Studies have suggested that physically inactive people have a 35 to 52 percent higher risk of hypertension.

Diabetes.   The adult-onset form of diabetes is less likely to occur in people who engage in regular physical activity and maintain an appropriate weight. Being overweight or obese increases the body's resistance to insulin and leads to high levels of blood sugar. To help prevent diabetes, don't gain excess weight. If you're already overweight, see your doctor for advice about beginning a program of regular physical activity to lose weight.

Osteoporosis.   Weight-bearing exercise—or activity that places physical stress on the long bones—is believed to help maintain or build bone mass. Athletes who place large amounts of mechanical stress on particular areas of bone in pursuing their sport have denser bones than the nonathletic population. The role of exercise in preventing osteoporosis remains under study.

Obesity.   Weight gain, and often obesity, is the result of taking in more energy (eating more) than you consume (burn up) in physical activity. Regular physical activity can help you achieve a caloric balance. For exercise to be effective in weight loss, a change in eating habits is also necessary. Obesity has been linked with several health problems, including hypertension, high blood cholesterol levels, diabetes, and low self-esteem.

Mental health.   A commonly reported benefit of regular physical activity is an improvement in mood and a lifting of mild to moderate depression and anxiety. People who are physically active also report a higher level of self-esteem than nonexercisers.

There is a growing body of scientific evidence demonstrating that people who exercise may live longer. A study by Dr. Ralph Paffenbarger of Stanford University followed nearly 17,000 male alumni from Harvard University and found that the more physically active grads actually lived longer. The ones who burned up at least 2,000 calories a week in physical exercise had a lower risk of death from heart attack.

Research is under way on the effects of exercise in preventing other illnesses and disorders, including colon cancer and abnormalities in the levels of lipids in the bloodstream. Research data that have appeared thus far on the relationship between physical activity and colon cancer indicate that exercise may reduce the risk of this disease by 50 percent. It is thought that exercise increases bowel motility and cuts the time that potential carcinogens linger in the bowel.

The Risks

Most injuries during physical activity are preventable. Injuries are usually the result of overdoing physical activity, dramatically increasing your exercise level without proper training, or using improper exercising techniques.

Studies are now being conducted to determine whether physical activity done regularly over a long period of time can cause osteoarthritis in the major weight-bearing joints of the hips and knees. Recent studies of long-distance runners weren't able to show a strong link between this exercise and osteoarthritis.

The other major concern surrounding exercise is the risk of sudden death while working out. There is a higher risk of sudden death—but it is greater for sedentary men (women were not included in this study) who suddenly undertake vigorous activity than for those who are regularly active. If we consider both the time during which they are exercising and when they are not, men who are physically active have a 60 percent lower chance of sudden cardiac death than sedentary men.

You can minimize the risk of injury. Before beginning any kind of physical activity or sport, warm up first and cool down afterward. Skipping your *warm-ups* and *cool-downs* is not only inefficient, it can be dangerous and lead to injury.

Warm-ups.   Warm-ups give your body a chance to gradually increase your heart rate and blood supply to the muscles. Cold muscles, which are less flexible, have a greater risk of becoming injured, and are also inefficient. A 5-to-10-minute period of warming up is generally adequate for a safe start.

One technique for warming up is the full-body, or general warm-up. Jogging in place or doing stationary cycling warms up your large muscle groups and helps raise the temperature deep inside your muscles. Before stretching or working with weights, do at least five minutes of general warm-ups. Unlike full-body warm-ups, specific warm-ups are a slower version of an activity you plan to do more vigorously. Some examples include slowly pedaling your bicycle for the first mile or doing a slow swimming crawl before beginning your pool laps.

Slow and gradual stretching is beneficial before a brisk walk or jogging. Stretching your hamstring, calf, and lower back muscles can help prevent tightness, cramps, and injury. Never bounce when stretching. Ease into each stretch in a gradual and relaxed fashion and hold the stretch for at least 10 seconds.

Cool-downs.   About 5 or 10 minutes before the conclusion of your activity session, gradually begin to slow down. If you're bicycling, pedal slowly for the last half-mile. If you're swimming or fast-walking, do your last lap or quarter-mile at a slower pace. Do another series of slow, gradual stretches to prevent tightness and cramping in your muscles.

It's extremely dangerous to stop exercising abruptly. The sudden stop can throw your body into disarray and cause your muscles to become painfully shorter and stiffer.

*   *   *

Fitness lasts only as long as you practice it. If you begin a program of physical activity and then drop out, your improved level of fitness soon disappears. Most important, physical activity is vital for people of all ages. As we get older, the value of physical activity may become even more significant in minimizing and decreasing the severity of many of the physical changes and problems that accompany aging.

3

Taking Care of Your Heart

Jonathan L. Halperin, M.D.

It's natural to assume that your heart will continue beating and delivering blood to every cell in your body right through to old age. And usually it does. But although the death rate from heart attack declined by 28 percent from 1977 to 1987, heart and blood vessel diseases remain the leading cause of death in the United States. Of the 976,000 people who lost their lives to cardiovascular disease in 1987, about one-fifth were under the age of 65.

For decades, medical scientists have been telling us that most heart attacks and strokes are preventable. Beginning in the 1960s, we learned how life-style habits count in keeping us healthy longer—with emphasis on better nutrition, more exercise, not smoking, and stress management. Now we know even more about controlling the risk of heart and blood vessel diseases such as atherosclerosis and hypertension.

Atherosclerosis

Atherosclerosis, the major cause of coronary heart disease, is the progressive buildup of fibers, cellular flotsam, calcium, and cholesterol fat on the inner lining of the blood vessel walls. These accumulations are called atheromas, or plaques, and are essentially clumps of fat, fibrous tissue, and cells that form inside arterial walls. Over time, these deposits may build until the blood vessel is so narrow that no blood can flow through the area. When partial or total blockage occurs, it can result in any of the following: the chest pain of *angina pectoris; peripheral vascular disease,* in which the blood vessels in the legs and feet are deprived of blood; a *heart attack,* which could be fatal. When atherosclerosis affects the blood vessels leading to the brain, a stroke may result.

Atherosclerosis isn't just globs of cholesterol clinging to the vascular pipes that make up your circulatory system. It's a complex, dynamic process that appears to involve the interaction of three ingredients: fats such as cholesterol; microscopic blood cells called platelets, which help the blood to form clots; and the smooth muscle tissue that makes up the blood vessel wall.

Medical researchers still haven't found the exact cause of atherosclerosis. However, it is thought that the disease begins with an injury to the inner lining of the four-layered artery. When this thin inner lining, called the endothelium, sustains damage, toxic substances in the blood apparently gain entry to the artery wall. These substances have access to the next layer, made of supportive collagen, which is exposed as a result of the injury. Blood-clotting platelets rush to the injury site and stick to the area to shield and protect it. This collection of platelets can congregate into a clot that eventually may prevent the blood from flowing through the artery.

The platelets also contain substances called prostaglandins, which can constrict the arteries and increase the tendency of blood to clot. Another substance in platelets—platelet growth factor—can induce the proliferation of smooth muscle cells. While smooth muscle tissue is a regular resident of the artery wall, the proliferation of this tissue produced by platelet activity is thought to be a forerunner of atherosclerosis. The ability of aspirin to interfere with the stickiness of platelets in this process is under investigation. (See page 76.)

It may be that the excessive growth of smooth muscle cells is similar to the rapid multiplying of cancer cells. These smooth muscle cells migrate into the artery wall and set down a network of connective tissue that becomes the foundation for the arterial *plaque.*

In a sense, a plaque is like a scab that forms on a skin wound. But unlike the scab that eventually sheds and gives way to new tissue, atherosclerotic plaques accumulate inside the artery wall. Cholesterol in the bloodstream and cellular debris contribute to the buildup that eventually bulges inward into the path of blood flowing through the artery. Atherosclerotic plaques may not produce any symptoms until the artery is almost totally occluded. If a blood clot tries to flow through this restricted passage, blockage can occur and result in a heart attack.

Risk Factors

Atherosclerosis begins early. By age 20, the characteristic raised fatty streaks of atherosclerosis are present in the arteries of most people, but they don't cause any symptoms. From then on, atherosclerosis may progress slowly or rapidly, depending on your life-style and medical history.

Since it's impossible to know whether you are on a fast track to atherosclerosis, protect yourself by knowing and controlling your *risk factors*—those hereditary and environmental factors that work for you or against you in terms of a healthy cardiovascular system.

There are two types of cardiac risk factors, those you can change and those you can't:

Major Modifiable Risk Factors
  • hypertension, or high blood pressure
  • blood cholesterol levels
  • cigarette smoking

Nonmodifiable Risk Factors
  • heredity
  • gender
  • age
  • race

Other risk factors also contribute to atherosclerosis, including *diabetes, overweight, physical inactivity,* and *stress.* While there is no clear evidence that controlling these modifiable risk factors can definitely reduce your risk of heart attack, most doctors agree that it is prudent to control these factors as much as possible.

The more risk factors you have, the greater your likelihood of developing coronary heart disease. You can't change your sex, age, or genes, but the modifiable risk factors are amenable to change—either on your own initiative, or with a doctor's help.

To get an idea of the risk involved, here's how the odds stack up in a 40-year-old man. If his blood pressure and blood cholesterol levels are normal, his chance of developing atherosclerosis is *1 percent* over the next eight years. If he has high blood pressure, his risk *quadruples.* Add cholesterol levels that are one-third higher than normal, and his risk rises to *17 percent.* In the presence of diabetes, the figure becomes *28 percent.* If he smokes, his risk rises to *46 percent.* When physical inactivity and a family history of coronary heart disease are added, the risk soars to *50 percent.*

Let's look at those factors you can't change:

Heredity.   Heart disease appears to run in some families. When heart attacks, stroke, and high blood pressure occur among family members who are in their 30s, 40s, and early to mid-50s, they are at high risk for developing heart disease. By knowing your family history, you can become aware if you have an inherited tendency toward heart disease and you can work to lower your risk.

Gender.   Men at all ages are at a higher risk of heart attack than women. But after menopause, women lose the protection that estrogen and the other female sex hormones seem to confer on them. It is not known whether estrogen replacement therapy after menopause is effective in reducing coronary heart disease. In fact, this hormone could have adverse effects in other areas, which would cancel any benefits to the heart.

According to the American Heart Association, women over 55 have a 10 times greater risk of heart disease than do younger women. And women over 65 are more likely to suffer high blood pressure and strokes than men.

Age.   The aging process itself does not cause coronary heart disease, but progression of atherosclerosis over the decades can gradually block an artery and cause a heart attack or stroke. As a result, 55 percent of all heart attack victims are over age 65. Of the men and women who die from heart attack, four out of five are over age 65. At the same time, some people live into their 80s and 90s without any signs of heart disease.

Race.   Blacks suffer from moderate high blood pressure at twice the rate of whites, and from severe high blood pressure three times as often. Death rates from high blood pressure and related heart disease before age 50 are about six times higher in blacks.

Since these factors are set at birth, we cannot change them. Instead we should turn our attention to those aspects of health that we can control: hypertension (high blood pressure), cholesterol levels, and smoking. We should also pay attention to such secondary risk factors as obesity, diabetes, physical inactivity, and stress.

Hypertension

High blood pressure, or hypertension, is the increased force that blood exerts on the artery walls as the heart muscle pushes it out into the entire circulatory system. If the pressure is consistently high and goes undetected and untreated, it can damage the arteries and force the heart to work harder. (The *tension* in hypertension is a reference to pressure, not to nervous tension.) Hypertension is a disease usually without symptoms, until it reaches its later course. For this reason, it is called the "silent killer."

Blood pressure fluctuates during the day. When some people visit a doctor and have their blood pressure measured, their readings become elevated and then drop back to normal after they leave the doctor's office. Because it occurs only in the presence of a doctor, this phenomenon has been called "white-coat hypertension." (However, many of these people were found to eventually develop high blood pressure.)

If your blood pressure has been normal in the past but shows an elevation during a checkup, your doctor will want to take several more measurements before confirming a diagnosis of hypertension.

In either case, treatment begins the moment that high blood pressure has been diagnosed. For the patient whose blood pressure needs to be followed up in two subsequent visits, the physician should begin to explain how hypertension can be controlled. Nonmedicinal therapies that may be used separately or in combination with drug therapy for hypertension include weight reduction, salt restriction, avoiding tobacco, modifying your diet, exercise, reduced alcohol consumption, and stress reduction.

Drug Therapy

Although drug therapy is the most widely used method of controlling moderate to severe hypertension, the medications often may cause some unpleasant side effects that may require a change in prescription (or can lead to dangerous noncompliance).

In the past, *diuretics* were most commonly used to control high blood pressure. Diuretics work by increasing the amount of salt and water excreted by the kidneys. When there is less salt, the body retains less water. The volume of blood is lowered and so is the blood pressure. Among the possible side effects of diuretics are weakness and muscle pains, as well as lowering of potassium levels and increases in blood sugar and uric acid.

Drugs called *beta-blockers* also help to reduce blood pressure. They block the stimulating effect of adrenaline on certain receptors in the heart and cause the heart to beat at a slower rate. Beta-blockers can produce side effects such as fatigue, depression, impotence, insomnia, cold hands and feet, and asthma attacks.

A group of drugs known as *vasodilators* dilate or widen the blood vessels, mainly the arterioles. By reducing the resistance of the blood flow, vasodilators reduce the heavy load on the heart produced by high blood pressure. Possible side effects of vasodilators include headache, dizziness on arising quickly, palpitations, and edema (retention of fluid).

Newer classes of drugs now are available for treating high blood pressure: *angiotensin-converting enzyme (ACE) inhibitors* and *calcium channel blockers*. Because these drugs may have fewer side effects than older drugs, they are often being used as first-line therapy in hypertension.

When medication is given for hypertension, it is essential to take it *as prescribed.* High blood pressure cannot be cured, but it can be con-trolled. If the drug you are taking to lower your blood pressure causes undesirable side effects, discuss it with your doctor. If you once were taking medication to control your high blood pressure but stopped on your own, consult a doctor to discuss the newer treatments. Your med-ication can be changed or perhaps the dosage can be reduced. With modern hypertension therapy, most people need not experience unduly unpleasant side effects.

Treatment of Mild Hypertension

Even mildly elevated high blood pressure requires treatment, but it doesn't necessarily have to be done with drugs. Making certain changes in your life-style may help lower your blood pressure, or at least make it possible for you to take a low-dosage antihypertensive drug with few, if any, side effects.

Many of these life-style changes are discussed throughout this book: quitting smoking, weight loss when necessary, controlling stress, modi-fying your diet, and getting regular aerobic exercise. Restricting your alcohol intake also is recommended.

More than two drinks a day can raise blood pressure. The reason for this remains unknown. We do know that when heavy drinkers quit alcohol, their blood pressure usually drops. However, consuming one or two drinks a day appears to have a negligible effect on blood pressure.

Measuring Blood Pressure

Blood pressure should be measured at least every two years in people with normal blood pressure. The measurement may be performed by a physician or by another qualified professional.

A sphygmomanometer is used to measure your blood pres-sure. The tester wraps an inflatable cuff around your upper arm and pumps enough air into it to halt the blood flow in the artery. A stethoscope is then placed over the artery so that the tester can hear sounds inside the vessel as the air is gradually released from the cuff. When the pulse returns, the number that appears on the gauge of the sphygmomanometer reflects the force with which your heart is contracting and forcing blood into the arteries—the *systolic blood pressure.* Immediately, more air is released from the cuff to obtain the second part of the reading—the *diastolic blood pressure.* The second number indicates the status of the resting phase between the heart's contractions.

While a blood pressure reading of 120 over 80 has been considered the textbook normal reading, what is truly "normal" varies. The 1988 Report of the National High Blood Pressure Education Program (NHBPEP) lists the following ranges and checkup timetable:

Systolic	Recommended Follow-up
Below 140	Recheck every two years
140–199	Confirm within two months
200 or over	Immediate drug therapy may be necessary

Diastolic	Recommended Follow-up
Below 85	Recheck every two years
85–89	Recheck within one year
90–104	Confirm within two months
105–114	Evaluate within two weeks
115 or over	Immediate drug therapy may be necessary

Sodium.   The role of salt or sodium as a contributor to high blood pressure remains under investigation. While salt doesn't appear actually to *cause* high blood pressure, it can increase blood pressure in susceptible people.

Your body needs only about 200 milligrams of sodium a day, yet most Americans consume 10 times this amount. The new RDAs call for a minimum sodium requirement of 500 milligrams a day—the equivalent of a little more than a quarter-teaspoon. There is little risk of salt depletion at this level, except under conditions of extreme heat when there may be excessive loss of body fluids.

It isn't known whether such preventive restriction of dietary sodium will lower blood pressure, but a few studies have indicated that sensitivity to salt increases with age. As your body ages, the kidneys seem to become less effective at excreting sodium. Get an early start on prevention by moderating your salt intake sooner.

Hypertension and kidney disease are much more prevalent in blacks than in whites. Blacks tend to have a hereditary type of high blood pressure called *low-renin hypertension*. Renin is a hormone produced by the kidneys that constricts or contracts the blood vessels.

A major research effort published in 1988 by the Intersalt Cooperative Research Group studied 10,000 people from 32 countries and confirmed that overall, salt intake has only a minor influence on blood pressure. As an example, black study participants from Mississippi had the fifth-lowest salt intake of the 52 groups, but the prevalence of high blood pressure in this group was the third highest of all those studied. There was no evidence that too much sodium causes high blood pressure or that decreasing your salt consumption will prevent hypertension.

Generally, heavy salt use can make your blood pressure rise if you already have hypertension; if you don't, salt isn't likely to cause high blood pressure.

A lifetime salt habit is hard to break, but you can reach for spices and herbs in place of salt when you cook. Use more natural flavorings, such as fresh garlic and onion, fresh lemon or lime juice. Salt substitutes are recommended with caution because the potassium they contain may be harmful to some people. Check with your physician as to whether you can safely use one of these salt substitutes.

Sodium, of course, abounds in numerous processed and convenience foods. Some over-the-counter drugs are loaded with sodium, especially antacids, stomach preparations, and certain antibiotics. If you are watching your salt intake, be sure to check the label for the sodium content (see Chapter 2 for labeling information).

Cholesterol

A modest 5 percent reduction in the mean cholesterol level of Americans could lower the incidence of coronary heart disease by 10 percent. So once you know your blood pressure, find out your blood cholesterol level. The rationale for cholesterol awareness is similar, because a high level produces neither signs nor symptoms. A simple blood test can detect high cholesterol. Treatment can not only halt the progression of atherosclerosis, but in some cases may decrease the arterial damage that's already occurred.

Cholesterol is necessary to sustain life. The delicate membrane surrounding each cell in your body needs cholesterol for maintenance, and your body couldn't produce your sex hormones without cholesterol. The problem lies in the fact that most of the cholesterol your body requires is manufactured in the liver. The food you eat provides the rest—but too often, far in excess of what you really need.

Cholesterol is a fatty substance that is technically called a lipid. Cholesterol travels through your bloodstream by attaching itself to at least two kinds of carrier protein. The first type of protein heads directly to areas on blood vessel walls and accumulates there until an atherosclerotic plaque begins to form. This is the "bad" cholesterol, which attaches to *low-density lipoprotein (LDL)*. The second type of protein actually corrals and hauls superfluous cholesterol from the bloodstream back to the liver for elimination. This "good" cholesterol is carried by *high-density lipoprotein (HDL)*.

A high level of protective HDL confers a lower risk of heart disease. But when LDL is elevated, the risk increases. Raising HDL in the blood is a far more difficult process than lowering total blood cholesterol or LDL. Exercise appears to maintain HDL at its current levels and may even raise it, although thus far no clinical trials in humans have proven that increasing HDL will necessarily lower your risk of heart disease. However, when a doctor assesses a patient's need for treatment, the level of LDL cholesterol is what serves as the key index for any decisions about therapy to lower cholesterol.

Total blood cholesterol should be measured every five years in all adults age 20 and over. By detecting high blood cholesterol levels early, you and your doctor can reduce your risk of coronary artery disease.

Triglycerides

Triglycerides are also lipids, or fatty compounds, that travel in your bloodstream as companions to cholesterol. Like cholesterol, triglycerides are produced by your body and obtained through your diet.

Your body either deposits triglycerides in its fat cells for future use, or else breaks them down right away to produce energy. The triglycerides hop aboard proteins called very-low-density lipoprotein (VLDL) that your liver releases into the bloodstream. Your body's tissues take what they need from the VLDL and the remainder stays in your bloodstream. If your liver doesn't pull the VLDL out of circulation for excretion, the remnants stay afloat and raise the levels of your "bad" cholesterol.

Much controversy surrounds the relationship between high triglyceride levels in the blood and coronary heart disease. When triglycerides are high, the levels of total cholesterol and LDL cholesterol are often high as well, and protective HDL cholesterol tends to be low. While a large number of people with coronary heart disease also have high triglyceride levels, there are other people who have elevated triglycerides and no sign of heart disease.

High triglycerides may contribute to other conditions or be consequences of certain life habits that indirectly encourage the development of atherosclerosis. For instance, diabetes, obesity, some liver and kidney diseases, metabolic disorders, and excessive alcohol intake may bring an increased risk of coronary heart disease.

Triglyceride levels vary depending on age and sex. Recommendations for desirable levels vary from 100 milligrams per deciliter to 140 if you are in your 20s, 150 for people in their 30s, 160 for those in their 40s, and 190 for those older than 50. A National Institutes of Health panel has classified triglyceride levels between 250 and 500 milligrams per deciliter as borderline elevations, although many doctors consider these values excessive. Levels above 500 milligrams per deciliter fall into the high category.

Dietary and life-style changes are first recommended to reduce high triglyceride levels. When the level of triglycerides fails to drop in response to these changes, drug therapy is usually prescribed.

Alcohol

There is no definitive information on the role of alcohol and its effects on cholesterol levels. Alcohol does not affect LDL cholesterol, but it may increase triglycerides and HDL cholesterol in some people. Whether the higher HDL level produced by alcohol can offer protection against heart disease is a matter of uncertainty and controversy. Moderate alcohol consumption of one to two drinks a day is not considered harmful. However, when alcohol intake surpasses the equivalent of eight ounces of wine, 24 ounces of beer, or two ounces of 100-proof whiskey, it poses a threat to several organs in your body. With such a narrow window of safety, it is obviously not recommended that anyone take up drinking in order to prevent coronary heart disease.

Finding Your Cholesterol Count

Cholesterol is measured in milligrams per deciliter.

The current National Cholesterol Education Program guidelines for *total blood cholesterol* are as follows:

Risk Classification	Total Cholesterol (mg/dl)
Desirable	Below 200
Borderline-high	200–239
High	240 and over

If your total cholesterol level is under 200, you should have another test taken in five years.

If your reading is over 200, it is borderline; a repeat test should be taken to confirm that the result is a true reflection of your blood cholesterol. Borderline levels call for an evaluation of your HDL and LDL profile and, possibly, changes in diet to lower your cholesterol. If you are borderline and have no other cardiac risk factors, annual cholesterol tests are recommended in addition to dietary change. Those who are borderline and already have heart disease or two cardiac risk factors should have a lipid profile. Since a high level of HDL confers protection, an individual with this reading would be handled as "normal."

A lipid profile includes calculated LDL and measured HDL and triglyceride levels. Cholesterol levels over 240 enter the high category and also require a lipid profile. The follow-up care for people with high-risk levels is based on their LDL levels.

When a lipid profile is necessary, the NCEP guidelines for LDL cholesterol are:

Risk Classification	LDL Cholesterol (mg/dl)
Desirable	Below 130
Borderline-high	130–159
High	160 and over

Reducing Cholesterol

Dietary Therapy

The first line of treatment for reducing elevated cholesterol levels is diet. The cholesterol-lowering diet recommended by the American Heart Association suggests that you limit fat intake to 30 percent of your total calories, with saturated fats accounting for less than 10 percent of this amount. Carbohydrates should make up 50 to 60 percent of your total calories. The remainder is protein consumption, which you should keep at 10 to 20 percent of a day's worth of calories. Confine your dietary cholesterol intake to less than 300 milligrams, or the equivalent of one egg.

The 1988 *Surgeon General's Report on Health and Nutrition* states that "although there are many determinants of blood cholesterol levels, no modifiable factor has been shown to influence cholesterol and LDL more profoundly than diet."

The surgeon general singled out *saturated fat*—fatty meats, high-fat dairy products, and the cocoa butter, palm oil, and coconut oil found in many commercially prepared and processed foods—as the number-one enemy of a healthy heart. Dietary cholesterol—which comes from the animal foods (such as red meats, organ meats, and dairy products) in your diet—also is important, but its effect varies in each person. Some people are highly sensitive to cholesterol in the diet while others are more resistant.

Drug Therapy

If dietary changes fail to bring down an elevated cholesterol level, treatment with drugs may be necessary. In some cases, one cholesterol-lowering drug may be used in combination with another to increase effectiveness or to lessen any side effects. However, these medications may produce undesirable side effects in some people.

The drugs *cholestyramine* (Cholybar, Questram) and *colestipol* (Colestid), for instance, may produce gastrointestinal symptoms such as constipation, bloating, nausea, and excess gas. Cholestyramine and colestipol can also interfere with the absorption of other drugs you are taking. But both of these drugs are effective in lowering LDL cholesterol levels and reducing the risk of coronary heart disease.

Nicotinic acid, or niacin, of the vitamin B family, has been used to decrease high LDL cholesterol levels. Nicotinic acid is considered effective in lowering cholesterol levels and safe for long-term use in appropriate people. Its major side effect is facial flushing. (Recent studies, though, have shown that delayed-release forms of niacin can damage the liver.)

Among the newer classes of drugs are *lovastatin* (Mevacor), which may produce side effects such as gastrointestinal distress, muscle pain, and possible liver damage. Because lovastatin gained FDA approval only in 1987, its long-term safety has yet to be ascertained.

Gemfibrozil (Lopid), a drug that is used to lower triglyceride levels, may be effective in increasing HDL levels but is not approved for routine use in lowering cholesterol. Studies are under way to evaluate the effects of gemfibrozil on heart disease risk reduction as well as to determine its long-term side effects. This drug commonly causes gastrointestinal symptoms and may lead to the formation of stones in the bile duct.

Probucol (Lorelco) is also under study for its ability to lower elevated LDL cholesterol. However, one concern about probucol is that it may lower the protective HDL cholesterol. Among its short-term side effects are abdominal pain, nausea, diarrhea, and excess gas. Probucol also may lead to aberrations of normal heart rhythm in some people. The long-term safety of probucol has not been established.

Cautions.   While blood cholesterol testing is a key factor in reducing your personal risk of heart disease, any testing must be performed at an accredited laboratory that meets current standards of accuracy and reliability.

The U.S. Preventive Services Task Force calls for discretion in the use of drugs to lower cholesterol, noting that "The efficacy of these agents has been demonstrated conclusively only in middle-aged men with serum cholesterol levels above 265 milligrams per deciliter. The use of lipid-lowering drugs in young men, women, or elderly persons with only mild to moderate elevations of serum lipids is of unproven clinical benefit."

Secondary Risk Factors in Heart Disease

Cigarette Smoking

Cigarette smoking is unsafe for a number of reasons (see Chapter 1); in the cardiovascular system, smoking fuels the fires of atherosclerosis.

With each inhalation, cigarette smoke carries nicotine and carbon monoxide, a main component of automobile exhaust, into the bloodstream. The carbon monoxide usurps some of the oxygen that should be delivered to your body's tissues. Nicotine increases blood pressure and makes your heart beat faster, thus forcing it to work harder and to require more oxygen. But a smoker's heart muscle gets carbon monoxide instead of oxygen.

Smoking is also a major risk factor in the narrowing of the blood vessels of the arms and legs, a condition called peripheral vascular disease. Nicotine constricts the blood vessels and impedes the flow of blood to the small arteries of the hands and feet.

When atherosclerotic plaques are present on artery walls, the components of cigarette smoke appear to promote the development of cholesterol deposits in these areas.

Obesity

By medical standards, when you are 20 percent or more over your ideal body weight, your risk of mortality increases—especially in relation to heart disease. Being overweight also increases the likelihood that other coronary risk factors are present, including high blood pressure, elevated blood cholesterol levels, and diabetes.

Interestingly, the *location* of fat on your body may have a bearing on your risk for heart disease. A man's waist measurement should not be larger than his hips. A woman's waist measurement should not exceed 80 percent of her hips. A big abdomen, or potbelly, typically seen in overweight men (and in some women) appears to be a riskier fat distribution than the pear-shaped torso, commonly seen in women with fatty thighs and buttocks.

Carrying extra weight puts a greater strain on your heart, too, because it has to pump harder to supply a larger body mass. A good starting point to reduce your risk of coronary heart disease is to begin a program of regular exercise and adopt a low-fat diet (see Chapter 2).

Diabetes

A disease in which the sugar level in the blood is elevated, diabetes is three times more likely to occur when you are overweight, although many other factors, including heredity, may trigger the disorder. Much blood vessel damage can result from diabetes: the large arteries can become more vulnerable to atherosclerosis and the small blood vessels, especially the capillaries that supply blood to the eyes, kidneys, and nerves, can become irreversibly damaged. Diabetics also tend to have elevated levels of cholesterol and other fatty substances in the bloodstream, called triglycerides. Blood pressure also may increase when diabetes is present.

Most cases of diabetes appear after age 40, in a form called Type II diabetes mellitus. This type usually does not require the use of insulin. To control Type II diabetes, doctors recommend changes in diet and an exercise program to control weight. However, if you already have developed eye, heart, or kidney disorders as a result of diabetes, undertaking an exercise program that is too vigorous may be harmful. Your doctor can assess how much exercise you can safely handle.

Physical Inactivity

While physical inactivity is not a clearly established risk factor for coronary heart disease, it is a risk factor for such related disorders as hypertension and obesity. If you are physically inactive, your risk of developing heart disease is double that of people who exercise regularly.

Regular exercise appears to reduce bloodstream levels of the fat triglyceride, as well as particles loaded with triglyceride, called lipoproteins. Following a workout, an enzyme, lipoprotein lipase, goes to work breaking down triglycerides in the bloodstream. Men who exercised but maintained their regular body weight had lower VLDL (very-low-density lipoprotein) and triglyceride levels when their blood was analyzed right after meals and again 12 hours after meals. (When VLDL levels are high, the risk of heart disease is greater.)

In addition to its effects on blood lipids, exercise also helps to lower weight, blood pressure, and the resting heart rate, and increases cardiac efficiency.

If you have not exercised for a long time, do not begin an exercise program until you have consulted a doctor. After a physical examination, your doctor can advise you about which exercises are best for your age and physical condition. (See Chapter 2.)

Stress

The way you respond to stress may influence your risk of coronary heart disease. The concept of the classic Type A personality was first introduced 30 years ago and described a person who was aggressive, ambitious, competitive, driving, impatient, irritable, and hostile. Some researchers have confirmed an association between Type A behavior and coronary heart disease, while others have not been able to do so.

More recent studies point to one component of the Type A profile that may be the most harmful to health: hostility. A hostile attitude shows up as anger, cynicism, mistrust, skepticism, or suspicion. Of course, just about everyone has an occasional episode of anger or hostile feelings. But when hostility becomes a constant way of thinking and experiencing the world, the risk of heart disease may be higher.

Researchers at Duke University Medical Center conducted a follow-up study of 118 attorneys who took a standard personality test called the Minnesota Multiphasic Personality Inventory (MMPI) as students. Over the years, it was found that those who had the highest scores on the test's hostility scale were 4.2 times more likely to have died from heart disease or other causes compared to their less hostile colleagues.

Another study involving medical school graduates showed that 25 years after taking the MMPI, the doctors who had scored high in hostility were about five times more likely to have suffered a heart attack or death from a coronary event. Though it's hard to prove cause and effect, overall, these doctors were 6.4 times more likely to have suffered a premature death.

Laboratory studies of people who were deliberately harassed when given mental tasks to solve showed dramatic increases in blood pressure when the people became angry. Meantime, blood pressure readings of the calmer participants remained normal. People who are anger-prone also may have a higher release of adrenaline and, accordingly, a stronger fight-or-flight response.

If your attitude falls into the hostile category it's best to learn how to relax by recognizing and canceling out antagonistic thoughts as soon as they begin to form and trying to imagine how the person who provoked you in the first place must feel. Being conscious of your consistent behavior patterns and instinctive reactions can help you change your attitude and may reduce your risk of heart problems (see Chapter 5).

Heart Disease: The Warning Signs

A 39-year-old man works 10- to 12-hour days, exercises occasionally, has a history of heart disease in his family, and shows no signs of coronary artery disease. Can he expect his coronary picture to change suddenly?

It's very possible. Atherosclerosis is progressive and may present no signs in the early stages. The chest pain of *angina pectoris* may develop or a heart attack (*myocardial infarction*) may occur because of the decreased supply of blood to the heart muscle. *Sudden death* may occur if the heart's electrical system malfunctions as a result of an *arrhythmia,* an abnormal rhythm of the heart.

As a coronary artery gradually becomes narrowed by atherosclerosis, it may become 70, 80, or 90 percent blocked, but still produce no symptoms. Then one of three events may occur: a blood clot may come by and become jammed in the narrowed area; a large section of plaque may break off the artery wall and close off the narrowed area it comes to; or a spasm of the blood vessel may cause it to squeeze shut. Each of these occurrences may cause an abrupt decline in the circulation of blood to the heart muscle.

How Your Heart Works

To get an idea of the size of your heart, look at your clenched fist. Inside your chest, slightly to the left of center, this fist-sized organ is a pumping station that keeps blood continuously coursing through your arteries and veins. Specialized cells inside the heart's pacemaker produce an electrical current that causes your heart to pump blood, by contracting, relaxing, and contracting again, 60 to 80 beats per minute. The range is even wider with activity, when your heart may beat more than 150 times a minute. In a single day, the average heart beats 100,000 times.

Composed mostly of muscle tissue called myocardium, the heart has four sections, or chambers, with one pair forming the right side and another pair making up the left side. The *right* side of the heart (the right atrium on top and the right ventricle below) accepts oxygen-depleted blood that already has circulated through the body, and pumps it to the lungs. Inside the lungs, carbon dioxide—one of the blood's waste products—is exchanged for fresh oxygen. The newly oxygenated blood travels back to the *left* side of the heart (the left atrium and left ventricle), which pumps it out to the body's network of blood vessels. The heart's chambers and valves coordinate perfectly in sound and motion to produce the rhythmic lub-dub that your doctor hears while listening to your heart through a stethoscope.

The many components of the heart and blood vessels are durable, resilient, and adaptable. Mechanical problems or infection can throw the heart into wild disarray, but for the most part, these conditions are rare. When cardiologists talk about

keeping the heart disease-free, they mean preventing atherosclerosis, controlling high blood pressure, and avoiding the damaging effects of inactivity.

Angina

If your heart muscle is hungry for blood, it may warn you by producing the chest pain of *angina pectoris*. Angina, a symptom of coronary
heart disease, is characterized by a heaviness or squeezing sensation in
the center of the chest, behind the breastbone. In some cases, the pain
may spread to the arms, especially the left arm, jaw, neck, or back. The
discomfort of angina usually occurs when increased demands are placed
on the heart, such as sprinting for a bus or climbing a staircase. The
heart requires an increased supply of blood and oxygen at this time, but
doesn't get it. This imbalance in supply and demand causes a condition
known as *ischemia*.

The pain usually stops within a few minutes. Rest generally relieves
angina. For chronic stable cases of angina, the drug *nitroglycerin* may
be prescribed to control the pain. However, if episodes of chest pain
become more frequent or severe and if they last longer, consult a doctor
immediately. Severe angina may be a warning sign that you are at great
risk for a heart attack.

Another form of angina, called *unstable angina,* is not as predictable
as angina. Episodes of chest pain occur frequently and often, even in the
absence of physical exertion or emotional excitement. Unstable angina
may also be a forerunner of a heart attack. Nitroglycerin, beta-blockers,
or calcium-blocking drugs may be prescribed to help quell the pain.
Drugs that prevent blood clotting may also reduce the risk of a heart
attack.

Silent ischemia occurs when there is an inadequate supply of blood
to the heart, but no anginal pain to let you know that your heart may
be in danger. Many people who have angina may experience episodes of
silent ischemia as well. Those who have silent ischemia are at increased
risk of heart attack, despite the absence of pain.

This form of silent angina often occurs at rest and it may be triggered
by emotional stress. The only way to detect silent ischemia is by undergoing an exercise stress test or wearing a 24-hour Holter monitor to record
the electrical activity of your heart. Both tests are expensive and are not
recommended as a screening method for people who have no symptoms
of heart disease. If you are at significant risk for developing heart disease,
though, your doctor may recommend such testing.

The main screening tests for coronary artery disease without symptoms include measurement of blood pressure and blood cholesterol. If a patient is a smoker, the doctor should provide counseling to stop smoking. Electrocardiograms (ECGs) are not recommended for men and women with no symptoms. Only if you are in a high-risk group, such as a man over 40 with two or more cardiac risk factors, or a high-risk male over 40 who wants to begin a vigorous exercise program, is an ECG suggested.

However, an ECG taken at rest may be entirely normal—even in people with severe forms of coronary disease. Any decision about further testing with exercise stress tests or any other methods remains a matter of discussion between the patient and his or her physician.

Heart Attack

When a heart attack occurs, the chances of surviving it, as well as the quality of life afterward, all depend on how much damage the heart muscle suffers during the episode. A heart attack, or *myocardial infarction,* can be fatal or severely disabling if emergency medical care is not available immediately.

Severe pressure, tightness, or a squeezing sensation in the center of the chest may be due to angina or heart attack. The crushing chest pain that radiates down the left arm is a classic sign of heart attack. Yet the same type of pain occurs when the esophagus goes into spasm. Indigestion and heartburn have symptoms that mimic the pain of angina and heart attack. Anxiety and pulmonary disease also may produce chest pain with such symptoms as dizziness and shortness of breath.

Since it's unreliable to diagnose yourself, take any symptoms of chest pain seriously. Chest pain that persists for more than a few minutes should not be ignored.

Warning Signs of a Heart Attack

- uncomfortable pressure, fullness, squeezing, or pain in the center of the chest lasting two minutes or longer
- pain spreading to the shoulders, neck, or arms
- severe pain, lightheadedness, fainting, sweating, nausea, or shortness of breath

(Not all of these warning signs occur in every heart attack. If some start to occur, don't wait. Get help immediately.)

Emergency Measures

- If you have chest discomfort that lasts two minutes or more, call the emergency rescue service.
- If you can get to a hospital faster by going yourself and not waiting for an ambulance, have someone drive you there.
- If you're with someone who is experiencing the signs of a heart attack—and the warning signs last two minutes or longer—act immediately.
- Expect a denial. It's normal for someone with chest discomfort to deny the possibility of something as serious as a heart attack. But don't take no for an answer. Take prompt action.
- Call an emergency rescue service or get the patient to the nearest hospital emergency room.
- If you are properly trained to give CPR (cardiopulmonary resuscitation), administer the technique if it's necessary.

Coronary Thrombosis

As many as 90 percent of all heart attacks are triggered by a fresh clot of blood, or *thrombus,* that has lodged in a coronary artery. Hence the name *coronary thrombosis* or *coronary occlusion.*

A smaller number of heart attacks are due to *coronary spasm,* in which the coronary artery contracts and then decreases or even halts the flow of blood to the heart muscle. The cause of coronary spasm is unknown. This disorder may occur in normal arteries as well as in those with atherosclerosis.

Since the role of blood clot formation in heart attack was confirmed in the early 1980s, several effective new therapies have become available to dissolve these life-threatening clots. When administered within a few hours after a heart attack, these *thrombolytic* therapies may be able to reduce the chance of death and disability from a major coronary event.

Drug therapy.   Doctors now have an array of substances available that can dissolve a lethal blood clot and improve the survival rate of a heart attack victim. But there is still much confusion and controversy over which drug is best for each individual patient.

The thrombolytic therapies include *streptokinase* (Streptase), a protein that the body makes naturally from streptococcal bacteria; *urokinase* (Abbokinase), a protein that is a product of urine; *tissue plasminogen activator,* or *t-PA* (Activase), which the body produces to dissolve blood clots when malignant melanoma cells are present. *Aspirin* helps to reduce clot formation in some people (see page 76).

T-PA, which is produced through genetic engineering, and the kinase drugs all work by dissolving fibrin, which forms the infrastructure of a blood clot. Streptokinase and urokinase may dissolve blood clots throughout the body, while t-PA appears to work specifically on the fresh clot in the coronary arteries. All three substances are effective, but each has its advantages and disadvantages.

The thrombolytic therapies present the risk of hemorrhage in people who are prone to abnormal bleeding. Thus they may be harmful to heart attack victims who have had a bleeding ulcer in the last two months, or surgery within the last two to six weeks, or a recent head injury. Other poor-risk candidates include people who have a history of hemorrhagic strokes or diabetic retinopathy. Pregnant women also may be at risk from clot-dissolving therapy.

Streptokinase reduces mortality from heart attack by about 25 percent. When given in combination with aspirin, streptokinase has reduced the death rate by 50 percent. But the drug may produce an allergic reaction in some patients. A person who receives streptokinase the first time may develop antibodies to the bacterial protein from which it is made. If the drug is given a second time, the antibodies may block its effectiveness and produce an adverse reaction.

T-PA appears to have a lower risk of bleeding. It also seems to produce no allergic reactions. Like streptokinase, it reduces heart attack mortality by about 25 percent.

In 1990, Italian researchers who compared the use of streptokinase and t-PA in 12,381 heart attack patients reported that both drugs were equally effective. The death rate, heart function, and rate of complications for patients in each study group were so similar that researchers considered the slight differences statistically insignificant.

Scientists in the United States say that further analysis of the long-term benefits of both drugs is necessary before recommending an across-the-board switch to the lower-priced streptokinase. Certain aspects of the study design have been criticized and some controversy surrounds the results. Currently, about two-thirds of heart attack patients in the United States receive t-PA.

Cost is a major consideration in choosing between the two drugs. The bill to treat a heart attack victim with streptokinase runs about $200; a person who gets t-PA must pay about $2,200.

Whichever therapy is used, time is of the essence. Ideally, treatment with the drugs, which are administered intravenously, should begin within minutes of the heart attack. Both drugs are most beneficial when given within the first five hours of a heart attack.

When anticlotting therapy is successful in stopping a heart attack in its tracks, it must be followed by the prompt use of *heparin* (Calciparine, Liquaemin), an anticoagulant, to prevent the formation of another clot. Success has also been reported with aspirin.

Angioplasty. This technique uses an inflatable balloon at the tip of a catheter to reach a blocked artery, flatten the plaque, and open up the clogged blood vessel. This procedure, which has become a commonly performed treatment following heart attack, has recently come under fire by some leading cardiologists as being costly, risky, and of negligible value in terms of long-term effectiveness.

The advent of the thrombolytic therapies and their ability to dissolve effectively potentially lethal blood clots has reinforced these arguments. One recent study showed that the difference in mortality was less than 1 percent after one group of heart attack victims was treated with only t-PA while another group received t-PA plus angioplasty.

Certainly, angioplasty is not always successful. In fact, when the blockage in the artery is extensive, coronary bypass surgery may be recommended instead. For many patients, angioplasty can be compared to plowing a road while it's still snowing; the blockage may return within a few months.

Coronary bypass surgery. Controversy also surrounds the routine performance of *coronary artery bypass grafts (CABG)*. In a bypass procedure, the diseased arteries are removed and replaced with a section of vein from the leg. While CABG may be necessary and useful for those patients with major blockage in one or all coronary arteries, others with less severe heart disease have been found to do just as well with medication.

Bypass surgery, however, may relieve the pain of angina. More important, when a bypass graft is performed out of necessity, it may extend the patient's life for a number of years. The grafts may become occluded by blood clots or develop atherosclerosis years later, just like the native arteries themselves. In some cases, repeat bypass surgery may be needed. For this reason, it is vital that you modify your life-style and practice heart disease prevention if you must undergo coronary bypass surgery. The operation is *not* a cure for atherosclerosis.

After a Heart Attack

An adjustment of attitude is one of the first steps toward a successful recovery. It's normal to experience anxiety and depression following a heart attack. Doubts about returning to work, resuming sexual activity, and enjoying your normal activities often cause worry and concern. Discuss these questions with your doctor so that a realistic schedule for your resumption of these activities can be made, and the natural healing process can take place.

The outlook for many survivors of heart attacks is excellent. Atherosclerosis has already announced its presence, so draw up a plan of secondary prevention. It may be possible to reverse some arterial damage and avoid another cardiac episode, which might be fatal.

Life-style changes include stopping smoking, losing excess weight, watching cholesterol, and increasing physical activity. Make sure you get medical clearance and a graded plan of exercise before undertaking any strenuous exercise; supervised exercise programs for people who have had heart attacks may be available in your community. Check with your local chapter of the American Heart Association.

Common Cardiovascular Conditions

Arrhythmias

An *arrhythmia* is an abnormality in heart rhythm. Some arrhythmias are irregular heartbeats, while others are regular rhythms that are either too fast or too slow. The occasional sensation of your heart skipping a beat is a normal occurrence. But in an arrhythmia, the skipped beat occurs repeatedly and eventually the heart may be thrown into electrical chaos.

Specialized cells inside the heart—an area called the pacemaker—emit an electrical signal that is conducted to each pumping chamber. When the signal is too fast, too slow, or too jumbled, the result is an arrhythmia.

Some arrhythmias may be due to smoking, too much caffeine, anxiety, and some medications; a change in life-style can alleviate the symptoms. Others may result from coronary heart disease, certain cardiac abnormalities, a heart valve disorder, or thyroid disease. When arrhythmias persist, certain drugs may provide relief. However, in some cases, surgical implantation of an electronic pacemaker may be recommended.

Mitral Valve Prolapse

Mitral valve prolapse (MVP) is a common abnormality of the heart valves. An estimated 6 to 21 percent of the adult population may have the symptoms of MVP. While it can cause chest pain, dizziness, palpitations, and shortness of breath, the actual disorder is often more uncomfortable than dangerous.

The mitral valve—so called because its doorlike flaps or "leaflets" are shaped like a bishop's miter or hat—is supposed to open in one direction to allow the one-way flow of blood into the left ventricle, the main pumping chamber of the heart. When MVP occurs, the valve's two leaflets may not close properly and may allow some backflow of blood. When this occurs, the blood flow is more turbulent and may sound like a heart murmur through a stethoscope. Physical examination and echo-cardiography, or ultrasound, are used to diagnose mitral valve prolapse.

One possible complication of mitral valve prolapse is the risk of *infective endocarditis,* or infection of the heart cavity lining and valves. If you have MVP and are going to the dentist for a cleaning or dental procedure, mention your mitral valve condition. Antibiotics will be given to you before and after dental work to prevent infection from bacteria.

Panic attacks and anxiety have been associated with mitral valve prolapse, especially when a person is in poor physical condition. MVP is found in about 50 percent of patients with panic disorder, but the connection remains unclear. Most cases of MVP do not require treatment. Occasionally, beta-blockers, especially propranolol (Inderal), may be used to control some of the symptoms of MVP.

Stroke

When blood vessels leading to the brain become blocked or are ruptured, the result is a *stroke.* This disruption in blood supply may cause irreversible damage to the brain and central nervous system within minutes. If the brain's nerve cells are deprived of oxygen, they die and cannot be replaced because nerve cells do not regenerate.

The same emergency measures for heart attacks also apply to strokes—urgent and immediate treatment is necessary. A stroke doesn't necessarily lead to a life of disability. Prompt treatment may lead to a full or almost full recovery.

Stroke, the third leading cause of death, behind heart attack and cancer, was responsible for 149,200 deaths in 1987. Most strokes are caused by a blood clot, or *cerebral thrombosis,* that gets lodged in an artery that is narrowed by atherosclerosis and thus impedes the flow of blood to the brain. A clot also may originate in the heart and travel through the arteries until it reaches an area too narrow for passage, in which case it is called an *embolism.* In another form of stroke, high blood pressure may damage small blood vessels and block the passage of blood. Hemorrhages also may cause strokes. An *aneurysm,* which is a weak section of a blood vessel that blisters outward, is also responsible for a number of hemorrhagic strokes.

Stroke risk factors.   The unmodifiable factors that boost the risk of stroke include age—the incidence of stroke in the 55-and-older population doubles in each upcoming decade; sex—men have a 30 percent higher incidence of stroke; race—blacks have a 60 percent greater risk of stroke than whites; diabetes—when coupled with hypertension, the risk of stroke is higher; prior stroke—increases the risk of another stroke; heredity—a family history of stroke increases the risk. Another risk factor is asymptomatic carotid bruit—an abnormal sound made by the blood flowing to the brain through a narrowing in the carotid artery in the neck. Turbulent flow of blood may point to an increased risk of stroke.

The most important risk factor for stroke that you *can* control is high blood pressure. Have your blood pressure checked every two years even if you have no symptoms of heart disease or stroke. If you already have a diagnosis of hypertension, follow your doctor's advice, take your medication regularly, and go for scheduled checkups. Cigarette smoking and elevated blood cholesterol levels also increase your risk of stroke.

Neurologists are investigating the effect of a new clot-dissolving drug on some forms of stroke. This agent, tissue plasminogen activator, has already been seen to produce dramatic results when administered right after a heart attack.

Warning Signs of Stroke

- sudden weakness or numbness of the face, arm, and leg on one side of the body
- loss of speech, or trouble talking or understanding speech
- dimness or loss of vision, particularly in only one eye
- unexplained dizziness, especially when associated with other neurologic symptoms

Ministrokes

An estimated 10 percent of all strokes are preceded by a phenomenon known as a ministroke, or *transient ischemic attack (TIA),* caused by a temporarily reduced blood flow to part of the brain. TIA symptoms are similar to those listed for a full stroke, except that they are temporary—as short as five minutes or as long as several hours. When the symptoms fade, the person experiencing a TIA returns to normal.

If you have had symptoms, report them immediately to your doctor, even though no stroke developed. Dietary and weight control adjustments may be necessary. Anticoagulant drug therapy may be prescribed. One medication that *may* benefit some people with TIAs is aspirin. Consult your physician for recommendations on whether you would benefit from taking aspirin on a regular basis (see page 76).

There is not enough evidence to support testing for carotid bruits (listening with a stethoscope at the neck) or for noninvasive testing (with ultrasound) for abnormal narrowing of the carotid arteries in people with no symptoms. All men and women should receive routine screening for high blood pressure and counseling on other factors for atherosclerotic disease.

Aneurysm

An *aneurysm,* or outpouching of an artery wall, may occur in the brain, the aorta, or other arteries. Similar to the leak in a tire tube about to undergo a blowout, this arterial leak may be slow and give some warning signs, or it may be sudden and shoot blood into the affected area. An aneurysm can cause a stroke or sudden death.

When there is a slow leakage of blood into the brain, there may be symptoms such as sharp headaches and neck pain. A sudden rupture of an aneurysm produces immediate and severe pain. An angiogram, or X ray that uses contrast media injected into an artery through a catheter, is used to diagnose aneurysms. Emergency surgery is required to stop the bleeding.

Peripheral Vascular Disease

Arteriosclerosis Obliterans

Arteriosclerosis obliterans, also known as "intermittent claudication," is a progressive hardening of the arteries in the various parts of the body. When it affects the legs, it may produce leg cramps or muscle fatigue after a person walks only a few blocks. Occasionally, pain may occur even at rest. Cigarette smokers and people with diabetes or hypertension are at increased risk for arteriosclerosis obliterans. In severe cases, skin ulcers or gangrene may develop and lead to the loss of the limb.

Routine screening for peripheral arterial disease in people without symptoms is not recommended. However, a thorough evaluation of patients with clinical evidence of vascular disease is in order.

Raynaud's Disease

When the small blood vessels of the fingers, toes, and tip of the nose go into spasm, a process occurs that halts the flow of blood to the area. The affected area (usually the fingers) first turns white from receiving too little blood, then blue from poorly oxygenated blood, and finally red as blood flow returns. This condition is called *Raynaud's phenomenon.*

In the primary form of this condition, exposure to cold typically can set off an attack of Raynaud's symptoms. Most people with this form of the disease have no underlying medical problems when diagnosed.

Other conditions are associated with the secondary forms of Raynaud's symptoms. These include such connective tissue diseases as lupus erythematosus, rheumatoid arthritis, and scleroderma, all of which may produce *vasculitis,* an inflammation of blood vessel walls that reduces blood flow. People who operate equipment or tools that vibrate also seem to be at risk for Raynaud's disease. It is estimated that about 5 percent of Americans have Raynaud's.

Usually people with mild forms of primary Raynaud's disease need no treatment. Others with more severe forms may be able to prevent their cold-related symptoms by dressing warmly during cold weather, including wearing mittens instead of gloves to protect their hands, and avoiding undue exposure to cold temperatures. When other disorders cause the secondary form of Raynaud's, medical treatment for the underlying condition is necessary. Therapy for secondary Raynaud's may include the use of vasodilator drugs, which can help to open the small blood vessels.

Varicose Veins

Varicose veins usually affect the large veins of the lower leg. The veins swell and bulge out from the surface of the skin. Pain may accompany the swelling. The causes of varicose veins include overweight, pregnancy, tight-fitting clothing around the waist, thigh, or upper calf, and heredity factors.

To relieve the pain and swelling, wear well-fitted elastic stockings, elevate the legs when sitting, and exercise to improve circulation in the legs. Avoid crossing your legs when sitting because this can impair circulation. Sometimes surgery to remove the vein may improve the appearance of the affected leg and, hopefully, decrease any local discomfort.

Thrombophlebitis

When a vein in the leg becomes inflamed and can cause a blood clot, the condition is known as *thrombophlebitis.* The condition is potentially dangerous because the clot may dislodge and travel, forming an embolus, or embolism. If the embolism lodges in the lungs, it could be fatal. Treatment consists of warm compresses, elastic bandages, rest, anti-inflammatory drugs, and anticoagulants. The prescription of anticoagulant drugs is intended to prevent new clots from developing and to allow the body's natural clot-dissolving mechanism to work effectively.

To help prevent this condition, avoid sitting or standing in one position for a long time and don't wear constricting clothing.

Aspirin

Nearly a century after aspirin was introduced to relieve pain, fever, and inflammation, medical investigators are taking a new look at the role of the nation's most popular analgesic in the prevention of heart attacks.

The newest potential of aspirin was discovered in the late 1960s, when researchers found that the drug could reduce the ability of minuscule blood cells called *platelets* to stick together and form clots. The sticky platelets promote clotting and help stop bleeding. At the same time, they can contribute to the formation of a blood clot that may be instrumental in triggering a heart attack or stroke if advanced atherosclerosis is present.

About 90 percent of all heart attacks are caused by blood clots that jam an artery and deprive the heart of its oxygenated blood supply. Aspirin, with its ability to interfere in blood clotting, would seem to be an excellent preventive against heart attack.

However, while doctors are encouraged by the results of recent studies showing that aspirin may prevent heart attacks in apparently healthy people, they also issue a strong note of caution. Aspirin is a powerful drug that can have a thinning effect on the blood if used improperly. Just as a dose of aspirin can increase the amount of time you bleed if you cut your finger, aspirin may cause major bleeding in the stomach, or even a brain hemorrhage if the right conditions are present. Only you and your doctor together can decide whether you are a suitable candidate for aspirin therapy.

Risks.   Aspirin's side effects can range from mild to serious, depending on the user. Anyone who begins taking aspirin on a regular basis is likely to find that there is an accompanying rise in the risk of other problems.

• *High blood pressure.* Have your blood pressure level checked before you consider a regimen of aspirin therapy. Uncontrolled high blood pressure is a leading cause of hemorrhagic stroke. Some people who are taking antihypertensive medication may not be deemed good candidates for aspirin therapy, since even a single aspirin a day may increase the risk of stroke. Discuss it with your physician.

• *Gastrointestinal bleeding.* Inflammation of the stomach lining, stomach ulcers, and gastrointestinal bleeding increase when aspirin is consumed regularly. Other symptoms may include heartburn, nausea, and abdominal pain.

• *Sensitivity to aspirin.* An allergy to aspirin may develop in some people who are sensitive. An allergic reaction can also produce shock.

• *Diabetes.* Diabetic retinopathy (in which the tiny blood vessels feeding the retina in the back of the eye leak blood) could theoretically become worse if aspirin use is excessive. Diabetes may increase the risk of complications with aspirin therapy in some people even if diabetic retinopathy is not present.

Research studies.   The U.S. Physicians' Health Study followed more than 22,000 male doctors aged 40 to 84 for nearly five years. Half of the participants took an aspirin every other day, while the other half took a placebo. The study's independent monitoring board decided to end the trial prematurely when a 47 percent reduction in heart attacks was noted among the aspirin-takers. However, there was a slight increase in the incidence of hemorrhagic strokes among the aspirin-takers.

Immediately before the study results were released in early 1988, a six-year study of more than 5,000 British doctors who volunteered to take aspirin was published. The British findings were in direct contrast to the American study: the aspirin-users had no drop in the rate of heart attacks. The occurrence of hemorrhagic stroke among aspirin-takers was slightly higher, as in the American study. However, the studies were different in design, dosage of aspirin, and the number of participants.

The select group of participants in these studies had no history of heart attack or stroke. They were also screened to eliminate any who had conditions that would reduce their tolerance to aspirin, such as ulcers, gout, and liver or kidney disease. It remains a question whether women and men from other professions and economic sectors would also benefit from such use of aspirin. Although the results showed that low-dose aspirin therapy can reduce the risk of heart attack in men without symptoms, it is premature to recommend the routine use of aspirin by the general population to reduce the risk of heart attack.

Who should take aspirin?   As a *preventive* tool in healthy men who have no history of heart attack but have coronary risk factors, the answer varies with each person. Based on current knowledge, low-dose aspirin therapy should be considered for men age 40 and over who are *at increased risk for heart attack and who have no known adverse reactions to the drug.*

Women who are premenopausal have a low risk of heart attack and have little to gain from aspirin therapy. Pregnant women especially should not take aspirin or any other drug without discussing it with their physician. A postmenopausal woman has an increased risk of heart attack and may benefit from aspirin therapy, especially if she has one or more coronary risk factors. But it's important to remember that none of the major aspirin studies has considered the drug's effects on women.

The appropriate dose of aspirin for platelet inhibition is in the range of one milligram per kilogram of body weight per day. That is the equivalent of about 80 milligrams of aspirin a day for the average 150-pound person (an 80-milligram dose of aspirin is about the strength of a baby aspirin).

Platelet-blocking effects have been demonstrated with doses as low as 40 milligrams of aspirin every other day, an amount equal to half of a baby aspirin. Although the adverse effects of aspirin, such as gastric irritation, are likely to be small at such a low dosage, further study is needed to determine the long-term safety of such an aspirin regimen.

Aspirin may help prevent clots in some people, but it's not a quick fix that you should rely on exclusively. Aspirin has no known effect on atherosclerosis, the underlying disease process that is responsible for most heart attacks. Aspirin is not a substitute for reducing your primary coronary risk factors, including cigarette smoking, uncontrolled high blood pressure, and elevated blood cholesterol.

Only after a physical examination can it be determined whether you are a good candidate for aspirin therapy. If you try to prescribe regular aspirin for yourself, you may prevent heart attack but increase your risk of serious complications—especially stroke.

4

Sexual Health

Peter A. Gross, M.D., and Thomas N. Wise, M.D.

Some Americans say they want better sex. Others would like more sex. Although it might seem that "doing what comes naturally" should be easy, unfortunately, the reverse is often true. Confusion and anxiety over such issues as sexual performance, desire levels, choosing and using contraceptives, and the fear of sexually transmitted diseases can make sex fraught with complications and some apprehension.

The sense of freedom brought about by the sexual revolution that swept the nation from the 1960s into the 1980s is being replaced by caution, conservatism, and at times even celibacy. Since the AIDS epidemic was first officially recognized in 1981, the pursuit of uninhibited sexual fulfillment has begun to lose its appeal as we learn to put the need for protection before that of pleasure.

Healthy Sexuality

Your sexuality is an integral part of you—whether you're young or old, single or part of a couple, sexually active or celibate. Although it's natural to be sexual, expressing your sexuality isn't always easy or comfortable. Often, the impulse is there, but expressing it may feel awkward or confusing.

"Having sex"—the euphemistic term for coitus or other genital contact—is a physical or erotic experience centered for the most part in your genital organs. It isn't the same as being sexual. Knowing how to perform sexually doesn't necessarily guarantee satisfaction in every sexual experience. Nor are regular, passionate experiences necessary ingredients in a healthy sexuality. Ironically, just when you think you know everything there is to know about sex, you realize you've still got a lot to learn. It takes a lifetime to learn about sex.

Sexual satisfaction begins with your own positive self-image. Feeling comfortable about your body and who you are and accepting this information without judging it is the basis of healthy sexuality.

Problems about sexuality and sex are often the result of ignorance, guilt, fear, insecurity, and negative attitudes. Many of us received negative or mixed signals from our parents or schoolmates about sex while growing up. After years of ignoring, fearing, or repressing our sexual feelings, sorting out what is supposedly "normal" and what is "abnormal" when these feelings eventually bubble to the surface may be difficult.

Sex researchers William Masters and Virginia Johnson described the normal-versus-abnormal quandary this way: " 'Normal' is frequently defined as what we ourselves do and feel comfortable about, while the 'abnormal' is what others do that seems different or odd to us." Since normality, like beauty, is in the eye of the beholder, we should stop the fruitless search for a standard against which to measure our sexuality.

Two common—and normal—practices that usually begin in childhood and continue throughout adult life are *masturbation* and *sexual fantasy*.

Masturbation.   Sexual self-stimulation is the most widely practiced form of sexual activity by men and women alike. Children and teenagers naturally gravitate toward self-pleasuring as they discover their bodies. Although many adults regularly masturbate, very few will discuss this ultimately private pleasure.

During the nineteenth century, physicians, parents, and the public believed that masturbation caused insanity and a host of physical ills. The shift in this line of thinking did not come until the 1940s, when medical authorities decided to drop masturbation from the dread-disease list. Toward the end of the decade, sex researcher Alfred C. Kinsey published his landmark report of interviews with thousands of men and women; among the surprising findings was the number of adults who admitted that they masturbated.

Even today, misconceptions and ignorance about masturbation are prevalent. But mental health experts consider masturbation a normal and healthy practice for people of any age.

Sexual fantasy.   When you let your imagination run free as you fantasize about sex in certain settings, during certain activities, or with certain partners, you are having a sexual fantasy. Typically, the content of your fantasy is acceptable as an imaginary adventure, but it's not necessarily something you'd want to act on in real life.

Sexual fantasies have their place in healthy sexuality. In the privacy and safety of your own thoughts, you can be playful, imaginative, outrageous, and anything else you'd like. Whether you depict a scene of anonymous sex, group sex, or extramarital sex, you can explore it and leave it when you're finished. Fantasizing doesn't mean you've been unfaithful to your partner. More likely, your fantasy may heighten your sexual desire.

Commonly, men and women have sexual fantasies during masturbation, as well as during sexual activity with another person.

Sexual fantasies can become a problem when the playful aspect disappears and you get so caught up in your fantasy that it replaces normal sexual activity. For instance, focusing exclusively on a fantasy that repeatedly uses a particular person or object can leave you dependent on this fantasy for sexual arousal. The intensity of a fantasy can also be a problem if it interferes with any aspect of your life or intrudes on normal sexual activity.

Sexual Relationships

If you can't fully experience your sexuality, you may suffer in terms of health and happiness. Although we don't know the rank order of sexuality in the overall scheme of human endeavor, it's pretty high on the list for many people.

Many people don't enjoy sex unless their relationship is intimate and sensitive, or unless their partner meets certain emotional needs or satisfies some kind of physical or psychological ideal. These people may inhibit their sexual feelings until they can find a desirable partner.

Sexuality is difficult to define. It's much like a force of energy that flows through each of our lives, ebbing and flowing depending on what is happening at the time. Sometimes it's subtle, other times it's intense and compelling. Occasionally, it's necessary to put sexuality on hold. To appreciate and use this power constructively, a good starting place is understanding, learning, and acceptance—of ourselves and others.

Problems with sexuality can lead to problems with sex. Anxiety and guilt frequently put a damper on sexual satisfaction. A personal problem, an inability to communicate, relationship difficulties, and physical illness also affect your sexuality. As you grow older, you may become concerned about the effect of aging on your sexual capability and enjoyment. But many men and women remain sexually active well into their 70s and 80s.

Building a satisfying sex life with your partner calls for understanding, communication, spontaneity, trust, willingness to take time, and a sense of fun with a goal of mutual pleasure. Intimacy is an added attraction—and an essential component—of any successful long-term sexual relationship. As you and your partner become intimate, you open the deepest part of yourselves to each other. It's true that doing so creates the serious risk that one of you will face the very real pain of personal rejection, but when two people truly desire to be intimate with each other it's likely to yield a bigger benefit: closeness, trust, mutual acceptance, and commitment.

Improving Your Sex Life

If your sex life has become less satisfying to you or your partner, you may be able to make some changes that will improve both attitudes and performance. The most commonly cited causes of sexual problems include:

- *boredom* with a sex life that has become routine and predictable
- performance *anxiety,* or worrying about each move to the point that you can't enjoy yourself
- *guilt* and sexual inhibitions, especially feelings of physical inadequacy or unattractiveness
- *myths* and misinformation about sex

Once you recognize that there's a problem, you and your partner may be able to solve it successfully on your own with some attention, caring, and empathy. Some recommendations:

- Be affectionate and tender with your partner in your words and actions. Affection should not be expressed solely as a prelude to having sex. It makes you feel close to each other in every aspect of your life together.
- If your needs aren't being met, express your concerns to your partner. Be clear and specific about what is bothering you. There's no place for blame or accusations here, so don't offer your opinion or criticism. Instead, express your feelings as you experience them. For instance, "I feel sad because we don't make love much anymore." Then ask how your partner feels about the subject. It's essential to be honest without hurting your partner's feelings or being critical.
- Spend time together. If you or your partner have heavy schedules, keep a log of your activities and time allocations for one week. Compare your time charts and try to reach an agreement about where you can make adjustments in order to have more time with each other.
- Don't allow your lovemaking to fall into a pattern. Try different

positions, times, and settings. If you're always the aggressor, encourage your partner to switch roles. Use sexual fantasy to spark your imagination.

• Recall the first time you made love with your partner. Approach each lovemaking session as if it were the first time you are touching your partner's body.

• Keep a little romance in your life. Small gestures like a candlelight dinner, a small surprise gift, or a love note can help make your relationship feel more alive.

• If your partner is in the mood for lovemaking and you're not, don't shut him or her off. You may notice a shift in your feelings and be glad that you didn't reject the offer.

• Don't adopt a rigid attitude. Remember that the idea is to enjoy the excitement and intimacy of sex, not to monitor your every move to see if you're doing it "right."

Frequently, you may encounter some temporary situations during which you feel sexually out of sorts. If you've been sick, fatigued, depressed, dealing with a lot of stress, experiencing grief over the loss of someone close, facing job pressures, or having family problems, it's normal for such feelings to depress sexual appetite. But if your problem lingers without any improvement, see your doctor. Certain medical conditions and even medications can cause sexual problems that often respond well to treatment.

Sexual Dysfunction

Problems with normal sexual functioning are common. A study by psychologist Ellen Frank of the University of Pittsburgh showed that among happily married couples, half of the men and 80 percent of the women reported some sort of sexual dissatisfaction or dysfunction.

For men, the most common dysfunctions are *erectile problems*—commonly known as *impotence*—and *premature ejaculation*. Women experience such dysfunctions as *lack of orgasm, vaginismus* (spasm of the vaginal muscles), and *dyspareunia* (pain during sex).

Medical science has developed an enormous amount of knowledge about these problems and how to treat them. You no longer have to suffer in silence. A variety of health care professionals are trained to treat these problems.

Sexual Problems in Men

Erectile dysfunction. Impotence is the inability to achieve or maintain an erection that is rigid enough for sexual intercourse. At some point in his life, practically every man has an occasional difficulty in getting an erection and that's perfectly normal. An actual erectile dysfunction may be an acute episode that lasts a few months and resolves on its own. Or it may be a case of chronic impotence, a stubborn disorder in men who have never been able to achieve a fully effective erection.

An estimated 10 million American men suffer from impotence. Alfred C. Kinsey reported that less than 2 percent of men experience impotence at age 40, whereas the incidence climbs to 25 percent by age 65.

During an erection, blood rapidly flows into the penis and causes penile swelling. When this change in blood circulation doesn't occur in the penis, neither does an erection. Physical illness, certain medications, and psychological factors can block an erection.

Among the physical factors, insulin-dependent diabetes is a leading cause of erectile dysfunction because it can eventually damage the network of nerves that make an erection possible. When the blood vessels are damaged from circulatory diseases, blood supply to the penis is insufficient. A hormonal imbalance can cause impotence, as well as such physical disorders as an injury to the spinal cord, severe liver or kidney disease, multiple sclerosis, and other neurological diseases.

Various drugs can lead to erectile dysfunction. Alcohol, which depresses the central nervous system, is a common cause of impotence. Some medications used to lower high blood pressure, antidepressants, sleeping pills, and antacids may produce erectile dysfunction in some men.

There are many possible psychological causes of impotence, including depression, constantly monitoring your sexual performance, a conflict in your relationship with your partner, sexual inhibition, a history of sexual abuse as a child, conflict over sexual preference, and fear of impregnating your partner or contracting a sexually transmitted disease.

If your impotency lasts more than three months, see your doctor. When a medication causes a loss of potency, talk to your doctor immediately. Usually the drug or the dosage can be changed. If the diagnosis indicates an emotional problem, you may be referred to a counselor or psychiatrist for short-term therapy. A physically caused erectile dysfunction may be treated with medication that is injected directly into the penis to increase blood flow.

One of the most underutilized treatments available—and also one of the most expensive—is the surgically implanted penile prosthesis. The different types of implants include one that remains in a semirigid position and another that can be mechanically inflated. About 25,000 American men receive penile implants each year. So far, a majority of the recipients report satisfaction. If you are considering this type of surgery, seek out a qualified urologist.

Premature ejaculation.   When a man reaches orgasm as soon as, or before, he penetrates the vagina, he experiences premature ejaculation. This common sexual dysfunction is thought to be a learned behavior that arises out of anxiety over sexual performance.

Behavior modification is an effective treatment for premature ejaculation. Minor tranquilizers may help too.

Sexual Problems in Women

Anorgasmia (lack of orgasm).   The most common sexual dysfunction affecting women is failure to achieve orgasm. Women who are anorgasmic fall into at least three categories: those who never have an orgasm under any circumstance, those who once were regularly orgasmic but now are not, and those who can't experience an orgasm with a certain partner or under some circumstances.

There are no clear data as to how many women are anorgasmic; it is thought that about 10 percent of American women have never experienced an orgasm.

It's important to note that a woman who has orgasms as a consequence of sexual stimulation, but not necessarily during intercourse, is not dysfunctional. Indeed, Masters and Johnson note that many women often need additional stimulation—such as stroking the clitoris—during intercourse in order to reach orgasm.

Only about 5 percent of anorgasmic women can attribute their dysfunction to a physical cause, according to Masters and Johnson. More often, the inability to achieve an orgasm may be due to a problem somewhere in the cycle of sexual response that begins with desire, leads to excitement, and concludes with the climax of orgasm.

In some cases, anorgasmia is due to poor communication between a woman and her partner. Women who feel uncomfortable with their sexuality may have long-held beliefs that sex is dirty and not an activity for a woman to enjoy. When such beliefs are the cause, the condition can be effectively treated with behavior modification.

Treatment for anorgasmia differs depending on the nature and the cause of the dysfunction. Sex therapists encourage a woman to explore her own body, especially the genital region, without feeling pressure to experience any kind of sensation. Erotic images or fantasies are encouraged. Eventually, self-stimulation of the clitoris may produce an orgasm.

Vaginismus.   When the muscles around the outer third of the vagina develop acute, painful spasms in response to your partner's attempt to insert his penis, the condition is known as *vaginismus*.

This disorder often has a physical cause—such as infection, a soft-tissue abnormality, or injury. The major emotional causes of vaginismus are fear and anxiety over sexual activity. Many women with this dysfunction are sexually responsive. They just cannot tolerate the idea or the reality of penile penetration.

Depending on the cause of the dysfunction, there are a range of treatments for vaginismus. Therapy includes learning special techniques for relaxing the vaginal muscles. Your physician may also give you a set of plastic vaginal dilators of increasing circumference that you use until you are comfortable inserting one that approximates the size of an erect penis.

Dyspareunia (painful intercourse).   An estimated 15 percent of women of all ages experience pain during intercourse on at least some occasions. The pain of *dyspareunia* can lead to avoidance of sexual intercourse as well as feelings of frustration and guilt on the part of both partners.

The most common physical causes of dyspareunia include vaginitis, pelvic infections, vaginal dryness (especially in postmenopausal women), allergic reactions to clothing, vaginal foams, and tampons. Trichomonas infections, which are easily passed back and forth between a symptom-free man and woman, can lead to painful intercourse.

Men can also suffer from dyspareunia, but the incidence is thought to be lower. The tip of the penis can become irritated from rubbing against the tail of an intrauterine device or the top of a cervical cap. Some men may develop an irritation from exposure to a contraceptive cream or jelly.

Treatment depends on the cause of dyspareunia. When the problem is due to infection, medications are prescribed. The hormonal shift that occurs in women during menopause may produce vaginal dryness. This problem can be effectively treated with an estrogen cream or hormonal replacement therapy (see Chapter 6). If an allergy is the problem, you may be advised to use a different product.

Sexual Therapy: Focusing on the Sensual

One of the most common techniques used to treat both the male and female dysfunctions are *sensate focus* exercises. These awareness exercises are designed to have you rely on your tactile sense to communicate with your partner in a sensual manner, with the emphasis on touching and with pleasure as a goal instead of orgasm.

Sensate focus is usually practiced as a three-step series of exercises. In the first phase, each partner takes a turn touching the other's body. The emphasis is on silent, sensual exploration, based on what you find pleasing to touch, not on what you think your partner would like. The only areas that are off limits are the genitals and breasts.

In the second phase, you and your partner can include the genitals and breasts in the expanded field of play. Sensual awareness and enjoyment are emphasized, with your goal being physical stimulation. At this point, you and your partner should find yourselves becoming more familiar with each other's nonverbal body language as you learn to communicate without words where and how you'd like to be touched. Penetration and orgasm are not included in phase two.

When you reach the third phase, you continue to enjoy the pleasures of the first two stages but now your enjoyment can include orgasm.

If you try these exercises, allow for enough time so that each stage can be practiced daily for a few weeks. The exercises are most effective when you devote enough time and effort to mastering one phase before moving on to the next.

Sexual Desire Disorders

The three phases of sexual response as defined by sex therapist Helen Singer Kaplan are desire, excitement, and orgasm. Persistent problems with the second and third phases are considered sexual dysfunctions, but when the first phase is blocked it may produce its own set of problems, known as *sexual desire disorders.*

These conditions of lowered sex drive may appear as either lack of interest in sex—*inhibited sexual desire*—or a fear of sex that borders on the phobic—*sexual aversion.*

It's not necessarily abnormal to be devoid of sexual interest, or *asexual.* Some people, by nature, have a lower sex drive (*hypoactive sexual desire*). If a couple is perfectly happy to have sex once a month, once a year, or never, there may be no problem—as long as both partners find this arrangement acceptable. But a discrepancy in desire between you and your partner can create frustration and distress.

Inhibited sexual desire (ISD).   Many people with otherwise normal sexual function may experience a lack of interest in sex. Often the reason is a low sex drive, stress, preoccupation with career, fear of intimacy or failure, guilt, hostility toward your partner, poor self-image, denial of sexual preference, or ignorance about sex and how to become sexually stimulated.

ISD may stem from a physical cause, such as a hormone deficiency, depression, certain prescription medications, alcoholism, kidney failure, drug abuse, or a chronic medical illness. In other cases, ISD may be the apparent but not the underlying problem. A man may be using a low sex drive as an excuse to mask an erectile problem, or a woman who doesn't have orgasms may claim a lack of interest in sex to avoid the frustration of heightened sexual tension that will be left unresolved.

If depression or a hormonal imbalance is responsible for ISD, medication may be able to correct the problem. Since most cases of ISD have both social and psychological components, resolving the problem calls for making personal changes to revitalize your relationship. After you identify the problem interfering with a healthy expression of sexuality within the relationship, you and your partner may be able to serve as your own sex therapists. If you keep encountering obstacles, you may want to contact a qualified sex therapist for help.

Sexual aversion. Sexual avoidance syndrome isn't a lowered sex drive, it's a phobia—or irrational fear—about engaging in sexual activity. Both men and women can suffer from sexual aversion for such reasons as having been sexually abused as children, growing up in a home where the attitudes about sex were negative, and feeling too much pressure from a partner with a higher sex drive.

Sexual aversion disorders respond well to sexual therapy. Patients who are extremely anxious or who experience panic attacks as part of their aversion disorder often receive medications that help reduce their anxiety. After the anxiety-lowering drugs have become effective, sex therapy is begun.

Getting Help

There are no prevailing professional or legal standards that govern the vast array of specialists who treat sexual problems. For this reason, be especially wary when seeking help.

Your primary care physician (or, if you are a woman, your gynecologist) may be able to recommend a specialist. If you don't have a primary care doctor, call the referral service of your local hospital or the nearest university-affiliated teaching hospital and request some recommendations. After you get these names, call and ask about training and qualifications. If a practitioner is vague or hesitant about discussing credentials, training, and experience, look for someone else.

Trust your instincts. But remember that it's normal to feel some discomfort during a first meeting with any person with whom you will be discussing so personal a problem. If you seem unduly uncomfortable, ask yourself why. Do you feel excessively awkward or embarrassed about the subject matter itself? Or does your gut feeling indicate that you really can't work with this therapist?

It's essential that you feel comfortable with the professional with whom you are working. The therapist should be at ease discussing sex, listen to what you are saying, and be able to offer observations, insights, and helpful information. A qualified, specially trained counselor or therapist must behave like a professional. For example, treatment for sexual problems never includes having sex with the therapist.

Some professional organizations publish lists of their members. Two such organizations are American Association of Sex Educators, Counselors, and Therapists, 435 North Michigan Avenue, Suite 1717, Chicago,

Illinois 60611, and Society for Sex Therapy and Research, c/o Center for Human Sexuality, University Hospitals of Cleveland, 11400 Euclid Avenue, Suite 200, Cleveland, Ohio 44106. However, a listing on these rosters doesn't guarantee the overall competence or the quality of the practitioner's work.

Sex and Illness

If you are acutely or chronically ill, your physical condition as well as your state of mind affects your sexual responses. The depression, anxiety, and sadness that often accompany a long-term illness are also bound to have a negative effect on sexual relationships.

Heart attack. Not that long ago, if you suffered a heart attack, your treatment plan forced you to stay in a hospital bed for about three weeks. The recovery period was lengthy, and anxiety over performing any kind of demanding activity—including sex—fostered a cardiac-cripple attitude. A year after the heart attack, most of these patients remained anxious and depressed. Many hadn't returned to their familiar way of life, although they were physically capable of doing so.

It should not be surprising, then, that few recovering heart attack patients had been counseled about sexual activity, despite the fact that most of them feared what effect the cardiac event would have on their sexual ability and their relationships.

Generally, after 8 to 12 weeks of recovery, intercourse can be resumed, depending on the severity of the attack and the recuperative progress. Doctors must provide some counseling to help allay the exaggerated fears of many heart attack patients about sexual activity. It's important that the attending physician ask the spouse or lover to join in on the discussion, and to answer whatever questions the partner has. It is not enough to have survived the heart attack. It is also necessary that you resume as much of your former life-style as you can prudently resume, and as soon after the attack as possible. If your own physician is too busy or too embarrassed to undertake this counseling, you might think of looking for another physician.

Cancer. When breast cancer is treated with surgery to remove the breast, it may lead to future sexual problems. Frequently, the difficulty stems from the change in self-image, anger, and feelings of discouragement or depression. Embarrassment over the scar from the mastectomy is common, sometimes to the point that feelings of shame may lead to a complete breakdown of sexual activity. Sexual difficulties that arise from a lack of self-esteem over losing a breast are far less likely to occur when a woman and her partner discuss the possible consequences to their sex life before the surgery and when they resume sexual activity soon afterward. Today, more treatment options are available, depending on the stage of the disease (see page 104).

Colorectal cancer or severe ulcerative colitis sometimes requires the removal of a section of intestine and the surgical creation of an opening—or stoma—to allow bowel wastes to leave the body. This surgically created opening and the appliances that come with it commonly lead to problems with sexual enjoyment because of fears of fecal waste leaking from the colostomy bag.

Although only a small number of men lose a testicle to cancer, this kind of loss can lead to serious self-image problems. In fact, there is no biological reason for losing the ability to perform sexually as a result of this kind of surgery. However, persistent fears over performance can lead to psychologically induced problems with erection.

Other illnesses.   Other patients with certain diseases or injuries that affect the central nervous system or the kidneys may undergo serious difficulties that often impair normal sexual function.

As stated previously, some disorders of the endocrine system are associated with sexual difficulties. Men who have received several years of treatment for insulin-dependent diabetes commonly develop erectile dysfunction decades after their diagnosis. Because the nerve damage caused by diabetes is permanent, a surgically implanted penile prosthesis is often used to restore many diabetes patients to sexual function. The effect of diabetes on women is not as well understood.

Underactivity of the pituitary, thyroid, and adrenal glands has been linked to lowered sex drive, erectile difficulties, and lack of orgasm.

Alcoholism often leads to sexual difficulties in both men and women. The larger the amount of alcohol consumed, the lower the likelihood of sexual arousal. Men who drink large amounts of alcohol are frequently impotent. Alcoholic women report lowered sexual desire, often with a lack of orgasm.

Drug abuse can lead to a variety of sexual problems. Even the regular use of tranquilizers can sometimes cause problems with desire, erection, and orgasm.

Premenstrual Syndrome

Premenstrual syndrome, or PMS, is a complex condition that baffles the women affected by it as well as their doctors. PMS is hard to define because its symptoms are so variable. This syndrome consists of physical symptoms that may also be accompanied by emotional symptoms during the two-week period before menstrual bleeding begins.

Estimates vary as to just how many women suffer from PMS. All women undergo certain hormonal changes that affect various body systems during their premenstrual days. Some may experience minimal symptoms, such as minor discomfort, while others suffer symptoms so severe that their ability to interact with other people in social or job settings is seriously impaired.

The cause of PMS remains elusive. For years, doctors, family members, and coworkers of PMS sufferers chalked up the problem to psychological causes. But PMS is not a psychiatric illness. We are learning more about its biological basis, with special attention to the role of hormones. However, emotional and social factors may also influence the severity of PMS symptoms, and some studies have linked PMS and depression.

More than 150 different symptoms have been associated with PMS. The most commonly reported complaints include:

Physical	*Emotional*
Headache	Irritability
Bloating	Mood swings
Breast pain or tenderness	Depression
Abdominal discomfort	Anxiety
Increased appetite	Lethargy
Food cravings	Difficulty concentrating
Change in bowel habits	Increase or decrease in sex drive
Fatigue	Lower self-confidence
Flareup of allergies, asthma, migraine, or epilepsy	Less interest in socializing

If you suspect that you have PMS, you may be able to find some relief by making a few life-style changes. Some women report that they are better able to cope with PMS once they identify their individual pattern of symptoms. You may prefer to come up with your own plan based on the following suggestions, or you may want to work with your doctor. Either way, there's no cure for PMS, but various life-style approaches and some medical treatments can make the condition more manageable.

First, you'll need to track all of the physical and emotional changes you experience during the two weeks before the onset of menstrual bleeding. Keep a diary of all your premenstrual symptoms for at least two or three months. If stressful events trigger your symptoms, be sure to make note of these.

Once you are aware of when your worst symptoms occur, you can use this knowledge to your advantage. For instance, if you tend to become irritable on certain days, you can try alerting your family in advance so they can understand and possibly even block some of the stress in your life.

The most popular self-help remedies include daily exercise, stress management techniques, and dietary modifications—especially cutting down on caffeine, sugar, and salt.

If these conservative methods aren't effective, and your symptoms continue to cause distress, your doctor may offer you drug therapy for a specific complaint. Diuretics often are prescribed for bloating and weight gain. When severe anxiety develops as a result of PMS, an antianxiety medication may be prescribed.

Vitamin B$_6$ therapy has been studied for its ability to relieve some PMS symptoms, but this treatment remains controversial and risky, because it may cause neurological symptoms in some users. Progesterone therapy and oral contraceptives also may be recommended, but the effectiveness of hormonal therapy has mixed results. PMS researchers at the New York State Psychiatric Institute and Department of Psychiatry at Columbia University's College of Physicians and Surgeons recently found that alprazolam (Xanax) may be helpful for the anxiety, irritability, and depression accompanying severe cases of PMS.

Infertility

If you and your partner have been trying to conceive a child without success for a period of 12 months, there's a chance that you may be infertile. The inability to conceive is a fairly common problem in the United States, affecting about 15 percent of the population.

When *infertility* occurs, it is a couple's problem—not just a male or female problem. Actually, about 40 percent of the time, doctors can trace the difficulty to the man, and in 40 percent of other cases to the woman. Both sexes share responsibility in the remaining 20 percent of cases.

Many people who think they are permanently infertile may be wrong. There are many causes of infertility, some of which are treatable. In some couples, the timing of sexual relations must be near perfect for a healthy sperm and egg to meet, unite, and go on to grow inside the uterus. In this case, a common solution is charting the fertile days of the menstrual cycle in order to schedule more sexual intercourse during this time. If it turns out that better timing can't correct the problem, your doctor may suggest a fertility workup to determine the cause of your difficulty.

In the male, infertility may be due to a problem in the sperm production or delivery system. The nondefective sperm count may be low, or the sperm may lack motility (the ability to move rapidly enough to fertilize the egg). Occasionally, the sperm is healthy and motile, but there is a physical blockage preventing its entry into the flow of semen.

There are many reasons for male infertility. They include an endocrine deficiency or abnormality, infection, an immune disorder, undescended testicles, or destruction of the sperm-producing cells by an earlier case of mumps. A scar from an infection caused by a sexually transmitted disease can permanently block the sperm transport ducts. When there are varicose veins, or *varicoceles,* in the scrotum, their presence may create extra heat and pressure on the reproductive passageways. Varicoceles usually can be surgically corrected.

Men who have a low sperm count often are advised to avoid tight underwear because it is thought to increase the temperature of the testicles and damage sperm production.

If you are female, your doctor will first want to confirm that an egg is being produced and released during each cycle. The Fallopian tubes are checked for blockages and all of the pelvic organs are examined for the presence of scar tissue from a past infection or illness. Your cervical mucus will be analyzed for consistency and quality. Occasionally, the mucus is so thick or acidic that it bars sperm from entering the uterus.

When a hormonal problem disrupts the cycle of ovulation, your doctor may prescribe medication to help resynchronize your cycles. If blocked tubes are the reason for infertility, they often can be opened by microsurgery.

About 5 percent of all infertility cases resolve themselves spontaneously—that is, after all the frustration and fertility workups, pregnancy finally occurs.

Alternative Techniques

If an extensive medical evaluation determines that you or your partner is infertile, you may want to consider some alternatives. One method is artificial insemination with your partner's sperm. Several advanced techniques are available at certain large medical centers, including *in vitro fertilization,* in which eggs are removed from the ovaries and fertilized in the laboratory with the man's sperm. Within about 48 hours, the fertilized egg grows into an embryo of about six to eight cells. At this point, doctors transfer the embryo back into the woman's uterus by means of a catheter. When IVF is successful, a normal pregnancy can follow.

Other alternatives include the *GIFT procedure* and *intrauterine insemination* (IUI). GIFT is an acronym for Gamete Intra-Fallopian Transfer and bears some similarity to in-vitro fertilization in that eggs are removed from the ovary and then replaced once they are fertilized. The main difference is that because the embryo is not left to grow in the laboratory before retransfer, the GIFT technique can be completed in a much shorter time.

Intrauterine insemination relies on hormonal stimulation of the ovaries in combination with artificial insemination inside the uterus. In IUI, the doctor uses a catheter to place the sperm in the uterus. This technique bypasses the cervix, which is the site of several problems causing infertility.

In-vitro fertilization and its alternatives are promising, but they may not appeal to everyone. Cost certainly is a factor. These techniques are expensive and they aren't available in all areas of the country. Each IVF program has a screening program that requires that participants meet certain criteria and follow certain protocols—something that many couples may find stressful. Finally, there are no guarantees that it will work.

Preventing Pregnancy

Numerous methods are available to prevent pregnancy, but there's no single contraceptive that offers in one product what every user of birth control wants: absolute reliability, combined with safety, convenience, affordability, and an absence of harmful side effects.

Choosing a contraceptive system or device from among those available is a matter of personal preference, and sometimes a decision influenced by religious beliefs. Also, health considerations may make certain contraceptives a poor choice for some women.

Until recently, no new contraceptives had been developed or introduced in this country (see page 103). Both the pill and the intrauterine device (IUD) have been modified several times over the last several years to improve safety and reliability, but these methods remain less than ideal choices for all couples.

Since every currently available method of contraception has its drawbacks, you'll most likely have to compromise when you choose a means of birth control. You may have to try different methods until you find one that best suits your personal needs.

When reference is made to a contraceptive's *failure rate,* it means the percentage of unwanted pregnancies occurring in all women using a particular method of contraception in the first year of use.

Oral Contraceptives

An estimated 10 million American women use *oral contraceptives—* a popular and almost 100 percent effective way to prevent pregnancy. The pill works by suppressing ovulation, or the release of an egg from the ovaries.

Oral contraceptives are available in different preparations. The form that combines synthetic versions of estrogen and progesterone is the most commonly used, and may be the most effective. A progesterone-only pill—called a "minipill"—is slightly less reliable than the combination pill. The minipill is usually reserved for use in women who have difficulty tolerating estrogen's side effects of nausea, headaches, or bloating. The pill must be taken every day in order to be effective.

The pill may also offer some degree of protection from ovarian cancer and endometrial cancer. Other benefits may include a reduction in the incidence of benign cysts in the breast, ovarian cysts, and pelvic inflammatory disease. The pill is also often prescribed to relieve severe menstrual cramps and heavy bleeding in some women. Certain drugs, such as some antibiotics and antiarthritis drugs, may decrease the effectiveness of the pill.

A number of side effects may occur in women who begin taking the pill, including breakthrough bleeding between menstrual periods, breast tenderness, nausea, headaches, and depression. Among the well-established disadvantages of the pill are its association with an increased risk of heart attack, stroke, and blood clots—conditions that normally rarely occur in women of childbearing age.

Studies released in 1989 raised anew the question of whether the pill increases the risk of breast cancer. However, earlier studies pointed to very little risk and researchers consider the newer data inconclusive. The National Cancer Institute is conducting a large study to learn more about the link between breast cancer and the pill.

Although the majority of women who take the pill experience few complications, there are some women who should not use any oral contraceptives. They include women with the following conditions:

- being a smoker over age 35
- the presence of blood clots in the lungs or legs
- suspected or known cancer of the breast or reproductive organs
- undiagnosed vaginal bleeding
- hepatitis or impaired liver function

Barrier Methods

Barrier methods work by barring sperm from entering the uterus or by destroying them with a spermicidal chemical. Among the barriers are the condom, diaphragm, cervical cap, vaginal sponge, and an array of spermicidal agents that may be used alone or together with one of these blocking devices.

When condoms and diaphragms are used correctly and consistently, their failure rate can be as low as 2 percent. But human error tends to drive the actual failure rate as high as 10 percent.

Condoms—the oldest form of male contraception—have never been popular with men. But the fear of sexually transmitted diseases is begrudgingly ushering in a change of preference.

When used to prevent pregnancy, condoms have an estimated failure rate of about 10 to 15 percent. As a barrier that offers protection from sexually transmitted disease, condoms are thought to have an equal rate of effectiveness. Condom failure usually occurs when the product slips off the penis or leaks. But it is probably human error that causes most of the problems. Incorrect use of a condom limits its effectiveness and increases the risk of exposure to both sperm and germs.

Condoms come in many varieties and strengths. Preference for features such as lubrication, reservoir tip, and color depend on the individual user. Most condoms on the market are made of latex, but "skin" condoms made from the intestines of lambs are also available. Although skin condoms are strong, and many users surveyed by *Consumer Reports* said that they produced a more pleasurable sensation, these natural membranes may be better used as contraceptives only. There remains a question as to whether skin condoms may be more porous than latex, thus creating the potential for the smaller AIDS and hepatitis-B viruses (see Chapter 7) to sneak through this permeable barrier.

Spermicides containing nonoxynol-9 as an active ingredient may offer additional protection against disease when used with a condom. Some condoms are available with a spermicide coating, but it may be safer to apply a vaginal spermicide as well. Spermicide should not be applied inside the condom because it may make the device slip off during sexual activity. The effectiveness of spermicides in anal sex is not known.

Whether you're male or female, if you're sexually active, be sure to keep an adequate supply of condoms. Use them consistently, *not* just some of the time.

Store the unopened packets in a dark, cool, and dry place. Heat, light, and exposure to the air can make them deteriorate rapidly. Condoms are not reusable. Use a new condom each time you have sex. Open the condom packet gently to avoid tearing. Place the condom on the erect penis *before* penetration or genital contact. Although condoms are fairly simple to use, they're also easily misused. Learn to use them the right way:

• Place the rolled condom over the tip of the *erect* penis. If you're using a condom that has a reservoir tip at the end to collect semen, be sure to squeeze out the air. For condoms without a reservoir tip, leave about a half-inch of space at the end and squeeze out the air. This creates room for the semen to collect following ejaculation.

• While holding the tip of the condom with one hand, use your other hand to unroll it down the length of the erect penis. (Uncircumcised men should pull back the foreskin first.)

• If you want additional lubrication, apply a *water-based* lubricant. Use a lubricating jelly, a spermicide jelly, or a personal lubricant. *Never* use an oil-based lubricant (petroleum jelly, baby oil, mineral oil, vegetable oil, cold cream, or a hand lotion) because it can weaken the latex in the condom.

• Right after ejaculation, hold the condom firmly at the rim and withdraw the penis while it is still erect. This will help prevent spillage of the contents.

• Keep a spermicidal agent on hand in case the condom leaks.

Diaphragms. A diaphragm is a shallow latex dome with a flexible metal ring that is inserted into the vagina to cover the opening to the cervix. Before inserting the diaphragm, you must coat the rim and inner part of the dome with a spermicidal cream or jelly.

A diaphragm, used correctly and conscientiously, is highly effective in preventing pregnancy. No long-term side effects or major health risks accompany its use.

The drawbacks of a diaphragm are that it must be fitted to your particular anatomy by a physician, nurse-practitioner, or family planning professional. It takes a little practice to learn to insert a diaphragm properly. If you insert the device several hours before sexual intercourse, you must apply more spermicide before having sex. The diaphragm must be left in place six to eight hours after intercourse. If you gain or lose weight, have pelvic surgery or a pregnancy, you're likely to need a new size diaphragm, so visit your doctor to see if you need to be refitted. Some women are allergic to the latex in the diaphragm or to an ingredient in a spermicide.

Cervical cap. The cervical cap looks like a large rubber thimble that fits over the cervix. When you use a cervical cap, you must coat the inner area with a spermicidal agent just as you do with a diaphragm. This device measures about half the size of a diaphragm and can be worn for a longer period of time.

Although European women have been using cervical caps for several years, the device has only recently been commercially available in the United States, following its approval by the FDA. It is recommended for use only in women who have normal Pap smears. After a woman uses the cervical cap for the first three months, she must return to her doctor for another Pap smear. If the second test detects any abnormal changes in the cervical tissue, then its use is discontinued.

The cervical cap has a somewhat higher failure rate than the diaphragm. The 15 percent failure rate is thought to be due to the difficulty entailed in inserting the cervical cap and the chance of dislodgement during intercourse.

Because this device can remain in the cervix longer, it allows for greater spontaneity because you don't have to disrupt your intimacy to dash out and insert a contraceptive before your lovemaking advances to intercourse. Among the disadvantages of the cervical cap are occasional difficulty getting the right size cap to fit you. Inserting the device may be tricky. If you leave the cap in place too long, it can create an unpleasant odor.

Contraceptive sponge.   The contraceptive sponge is a soft, disposable spongelike device made of polyurethane foam that fits inside the vagina. The sponge contains its own supply of spermicide (nonoxynol-9), which continuously releases its sperm-killing properties over a 24-hour period. This device works by covering the opening to the cervix, trapping sperm, and killing sperm.

The failure rate of the sponge ranges between 10 and 20 percent— much higher than other barrier methods. The advantages of the sponge are its safety and relative ease of insertion. No custom-fitting is necessary. It can be purchased over the counter. Because it is effective for 24 hours, it doesn't interfere with spontaneity in sexual intercourse. However, it must remain in place for at least six hours after intercourse.

The downside of the sponge is that it may produce itching, soreness, vaginal discharge, or a disagreeable odor. Some women may experience an allergic reaction to the product. The major risk involved in using the sponge centers on the slight possibility that it can increase the risk of toxic shock syndrome (see page 117).

Spermicides.   A sperm-killing agent in the form of a foam, cream, or gel inserted very high in the vagina can be used alone to prevent pregnancy. But when a spermicide is used without the added protection of a condom, diaphragm, or cervical cap, its failure rate can climb as high as 18 percent.

Spermicides require no prescription and are readily available over the counter. They have no known adverse side effects, with the exception that some users may be allergic to certain ingredients. Spermicides that contain nonoxynol-9 as an active ingredient also offer the added benefit of protection from some sexually transmitted diseases.

A major drawback of spermicides is that they are messy and can be a nuisance because they must be inserted just before sexual intercourse.

Vaginal suppositories also prevent pregnancy, but they may be less effective than a spermicide if used without any other protection. The major potential disadvantage is that if a suppository fails to melt fully or foam inside the vagina before you begin intercourse, you don't have adequate protection.

Intrauterine Devices

The *intrauterine device* (IUD) is considered to be close to par with the pill in terms of its effectiveness in preventing pregnancy. An IUD is a small plastic or metal device that is medically inserted in the uterus to prevent a fertilized egg from implanting in the uterine wall.

During the early marketing of IUDs in the 1960s and 70s, these devices were available in several different designs and materials. By the mid-1980s, fearing lawsuits, virtually every IUD manufacturer had withdrawn its product from the U.S. market.

The sole remaining IUD, a progesterone-releasing device that must be replaced once a year, recently gained a competitor when the FDA approved a new copper-containing IUD that retains its effectiveness for four years.

The major advantage of IUDs is their convenience. Once an IUD is inserted, you don't have to do anything else. Although IUDs are highly effective as a contraceptive, 1 to 3 percent of all women who use them become pregnant.

A woman using an IUD has an increased risk of certain complications:

- increased menstrual bleeding and cramps
- infections, especially pelvic inflammatory disease, which can result in scarring of the Fallopian tubes, sterility, and even death
- perforation of the uterine wall
- ectopic—or misplaced—pregnancy, in which the fertilized egg is implanted in the Fallopian tubes. This condition can cause severe internal bleeding.

Studies indicate that women who receive IUDs are at a higher risk of infection during the first four months following insertion.

During the first several months after insertion of an IUD, there's also a chance of expulsion from the body. It's possible to expel your IUD, not notice that it's missing, and become pregnant. Ask your doctor to show you the proper technique for checking the length of the string that forms the "tail" of the device.

A small number of women with IUDs may experience cramps during orgasm as a result of uterine contractions around the area where the device is located.

IUDs are not recommended for women who have more than one sexual partner. This is because in many sexually transmitted diseases infection is aided by the presence of the IUD. Women who have never borne a child, but may wish to become pregnant sometime in the future, are usually advised to find another method of birth control.

Higher-Risk Methods

If religious restrictions, health concerns, or your personal preferences find you ruling out the pill, an IUD, or any of the barrier methods of birth control, only two choices remain: the rhythm method and withdrawal (coitus interruptus). Both methods offer less protection than other forms of contraception.

Rhythm method, or periodic abstinence. The practice of abstaining from intercourse during the fertile time of the menstrual cycle, known as the *rhythm method* of birth control, is a natural method of contraception. In theory, the only device you need is a calendar. But in reality, no woman can be assured of regularity with her menstrual cycle. For this reason, the rhythm method has a high failure rate, 25 percent.

A woman's fertile days—or unsafe period—begin about three days before and last about three days after ovulation (the release of an egg from the ovaries). Ovulation itself occurs about 14 days before menstruation. The key to natural birth control methods is *fertility awareness*; you must precisely calculate your time of ovulation. There are four different ways of determining your fertile days and your "safe" days:

• The calendar (rhythm) method, which requires that you keep accurate records of your menstrual cycles for at least 12 months. This is the least reliable of the periodic abstinence methods because in many women the cycle varies widely from month to month. Even among the most regular women, there is some variation.

There is a formula that some women use to calculate their least-safe days: to determine your first fertile day, subtract 18 from the number of days in the shortest menstrual cycle of the previous six to nine months. To find your last fertile day, subtract 11 from the number of days in your longest menstrual cycle. If, for instance, you calculate that your shortest cycle was 25 days and your longest totaled 30 days, your figures should look like this:

$$25 - 18 = 7 \quad \text{(first fertile day)}$$
$$30 - 11 = 19 \quad \text{(last fertile day)}$$

Days 7 through 19 are the 13 days during which your calendar indicates you should abstain from intercourse.

• The temperature method, in which you take your temperature on a basal thermometer the first thing each day and record it on a chart. The chart is later used to help determine your ovulation pattern.

• The cervical mucus inspection method, in which you look for specific changes in the consistency of the cervical mucus over a period of several menstrual cycles. When the clarity, texture, and elasticity of the mucus reach a certain stage each month, it indicates that ovulation is about to occur. A woman can detect a change in the mucus as much as 5 days before ovulation.

• The combination, or sympto-thermal method, which calls for monitoring both basal temperature and the cervical mucus.

If you choose to use either of these methods or a combination, seek a health professional or another user who can explain the method and the techniques involved clearly and concisely.

The advantage of natural contraception is that it is safe and inexpensive. The major drawback is that in any one year 20 percent of those who use these methods will have a pregnancy. A woman must be conscientious, if not meticulous, in monitoring her ovulation patterns. Her sexual partner must be supportive and willing to cooperate. Some couples may feel frustrated because they must avoid sexual intercourse during the unsafe days.

Coitus interruptus. *Withdrawal,* or pulling out the penis from the vagina before ejaculation, is an extremely unreliable method of contraception. Even if you try to time it perfectly, this method can fail. If only a few drops of semen enter the vaginal opening, or a few sperm are in the fluid secreted before ejaculation, it can result in a pregnancy. Besides having a high failure rate—about 24 percent—the withdrawal method can detract from the spontaneity and enjoyment of intercourse because both partners must be prepared to shift the focus of their attention at the very moment the activity becomes most intensely pleasurable for the male, and maybe for both.

Douching. Douching after intercourse doesn't even qualify as an effective way to prevent pregnancy. By sending a stream of pressurized liquid into your vagina, you may flush some sperm out while sending others higher into your uterus. Active sperm are strong swimmers and can reach the uterus in less than two minutes following ejaculation.

Sterilization

A man or woman who decides to undergo surgical *sterilization* must first be certain that he or she will not in the future want any—or any additional—children. Once you become sterilized, the results are considered permanent. Although it is sometimes possible to reverse sterilizations by microsurgery, reversal procedures are difficult and expensive, and their success cannot be guaranteed.

The two methods of sterilization are *vasectomy* for men, and *tubal ligation* for women.

Vasectomy. Your doctor (usually a urologist) can perform a vasectomy during an outpatient visit that lasts about 30 minutes. After administering a local anesthetic, the physician makes two tiny incisions on either side of the scrotum. The doctor then lifts out the vas deferens—the tube that carries sperm from the testicles to the penis—and clips and seals the ends on both sides, so that sperm cannot enter the semen during ejaculation.

A newer variation on the conventional procedure is the so-called no-scalpel vasectomy. In this method, the doctor uses a special instrument to make a tiny puncture hole to lift out the vas deferens instead of making an incision with a scalpel. This procedure takes less time and the recovery is quicker than with conventional surgery.

The effects of a vasectomy are not immediate, however. Active sperm may remain in the testicles as long as two to three months after the procedure. To prevent conception during that period, an alternate form of birth control must be used until a semen analysis shows that the sperm are gone.

Vasectomy is considered a safe, simple, and effective procedure. There may be minor pain and discomfort for a few days after the surgery, but the procedure carries a very low incidence of infection. A vasectomy doesn't interfere with erection and ejaculation, nor does it affect overall health.

Tubal ligation.   Tubal ligation (literally "tying the tubes") is a general term for female sterilization. The procedure entails cutting, blocking, or sealing the Fallopian tubes so that sperm and egg cannot unite. Once sterilization surgery is performed, it becomes effective immediately. The surgery doesn't affect sexual desire or your ability to have sexual pleasure, your menstrual cycles, or hormone production. Some women, however, have reported irregular menstrual cycles, painful periods, and pelvic discomfort after a tubal ligation.

There are various tubal ligation procedures available today:

• *Laparoscopy*. Following administration of a local anesthesia, your doctor makes one or two small incisions in your abdomen. The physician then introduces a laparoscope, a specially lighted instrument that may also be used to cut and electrically burn, or cauterize, the ends of the tubes.

• *Minilaparotomy*. A minilaparotomy requires a small incision just above the pubic bone, slightly above the hairline. After using an instrument to draw the tubes up through the incision into direct view, the physician then ties and cuts the ends. When the tubes are closed, they are put back in place.

Major complications are relatively rare with laparoscopic and minilap techniques. However, there is a slight risk of heat injury from the cauterizing instrument, perforation of internal tissue or organs, and internal bleeding.

• *Colpotomy* or *culdoscopy*. A tubal ligation performed through the vagina, this method of sterilization is performed less often today because of refinements in laparoscopic and minilap techniques.

Sterilization is a popular method of birth control for married couples in the United States. But, for your own protection, it isn't possible to just walk into your doctor's office or a clinic and walk out surgically sterilized. The federal and state governments require that you know fully the risks, benefits, and consequences.

After your doctor explains the risks, possible side effects, and the irreversible nature of sterilization, you will be asked for your written informed consent. Doctors or health professionals are not permitted to obtain your consent while you are in labor, having an abortion, or under the influence of alcohol or drugs. There is a waiting period of 30 days after you give your consent in writing before a sterilization procedure is performed.

New Contraceptives

In early 1990, a panel of experts convened by the National Academy of Sciences cited a three-decade lag behind Europe in birth control research and in the development of contraceptives. The Committee on Contraceptive Development's report called on the federal government to revise its procedures for evaluating new contraceptives and to shield manufacturers from product liability lawsuits.

Many European countries offer an array of advanced contraceptive methods, some of which are thought to be safer than the pill because they offer lower doses of hormones. Among these are implantable contraceptives that are placed under the skin and release hormones over a period of time, spermicidal agents with antiviral ingredients, reversible male and female sterilization, a contraceptive vaccine, and transdermal skin patches that interrupt sperm production without affecting male libido.

In 1990, the FDA approved the use of a long-lasting birth control implant for women that is surgically inserted under the skin, usually in the upper arm. Called *Norplant,* this method relies on the slow release of hormones into the bloodstream from tiny silicone tubes that contain progestin.

Clinical trials have shown Norplant to be highly effective, with a failure rate of 1 percent for a period of five years. Menstrual irregularities, including longer periods and spotting, are the major side effects of this contraceptive. The implant's long-term safety remains unknown.

A type of birth control pill known as the morning-after pill, approved for special prescription use in France, has already garnered much attention here and worldwide. When the discovery of RU 486, which works by inducing abortion, was first announced in 1988, it unleashed a storm of antiabortion protests. RU 486—a synthetic antiprogesterone known as mifepristone—faces many political as well as scientific obstacles that make its introduction into the United States impossible at this time.

Abortion

About 1.5 million abortions are performed annually in the United States. Although abortion is neither a contraceptive nor a means of family planning, it is often used as a form of birth control for unwanted pregnancy. This method of early termination of pregnancy is legal and safe if performed by qualified practitioners.

The type of abortion procedure likely to be performed depends on the stage of pregnancy. The earlier the stage, the lower the risk of complications. The laws in your state may govern pregnancy termination from the 13th to 24th week of pregnancy. The procedures used include:

Vacuum aspiration abortion.   This procedure can be done until the 12th week of pregnancy. It involves widening the opening of the cervix and inserting a small vacuum tube in the uterus to suction out the contents.

Dilation and curettage (D&C).   Also used in first-trimester pregnancies, a D&C involves scraping the uterus lining with a blunt metal instrument called a curette until all of the contents are removed. The D&C, which was widely used before the introduction of the vacuum method, tends to cause more discomfort and bleeding than vacuum aspiration.

Dilation and evacuation (D&E).   The safest procedure used during the early part of the second trimester (13th to 24th week of pregnancy) is dilation and evacuation. A D&E uses both vacuum methods and removal of the contents with special instruments.

Saline injection.   This is the most common method used during the second trimester. Under local anesthesia, a hollow needle is inserted into the abdomen to remove some amniotic fluid. This is replaced by the same amount of a saline solution. Within several hours, uterine contractions develop and the contents are expelled. In some cases, prostaglandins may be injected instead of saline.

Cancers of the Reproductive System

Women: Breast Cancer

The discovery of a painless lump in the breast immediately triggers thoughts of *breast cancer*. If you detect a lump, it is reason for a visit to your doctor. Although most of these lumps turn out to be noncancerous, prudence as well as peace of mind call for prompt professional evaluation.

Experts agree that mammography is the most effective method for detecting early breast cancer. There has been controversy, however, over the age at which this test should start to be performed on a regular basis. It's known that the risk of breast cancer increases with age, but the question has long been: at what patient age should mammograms become a routine part of periodic checkups?

Some groups have recommended that only women over 50 obtain annual mammograms. But others, such as the American Cancer Society and the National Cancer Institute, call for periodic mammograms between ages 40 and 49. In 1989, researchers analyzing data from a 1960s study of the effect of routine mammograms for women between 40 and 49 found that yearly screening led to a significant reduction in mortality from breast cancer.

The American Medical Association's Council on Scientific Affairs now recommends that asymptomatic women aged 40 to 49 get a mammogram and clinical breast exam at one- to two-year intervals. Beginning at age 50, mammography should be performed yearly. Women should also get a baseline mammogram between ages 35 and 40 for doctors to use for later comparison. All women should get periodic breast examinations between ages 20 and 40.

Risk factors.   If you are taking oral contraceptives, or have a positive family history for breast cancer, it's prudent to seek an annual clinical breast examination.

Age is a leading risk factor, followed by a family history of breast cancer; a previous episode of the disease; first childbirth after age 30 or no pregnancy; and early onset of menstruation or menopause. A diet high in fats and moderate alcohol consumption may increase the risk.

For many years, it was thought that women with so-called *fibrocystic disease* had an increased risk of cancer. Now we know that fibrocystic disease is an imprecise term and that lumpy, painful breasts don't increase your risk. A much less common condition, called *hyperplasia,* indicates the growth of abnormal but benign cells in the breast tissue. Hyperplasia points to a higher risk of cancer in some women and requires regular checkups to monitor any changes.

Diagnosis and treatment.   Early detection is the key to treating breast cancer. The three screening methods include mammography, a medical examination, and breast self-examination (BSE).

BSE, which is simple, safe, and easy to perform once you have been properly trained, has a notoriously poor record in terms of compliance. The Task Force reports that women who received a 30-minute training session in BSE improved their ability to detect lumps. When a doctor or health professional instructs a woman on the proper technique for BSE, she is more likely to perform this simple exam. Yet one drawback of BSE is that it can lead to an increased number of false-positives—and can cause unnecessary anxiety and medical expense.

If a biopsy determines that a breast lump is cancerous, several treatments are available. A *lumpectomy* involves removal of the cancerous lump and the surrounding tissue. A *mastectomy* is the surgical removal of the breast. The size and location of the tumor are important factors in determining which type of surgery to perform. Studies have indicated that women who undergo a lumpectomy with removal of the lymph tissues along with radiation therapy have similar survival rates to those opting for a mastectomy. Chemotherapy and hormone manipulation therapy are also used to destroy cancer cells.

In 1990 a panel of experts convened by the National Institutes of Health (NIH) to review the treatments for early-stage breast cancer concluded that breast conservation surgery—lumpectomy and radiation therapy—is as effective as a total mastectomy.

The consensus statement called breast conservation treatment preferable for most women with Stage I or Stage II cancer (see below), noting that the survival rates equal those for total mastectomy. When the cancer is diagnosed at these two stages, it has not spread beyond the breast or nearby lymph nodes.

In the past the standard treatment for breast cancer was a *radical mastectomy,* in which the breast was removed as well as the underlying muscles and surrounding lymph nodes. Other choices of treatment are now available, depending on the size and metastatic activity of the tumor, as well as the type of cancer. If a doctor recommends a radical, seek a second opinion.

Note: A "preventive mastectomy" is not *the standard treatment for women who have "fibrocystic" breasts.* If you experience painful, tender, swollen, or lumpy breasts, these symptoms don't necessarily mean that you have a disease that requires surgical treatment.

Stages of breast cancer.   Doctors take a variety of information into account when classifying the four stages of breast cancer, including the size of the tumor, the presence of cancer cells in the lymph nodes under the arms, and whether the tumor cells have spread (metastasized) to other parts of the body. The clinical stages include the following:

Stage I tumors measure less than two centimeters (under three-quarters of an inch). At this stage, the lymph nodes are free of cancer cells. It may be possible to feel the tumor. Five years after diagnosis, 80 percent of the women who received treatment are still alive.

Stage II tumors are either zero to two centimeters with positive nodes, or two to five centimeters (three-quarters of an inch to two inches) with positive or negative nodes. The lymph nodes under the arm are not usually palpable and may be negative or positive. In the past, 65 percent of the women who were treated survived five years. Women in this group now may be treated with chemotherapy, which is likely to improve their survival rate.

Stage III cancer is characterized by a lump larger than two inches with positive lymph nodes or signs such as swelling, ulceration, or attachment to the chest wall. Usually, the tumor cells have not spread elsewhere in the body. About 40 percent of women treated survive for five years.

Stage IV cancer has metastasized. Although the tumor may respond to treatment, a stage IV tumor is usually not curable. Only 10 percent of the women diagnosed at this stage are still alive after five years.

Breast Self-Examination

Because lumps grow slowly until they are noticeable, groups such as the American Cancer Society recommend that you perform regular breast self-examination (BSE) as an adjunct to your routine screenings.

BSE is best performed at the end of your menstrual cycle. If you have stopped menstruating, pick a certain day of each month on which you can routinely examine your breasts. To do BSE, follow these steps:

- Lie down. Place a pillow under your right shoulder. (If you have large breasts, hold your right breast with your right hand while performing the exam with your left hand.)
- With the sensitive pads of your middle three fingers, use a rubbing motion to feel for lumps.
- Press firmly so that you can feel the different breast tissues.
- Be sure to examine the adjacent breast tissue of the chest and the area along the armpit.
- There are three BSE patterns that many doctors and women prefer. There is a circular pattern, a vertical strip pattern, which simply involves inching your finger pads up and down the breast, and a wedge pattern, in which you visually divide the breast into pielike wedges for examination. (See illustration.)
- After you examine your right breast, use the same technique for your left breast. A woman with small breasts should devote two minutes to examining each breast. If your breasts are larger, the examination will take a minute or two longer.
- Upon completing your examination, sit or stand in front of a mirror—first with your hands on your waist and then with your arms raised—and look to see if there has been any change in size or contour, or if one breast is lower than

the other. Note whether there is any puckering or dimpling of the skin. Gently squeeze the nipple to see whether there is any sign of discharge.

• If you notice any changes, consult your doctor promptly. By becoming familiar with your breast tissue, you are more likely to notice when an abnormal change has occurred.

Ovarian Cancer

Early detection of *ovarian cancer* is difficult because the signs and symptoms are relatively vague, what physicians call "nonspecific." As malignant cells grow on the ovaries, a condition called ascites—the accumulation of fluid in the abdomen—often occurs, giving the abdomen a swollen appearance. The stomach discomfort, gas, and bloating that accompany ovarian cancer are commonly attributed to digestive prob-

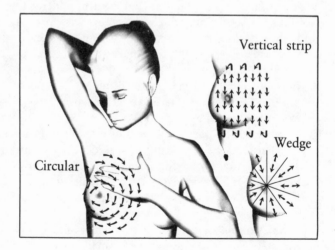

Breast Self-Examination. *Courtesy of the American Cancer Society, Inc.*

lems. Often, the suggestion of ovarian cancer comes so late that the disease has spread.

A routine annual pelvic examination is important because it allows your doctor to check the size and character of your ovaries. If there is an abnormality, additional tests are performed.

Ovarian cancer occurs less commonly than uterine cancer, but carries a higher mortality risk. The risk increases with age, especially for women over 60. Other important risk factors include a previous bout of cancer, never bearing a child, and a family history of ovarian cancer.

Depending on how far the cancer has advanced at the time of diagnosis, your physician may choose any one or more of several treatment options, including surgery, radiation therapy, and chemotherapy.

Cervical Cancer

All sexually active women are at risk of *cervical cancer,* especially those who have no access to good health care, have multiple sexual partners, or have been sexually active from an early age. A history of viral genital infections, especially genital warts and possibly herpes simplex virus, may increase the risk of cervical cancer. The good news is that this type of cancer is highly responsive to treatment when it is detected early.

The incidence of invasive cervical cancer has been decreasing for several years thanks to increased public awareness and the availability of Pap tests. When a Pap smear detects abnormal changes (dysplasia) in the cells that line the cervix, there is a risk that the condition could lead to cancer. Early treatment with laser, heat, or freezing therapy is usually successful in arresting the condition.

It is recommended that women who are sexually active get an annual Pap test or begin screening at age 18. Women who are not in a high-risk group are advised to return for a Pap test every one to three years after they have two consecutive normal tests.

When cervical cancer is not detected until it has reached an advanced stage, treatment may be with radiation therapy or a hysterectomy (removal of the uterus), and sometimes removal of the ovaries and Fallopian tubes.

Pap Smears

The Pap smear—one of the most commonly performed laboratory tests—is highly sensitive and reliable when properly done. Unfortunately, there's a chance that a poorly skilled laboratory may fail to pick up cell abnormalities that are present and give you a false-negative reading. Ask your doctor about the laboratory that will analyze your sample, and if it is accredited by the American College of Pathology or the American College of Cytology. If it isn't, don't be afraid to insist that your doctor use a laboratory that is.

Uterine Cancer

Cancer of the lining of the uterus, known as *uterine* or *endometrial cancer,* is one of the most common cancers of the pelvic area to affect women. The primary risk factors for endometrial cancer include a history of infertility, infrequent ovulation, long-time use of estrogen therapy after menopause, and obesity.

Endometrial cancer often tends to strike women who have already passed menopause. The symptoms include vaginal bleeding in postmenopausal women. However, younger women who are still menstruating also can develop endometrial cancer. Typical symptoms are heavy menstrual flow, bleeding between periods, and unusual vaginal discharge.

If you develop any of these symptoms, see your doctor. In some cases, a dilation and curettage (D&C)—or scraping of the uterine lining—may be recommended. If the condition is cancerous, treatment may include radiation therapy or a radical hysterectomy, or both.

Men: Cancer of the Testicles

Men between the ages of 15 and 35 have the highest risk of developing *testicular cancer.* Although cancer of the testicles is relatively rare, it is a leading cause of cancer deaths among men in their 20s and 30s.

There are certain factors that place some young men at a higher risk of developing the disease. Men who are born with undescended or partially descended testicles have a much higher risk. A family history of the disease is another key factor. Men with cancer of one testicle are at increased risk of developing the disease in the other one.

When cancer cells are present in the testicles, they can spread rapidly to other parts of the body. For this reason, the cancer-affected testicle is removed. In more advanced cases, radiation therapy or chemotherapy is also administered.

Early symptoms include slight swelling of the testicle and a small, painless lump that can be detected only by periodic examinations. The testicle may begin to feel heavy. Among the later-stage symptoms are pain in the groin or lower abdomen. (For information on prostate cancer, see Chapter 7.)

Testicular Self-Examination

Men who perform a testicular self-examination once a month may have a better chance of detecting any suspicious lumps early enough to seek treatment.

The best time to perform your examination is after taking a warm shower or bath because this is when the skin around the scrotum is the most relaxed.

While holding the testicles with both hands, gently roll each testicle between the thumb and fingers of your hands. You should spend three minutes doing your self-examination. With practice, you'll be able to recognize the feel of the normal structures inside the testicle, such as the epididymis. If you notice any changes—such as a lump or swelling—see your doctor as soon as possible. Not all lumps are cancerous, but only your doctor can make a diagnosis.

Sexually Transmitted Diseases

If you are sexually active, not in a monogamous relationship, and fail to take precautions—you have a good chance of getting a *sexually transmitted disease* (STD). Infections that result from sexual contact are on the rise. Some of these diseases produce mild or no symptoms, while others can cause disability, infertility, birth defects, and even death.

It takes intimate person-to-person contact to spread most of these germs. These bacteria and viruses thrive in the moist surfaces inside the sexual regions, including the vagina, the urethra in men, the anus, and the throat. Having genital, anal, or oral sex with someone who is infected puts you at high risk of catching an STD yourself. Although sexual transmission is the primary route of these infections, some nonsexual activities also play a role in the spread of STD—for instance, using a towel that contains the freshly shed herpes virus.

Preventing any STD, including AIDS, begins with limiting the number of your sexual partners. If you and your partner are new to each other, talk before you have sex. Ask about past partners and lovers as well as previous exposure to any STDs. Your partner may find it difficult to be candid, or may be completely honest. You may feel awkward bringing up the subject, but in any case, it's dangerous not to ask about this person's sexual history. Insist on using a condom. If neither of you is prepared, defer having sex until a condom is available.

If you notice that your partner has any sores, unusual discharge, strange bumps, or irritation from itching in the genital area—proceed with caution. If there are open sores from a herpes infection, for instance, avoid sexual activity until the sores heal.

Gonorrhea

Gonorrhea is one of the most frequently occurring bacterial infections in the United States, with more than one million cases reported each year. Gonococcal bacteria usually infect the urethral tube in men, and the cervix in women, although the throat and anus also may be affected in anyone practicing oral and anal sex. Most cases of gonorrhea occur in teenagers, young adults under 25, single people with multiple partners, and homosexual men.

Infection with gonorrhea may present no symptoms or such mild symptoms that it is difficult to notice, but easy to transmit to sexual partners. When there are symptoms, they have the following characteristics: men may develop painful urination associated with urethritis, an inflammation of the urethra. They may also notice a yellowish discharge. Women may develop increased vaginal discharge, discomfort of the lower abdomen, abnormal vaginal bleeding, and painful and frequent urination. These symptoms tend to appear from three days to two weeks after exposure. A gonococcal infection of the throat may produce a sore throat. If the anal canal is infected, there may be pain during bowel movements and a rectal discharge.

If you suspect that you have gonorrhea, see your doctor. Diagnosis includes carefully taking a sample of the discharge and making a culture for analysis. If the culture is positive, your doctor will prescribe an antibiotic. Because genital chlamydia often accompanies gonorrhea, you may receive medications to treat both problems. Some strains of gonorrhea have developed resistance to penicillin, so other antibiotics may be used to fight the infection.

Early detection of gonorrhea can prevent a number of complications. Untreated men can develop urethritis, prostatitis, and a narrowing of the urethral canal. Women who go untreated are at high risk of getting a painful condition called salpingitis, or *pelvic inflammatory disease* (PID)—which often causes infertility. Pregnant women infected with gonorrhea may have more difficult deliveries. They also risk bearing an infant with gonococcal conjunctivitis, which can lead to blindness if not treated. In a small number of cases, bacteria may enter the bloodstream and spread throughout the body, infecting the skin, joints, bones, and tendons.

Nongonococcal Urethritis (NGU)

Nongonococcal urethritis, an inflammation of the male urethra, is a far more common sexually acquired infection than gonorrhea. As its name indicates, there is no relation to the gonococcus family of bacteria. Other virus organisms, especially *Chlamydia trachomatis* and *Ureaplasma urealyticum,* are thought to account for most cases of NGU, sometimes called nonspecific urethritis.

Diagnosis of NGU may be difficult because signs and symptoms are often absent. Men who notice a urethral discharge and experience painful urination can easily mistake it for gonorrhea. When women have symptoms, they include painful, burning, and frequent urination.

Chlamydia. The *chlamydia* organism causes an estimated 3 to 4 million genital infections annually in this country. Because chlamydia is largely without symptoms, it typically escapes detection until complications develop in the male and female reproductive systems.

Men with chlamydia often develop NGU or *epididymitis,* an infection of the epididymis, or tube that runs inside each testicle. Fever, swelling, tenderness, and pain in the scrotal area are the main symptoms.

Infected women develop a cervical inflammation called *cervicitis.* But if the chlamydial infection spreads up into the endometrial lining of the uterus, or even farther into the Fallopian tubes and ovaries, it can produce a range of serious complications. About one-quarter to one-half of the annual 500,000 cases of pelvic inflammatory disease (PID) are a direct result of chlamydial infection. PID often results in female infertility and ectopic pregnancies (those that occur outside the womb).

A pregnant woman who has chlamydia of the cervix can transmit the infection to her fetus during delivery. Infants who are born to mothers with chlamydia can develop such infections as conjunctivitis, nose and throat infection, and pneumonia.

Ureaplasma urealyticum. The *Ureaplasma urealyticum* organism may be transmitted with chlamydia or may travel alone. In any case, ureaplasma—which belongs to a group of mycoplasma microorganisms classified as neither bacteria nor virus—is thought to be responsible for many of the NGU cases not caused by chlamydia. This cellular parasite often inhabits the male and female genital tracts without producing any symptoms.

Since a large number of chlamydia and ureaplasma infections are asymptomatic, it is recommended that physicians make direct cultures for chlamydia for high-risk patients without symptoms. This includes adolescents and young adults and those with multiple sexual partners. Pregnant women who are under 20, economically disadvantaged, and who have had more than one sexual partner also should be cultured at their first prenatal visit to a physician. All newborn infants should receive topical application of ophthalmic antibiotics immediately after birth to prevent conjunctivitis.

Chlamydia and ureaplasma are usually diagnosed by the process of elimination. If a direct culture does not indicate gonorrhea, then further tests will be taken. For chlamydia, cultures remain the diagnostic tool of choice. Treatment with antibiotics usually is successful. If you receive a prescription for antibiotics, it is important that you continue to take the medication for the length of time prescribed, even if symptoms subside.

Syphilis

Syphilis is back on the rise in the United States. At the beginning of 1990, the prevalence of this serious infectious disease had hit a 40-year high.

Syphilis is caused by a spirochete, or spiral-shaped bacterium, that spreads through sexual contact as well as through contact with the open sores that may be present on the skin and mucus membranes. Syphilis occurs in three separate stages, each with its own symptoms. If it goes undetected and untreated, it can damage the heart, nervous system, and other organs. Unfortunately, it often does go undetected because its first symptoms will disappear even without treatment, lulling the patient into a false sense of well-being.

In the *first* or *primary* stage, a painless sore known as a chancre (pronounced shan-ker) appears at the site of contact with the *Treponema pallidum* organism. Usually, the chancre occurs in the genital area, the rectal area, in the mouth or on the lips anywhere from three to 90 days after exposure, although the average is 21 days. In women, the chancre may be hidden deep inside the vagina or cervix. The sore disappears after several weeks, whether it is treated or not. There also may be swelling of the lymph nodes that are nearest to the chancre.

The *secondary* stage begins about two to eight weeks after the chancre first appears. By then, the spirochete bacteria have spread throughout the body. You may experience flulike symptoms, such as fever, headache, malaise, aching joints, and sore throat. Swollen lymph nodes are typical. Usually, there is a skin rash that may consist of raised red bumps that do not itch. The palms and soles of the feet are common sites of syphilitic skin rashes. Infectious flat-topped bumps called *condyloma lata* often develop in warm, moist areas of the body such as the genital and anal regions. These secondary symptoms eventually subside. If the syphilis remains untreated, the bacteria may remain latent, producing no symptoms but silently damaging the internal organs.

By the time you enter the *tertiary* or last stage of syphilis, you are no longer infectious to others. This highly destructive stage of the disease can cause such crippling disorders as heart disease, paralysis, brain damage, and the development of nodules called gummas in virtually any part of the body.

To diagnose syphilis in the first stage, your doctor will order a blood test. Second-stage syphilis is diagnosed by the symptoms you present in conjunction with a blood test. Syphilis is treated with penicillin, but if you are allergic to this drug, another antibiotic can be prescribed. Third-stage syphilis requires an even more vigorous treatment course with penicillin.

It is recommended that physicians routinely screen anyone in a high-risk group for syphilis, such as homosexual men, prostitutes, people with multiple partners, the contacts of people who have active syphilis, and pregnant women. If a pregnant woman transmits syphilis to her fetus, the bacteria can cause severe permanent damage to the infant.

Genital Herpes

The most common cause of genital ulcer disease in the United States is herpes simplex virus. Unlike gonorrhea and syphilis, which are responsive to antibiotics, herpes cannot be cured. Medical science can offer nothing more than treatment to suppress the symptoms.

Genital herpes, typically caused by herpes simplex virus type II, usually occurs in the genital region (for information on herpes simplex virus type I, see Chapter 7). Herpes is a highly infectious viral organism that can spread during vaginal, anal, or oral sex. Touching an active genital sore and then touching the eyes, nose, mouth, or skin can spread the infection to those areas.

The initial attack of herpes is often the most severe. It usually occurs two to 12 days after exposure. The first sign may be a tingling or itching sensation that lasts a few hours, followed by pain or a feeling of pins and needles. Fever, malaise, swollen lymph nodes, and loss of appetite also may occur. Small red patches erupt on the infected area, then soon change to fluid-filled blisters. When the blisters rupture, they leave shallow ulcers that either ooze fluid or bleed active virus that is highly contagious. Within a few days, a scab forms over the area and healing takes place over the next eight to 10 days.

Once you contract the herpes virus, it remains dormant in the nerve cells at the base of the spine. Some people never develop another outbreak, but most have recurrent attacks that often are less severe than the first episode.

Diagnosis is by viral culture. The antiviral drug acyclovir (Zovirax) is effective in reducing the duration and the symptoms of a first attack. Sitz baths may help relieve the pain. For people who experience frequent and severe recurring attacks of genital herpes, oral acyclovir can be effective in preventing these attacks. But the drug is most beneficial when it is taken at the first sign of symptoms.

Women who contract genital herpes may have an increased risk of developing cervical cancer. For this reason, those who have genital herpes must be sure to have regular Pap smears to check for any abnormal changes.

It is recommended that physicians conduct screening for genital herpes in pregnant women with recurring infections, an active episode during pregnancy, or sexual partners who have herpes. Pregnant women in an active stage of herpes can pass the infection to a newborn during vaginal delivery, causing brain damage, blindness, and death. If herpes flares up during the time of delivery, doctors will usually perform a cesarean section.

Genital Ulcer Syndrome

The herpes simplex virus is the most common cause of *genital ulcers* in the United States but sometimes is confused with other STDs that produce similar symptoms. Syphilis in the primary stage produces a painless ulcer, but if another infection is present, it could mimic the painful ulcers of herpes.

Three relatively uncommon sexually acquired diseases that cause genital ulcers have begun to show an increased incidence in the United States:

• *Chancroid.* This bacterial disease appears one day to several weeks after exposure, but the average is usually five to seven days. It often produces swollen lymph glands, along with the painful ulcers. Treatment is with antibiotics.

• *Lymphogranuloma venerium.* A strain of the chlamydia organism is responsible for this STD. After an incubation period that can range from a few days to a few weeks, some victims develop small, shallow genital ulcers that heal rapidly. The lymph nodes may become tender and enlarged. Antibiotics are effective against this infection.

• *Granuloma inguinale.* Although rare in the United States, this STD is common in other parts of the world. After an incubation period of one to 12 weeks, one or more nodules appear under the skin and then develop into painless ulcers. They can spread to other body sites such as the head, liver, and bones. Treatment is with antibiotics.

Vaginal Infections

When infection enters a woman's lower genital tract and causes irritation and inflammation, the condition is called *vaginitis.*

Although vaginal infections often are acquired through sexual activity, this is not always the case. For the vaginal environment to remain healthy, there must be a balance of acidity and alkalinity. Any number of things can upset this delicate balance, including douching, birth control pills, antibiotics, hormonal changes, pregnancy, diabetes or a prediabetic condition, and local irritation from trauma or a tampon. Most vaginitis results from infection with bacteria, fungi, parasites, and injury or irritation of the vaginal tissues.

Gardnerella vaginalis. This bacterial infection is also called non-specific vaginitis. Symptoms include an odorous, creamlike or grayish discharge. There is usually no itching, pain, or burning. Treatment is with metronidazole (Flagyl) or other antibiotics.

Trichomonas vaginalis. This parasite, known by its abbreviation "trich," is usually transmitted during sexual intercourse, but also can be passed on through contaminated towels or douching equipment. Sometimes, trich has no symptoms. When men are infected, there may be a slight discharge from the penis (although most men have no symptoms at all). Women tend to develop itching or swelling of the external genital area and have painful urination. A classic symptom of trich is a profuse foamy discharge that may have a foul odor. Metronidazole (Flagyl) is prescribed for trich. Because a woman can become reinfected if her male sexual partner carries the trich organism, it is advisable for the man to receive treatment at the same time.

Candida albicans. The yeast fungus Candida albicans is also known as monilia or simply as a yeast infection. When the normal acid/alkaline balance of the vagina is off, the yeast that normally inhabits the area may proliferate and produce an infection. Candidiasis is not considered a sexually transmitted disease. Symptoms include vaginal itching, an odorless thick white discharge, and pain during sexual activity. Creams and vaginal suppositories containing antifungal agents such as miconazole (Monistat) or clotrimazole (Gyne-Lotrimin) are used to treat candidiasis.

Women may be able to avoid vaginal infections by taking these simple measures: keep your external genital area clean. Dry yourself carefully after bathing. Wear cotton underpants instead of synthetic materials that don't breathe. Avoid pants that are tight-fitting in the crotch. Wipe from front to back after a bowel movement. If you use tampons, be sure to change them regularly. Make sure your sexual partners are clean before you begin lovemaking. If your partner has an infection, use a condom, or delay sexual activity until it heals. Avoid using any irritating vaginal sprays.

Toxic shock. Tampon use has been linked with a rare but serious disease called *toxic shock syndrome* (TSS), which often begins when

Staphylococcus aureus bacteria enter the vagina. The staph bacteria produce a toxin that enters the bloodstream and causes system-wide illness. Most cases of TSS have been linked with a vaginal infection; others have resulted from an infection in a wound following surgery.

The symptoms of TSS begin abruptly with a high fever, usually accompanied by nausea, vomiting, and watery diarrhea. A rash resembling sunburn appears within a few days, often on the palms or on parts of the trunk. The tongue may become red and swollen, and you may feel dizzy or faint a few days after noticing the first symptoms. This last symptom can indicate low blood pressure, one of the disease's serious problems. Sudden, severe drops in blood pressure can result in shock. With proper treatment, the symptoms disappear within seven days to a week.

Although some cases of TSS are mild, others can produce such complications as gangrene in the fingers or toes if blood flow to these areas is halted as a result of lowered blood pressure. Prompt and proper treatment with antibiotics and removal of the source of the staphylococcus can relieve the symptoms of TSS. Menstruating women who have experienced TSS should avoid using tampons, because the disease has a tendency to recur.

Genital Warts

When adults develop warts in the genital or anal area, it is usually the result of sexual contact. These warts are caused by the *human papilloma viruses* (HPV) family. Scientists have identified more than 50 different types of papilloma, including the condylomata acuminata, which is responsible for venereal warts. At least two types of papilloma virus have been associated with cervical cancer.

Occasionally, genital warts are visible on the external genitalia. They usually appear a month or two following exposure to the virus. If you notice small bumps that resemble the florets of a cauliflower on your sexual partner's genitals, avoid direct contact because these warts are contagious. Often, the papilloma virus gives no telltale signs of its presence. Warts that can be detected only by magnification may be hidden inside the female genital tract and escape notice until a Pap smear detects their presence.

The Centers for Disease Control estimate that about one million new cases of genital warts occur each year. Genital warts are treated by removal, usually through cryotherapy (freezing the area with liquid nitrogen). If you receive treatment for genital warts, make sure that your sexual partner is treated as well. Otherwise, you're likely to become reinfected. The role of HPV in cervical, penile, and rectal cancer is not fully understood.

Pubic Lice and Scabies

One species of louse that infests humans is called Phthirus pubis, popularly known as "crabs." These parasites are transmitted to hair in the genital and anal area by sexual contact. When *pubic lice* infest a hairy region, they cling to the hair shaft, feeding off blood vessels in the skin. After female lice lay their eggs on a hair shaft, the white pods from their eggs (nits) are often visible.

There usually are no symptoms until several weeks after the lice have invaded. Itching and redness often occur as a reaction to the parasites' saliva. Small gray patches that don't itch may develop around the infested area. Washing with regular soap and water will not eradicate lice. Your doctor can prescribe a preparation containing an insecticide that you apply to the affected area.

Microscopic mites are responsible for *scabies*. Female mites burrow into the outer layer of skin and deposit their eggs into what becomes a series of tunnels. The skin over the tunnels becomes slightly elevated and may appear as raised gray lines on the sides of the fingers, wrists, elbows, nipples, and penis. Small red bumps or blisters may occur on the abdomen, thighs, and buttocks.

Within two to six weeks after exposure, intense itching develops. Treatment is with a lotion or cream containing lindane. While you can pick up the mites through sexual contact, there are other nonsexual routes of transmission, including sharing a bed, clothing, or a towel with an infested person.

Pelvic Inflammatory Disease

Pelvic inflammatory disease (PID) is a chronic infection of the upper female genital tract and a leading cause of infertility in women. An estimated one million women develop PID each year.

PID, also called salpingitis, affects the endometrium, Fallopian tubes, and ovaries. Infection begins when microorganisms enter the upper reproductive tract, usually through sexual activity. Most of these cases stem from exposure to chlamydia or gonorrhea. A smaller amount of PID is due to nonsexual activity, such as childbirth, invasive medical procedures, and exposure to *E. coli* bacteria. Women who use an intrauterine device for contraception have a higher risk of PID.

Because the symptoms of PID vary in severity, diagnosis may be difficult. Lower abdominal pain and tenderness, along with fever, are the classic hallmarks of PID. Sometimes there may be no symptoms, or a range of other symptoms, including increased vaginal discharge, irregular vaginal bleeding, loss of appetite, nausea, and vomiting.

Early detection and treatment of PID can help prevent permanent damage to the reproductive system. PID has many serious complications: destruction or scarring of the Fallopian tubes from infection, a high risk of becoming infertile, ectopic pregnancy (one that occurs outside the uterus), inflammation of the lining of the abdominal cavity, and chronic pelvic pain.

When PID is the diagnosis, antibiotics are prescribed. Your sexual partner must be tested for the presence of the infection as well; otherwise, reinfection could occur. The greater the number of episodes of PID, the greater the risk of tubal scarring and infertility.

Acquired Immunodeficiency Syndrome (AIDS)

AIDS (acquired immunodeficiency syndrome) didn't even have a name when the virus-caused disease first surfaced in the late 1970s. Because uncommon infections and rare cancers began appearing in homosexual men who had developed severe deficiencies of the immune system, doctors called it GRID, for gay-related immune deficiency.

Although homosexual men were the first documented group of AIDS victims, the circle of infection now extends far beyond, to include intravenous drug users, hemophiliacs who received an AIDS-contaminated blood transfusion, unborn infants whose mothers harbor the virus, and a growing number of heterosexual men and women.

The history of AIDS is short, but its incidence has increased in epidemic fashion. In the spring of 1990, a report issued by the Centers for Disease Control (CDC) said that 132,510 cases of AIDS had been diagnosed in the United States. An estimated one million Americans are already thought to be infected with HIV—the human immunodeficiency virus.

The CDC projects that, by 1993, the annual number of new AIDS cases will rise to 61,000 and 98,000. (The estimates include two figures to adjust for both the diagnosed and unreported cases of AIDS. The CDC reaches the second number by adjusting the first figure upward by 18 percent.) By the end of 1993, between 390,000 and 480,000 new cases of AIDS are expected to be diagnosed, according to CDC estimates. Current projections forecast that AIDS will have claimed 285,000 and 340,000 lives for the period through 1993.

Transmission.   The HIV virus is too fragile to be passed along by shaking hands, sneezing, sharing a glass, or eating food prepared by someone with AIDS. It requires intimate contact with body fluids—including semen, blood, blood products, and vaginal fluid—for the AIDS virus to enter the body. Although small amounts of the virus have been found in the saliva of AIDS carriers, there is no scientific evidence that the AIDS virus is transmitted by saliva. The main routes of transmission now are sexual intercourse and sharing needles used for intravenous drugs.

There is a very small risk of acquiring the AIDS virus through a blood transfusion. But the chance of receiving blood contaminated with a hepatitis virus is higher. If you are planning to have elective surgery, ask your doctor about an autologous transfusion (donating your own blood in advance).

The HIV virus belongs to a class of viruses known as human retro-viruses, which have the ability to incorporate their genetic material into that of the human cells they enter and permanently alter them. When the virus gets into the bloodstream, it invades the immune system's white blood cells, called helper T-cells. After the HIV virus makes copies of itself, it destroys the T-cells, thus weakening the body's immune defenses and making it difficult for the victim to fight off the most routine infections.

Medical researchers cannot explain why some people who are exposed to the HIV virus don't become infected while others develop the infection more readily. It appears that the more often you are exposed to the HIV virus, the higher your risk. So, if you frequently have sexual contact with a partner or partners who may be infected, you have an increased chance of becoming infected yourself.

Based on averages of several studies of the female partners of infected men, the chance of infection from a single act of unprotected sexual intercourse can range from one in 100 to one in 500. But the risk depends on the type of sex involved:

- If you are the receptive partner in anal sex, you are at higher risk. This is because the fragile lining of the rectum is extremely vulnerable to tears, and the infected semen remains in contact with the rectal tissues for a longer period of time than it does in vaginal intercourse.
- If you or your partner have sores on your genitals, you may have an increased risk of infection.
- Having repeated unprotected sex with an infected person increases the risk of developing the AIDS virus.
- Genetic factors may also make a difference in your ability to fight off infection, or to be less resistant.

Once the HIV virus gains access to the bloodstream, it remains there silently until the symptoms of AIDS develop. After exposure to the virus, it usually takes three months to a year before the blood produces antibodies that can be detected in a blood test. In a small number of cases, it may be as long as four years before HIV antibodies begin to form.

The incubation period—the time between first becoming infected and developing symptoms—seems to average about eight years, although it can be shorter or longer.

Signs and symptoms.   Depending on how the HIV infection progresses through the body, it's possible to be silently infected without symptoms until years later, when it becomes a full-blown case of AIDS. In this instance, the HIV virus is slowly attacking the immune system, but you may not be aware of anything unusual, except minor problems, such as a white coating on the tongue (thrush).

Some people develop symptoms resembling mononucleosis six days to seven weeks after infection. Fever, sweating, aching muscles and joints, malaise, and swollen lymph nodes may last for two to four weeks. After the symptoms of this seemingly minor illness disappear, you may feel healthy for months or years.

Others progress from having no symptoms to a stage called ARC (AIDS-related complex). ARC is characterized by swollen lymph glands in more than one location, fever, rapid weight loss, fatigue, diarrhea, and night sweats. Skin rashes may also develop.

By the time the HIV virus has crippled the entire immune system, it heralds the final stage of infection: full-blown AIDS. At this point, opportunistic infections are free to run rampant in all body systems and organs. The list of infectious complications of AIDS draws representatives from every major category of organism.

Viruses attack the body, including hepatitis B, herpes simplex virus, cytomegalovirus, and Epstein-Barr virus. Bacteria such as pneumococcus cause pneumonia, and salmonella bacteria produce severe diarrhea. One of the most commonly occurring opportunistic infections is pneumonia caused by pneumocystis carinii, which is caused by a protozoan. Fungal infections are common, especially candida. Unusual cancers such as Kaposi's sarcoma, characterized by raised purple patches resembling bruises that develop on the skin, strike many homosexual AIDS victims. Death usually occurs within two years after the development of full-blown AIDS, although this period can be prolonged now because of new medications.

Diagnosis.   The only way to know if the HIV virus has entered your bloodstream is to get a blood test. The test itself is simple, but the issues and decisions that accompany testing are often complex—especially those regarding the results.

It is recommended that doctors offer testing to men and women who seek treatment for a sexually transmitted disease, and to those at risk, including homosexual and bisexual men, intravenous drug users, women whose current or past sexual partners are HIV-infected, bisexual, or IV-drug users, pregnant women who are at high risk, and anyone who had a blood transfusion between 1978 and 1985. Blood transfusions performed after 1985 carry a very small (but not a zero) risk of transmitting HIV.

Your physician must get your *informed consent* before performing the AIDS test. In many states, it is illegal to perform AIDS testing without informed consent. Your physician should also offer counseling before the test regarding such concerns as its purpose, the meaning of positive and negative results, the measures that will be taken to assure confidentiality, and the need to notify your sexual contacts who may be at risk.

The test has its limitations. Instead of detecting the virus itself, the test seeks out antibodies that the body produces when infection is present. Depending on when this test is administered, it may be negative today, but positive next month or next year. That's because the virus usually takes a certain period of time to establish itself and provoke antibody production—in medical jargon, to *seroconvert* to positive status.

The test for HIV is a two-step procedure. First, a sample of your blood is drawn for an antibody-detection test called ELISA (enzyme-linked immunoassay). This highly sensitive test was originally designed to detect the HIV virus in the nation's blood supply. The test, however, is not 100 percent accurate.

One problem with ELISA's sensitivity is that it may produce a false-positive result, meaning that a person not infected may be erroneously labeled positive. False-positive test results may be due to such conditions as multiple pregnancies, alcoholic liver disease, cancer, and various immune disorders and allergies.

A report that your test is negative may mean that you are infection-free with no signs of the virus in your body. Or it may mean that the HIV virus is in your bloodstream but has been there too short a time to have stimulated antibodies to form. A third possibility is that the test missed antibodies that may have been present. If you recently engaged in high-risk activity and have had a negative test result, it's wise to have the testing repeated after a period of time.

When the ELISA test comes back clearly positive or gives borderline results, it is repeated. If the second ELISA test reads positive or indeterminate, the process goes into the second step—the Western blot (WB)—to confirm the results. In cases where the WB is indeterminate, it may mean that seroconversion to positive is about to occur. It also could signify that other antibodies in the blood are causing a reaction and giving a false-positive reading. Some uninfected people remain in an indeterminate status for months.

Testing positive.   If your first run of tests comes back positive, get another test to confirm the initial diagnosis. Your doctor will ask you for a fresh sample of blood for analysis.

A confirmed positive result doesn't mean that you have AIDS. It indicates that you are *seropositive* for HIV, or have antibodies to the virus in your bloodstream. Scientists believe that most people who carry the HIV virus will eventually develop AIDS. Although you may feel and look healthy, you are now infectious to your sexual partners.

It is devastating to find out that you have tested positive. Telling others the news may lead to lost jobs, housing problems, and loss of health insurance. Be selective in sharing this personal information in order to protect yourself. But you *must* be responsible. You need to protect others with whom you may have, or may have had, intimate sexual contact.

If you are HIV-positive, here are some general guidelines:

• Abstain from sexual intercourse, or use condoms consistently each time.

• Be aware that immunization shots that contain live viruses may harm you because your immune system is weak. Check with your doctor first.

• Do what you can to stay healthy. Eat nutritious meals. Exercise regularly. Get enough rest. Avoid cigarette smoking, drugs, and heavy use of alcohol. Find effective ways to reduce stress.

• Be wary of any claims for unproven or unorthodox remedies. There is no known cure for AIDS. If you keep yourself as healthy as possible, medications designed to slow the progress of the disease will have a better chance to work in your body.

• Tell your sexual partners—past, present, and future—that you tested positive for the HIV virus. If they have had any intimate sexual contact with you, they have increased their risk of infection. If you can't tell them yourself, discuss it with your doctor or local public health department. A department representative will tell them that they may have been exposed to the AIDS virus while keeping your identity confidential.

• Don't do anything that could infect another person. Abstain from sexual activity that involves the exchange of body fluids. Use condoms, and use them carefully and properly. Condoms are not an absolute preventive, but they do reduce the risk of HIV transmission when used correctly.

• Don't donate blood, sperm, or sign an organ donor card.

• If you are a woman of childbearing age, refrain from getting pregnant. An infant born to a mother infected with the virus has a high likelihood of getting the disease by transmission from the mother. Pregnancy also alters the normal immune response in women and may accelerate the course of the disease in the pregnant mother.

• Before you do anything, talk to your primary care physician or call the toll-free National AIDS Hotline at 1-800-342-AIDS for information on how to contact an adviser in your area. Your doctor or a specially trained counselor can help you to decide whom to tell about your test results and when to tell them.

Treatment. There is strong evidence that the antiviral drug zidovudine, popularly called AZT, can delay the onset of symptoms of AIDS in those who test positive for the virus. In the past, the drug was given only when a person's T-cell count fell below 200—a level considered too low for the immune system to fight off infection. The FDA now recommends smaller doses of zidovudine in newly diagnosed people who feel healthy, have no symptoms, and have T-cell counts under 500. (A normal T-cell count ranges between 600 and 1,200.)

AZT, the only FDA-approved drug for the treatment of HIV infection, is very expensive: the recommended low dose of 500 to 600 milligrams a day can cost up to $2,700 a year. Now that early treatment of the infection with AZT has the FDA's blessing, it should be easier for those covered by insurance to be reimbursed.

Although AZT is effective in slowing the progress of the HIV infection and can increase one's sense of well-being, it has some serious side effects—notably anemia. However, there are fewer side effects when the drug is given at the lower dosage.

Several promising new drugs are currently under investigation for their effectiveness and safety in the treatment of AIDS. The FDA now has a system that speeds up the testing time of certain new drugs that are under study in clinical trials so they will get to patients faster.

Because it is a disease without a cure, AIDS is open territory for quackery. Many unorthodox practitioners promote a variety of unproven products and remedies that claim to strengthen the immune system. The list of nostrums includes pond scum, the food additive BHT, injections of hydrogen peroxide, and a chemical used in processing photographs. Unproven treatments not only foster false hope, they may accelerate your infection when other more effective drugs that can help slow it down are not used.

5

Mental and Emotional Health

Thomas N. Wise, M.D.

The idea of a sound mind in a sound body has been around since the time of Hippocrates. Although the role that the mind and the emotions play in sickness has been long studied, we are only beginning to understand how both serve as major contributors to a sense of well-being and bodily health.

It's long been conceded that attitude plays a role in good health. Having a sense of control over your life—in your job, what you eat, how you spend your leisure time, whether you're happy with your life—is essential to feeling well. Giving up control is demoralizing and often leads to stress, anxiety, or depression.

There are plenty of other events that take the joy out of life. External pressures, low job satisfaction, family demands, a dependency on alcohol or drugs, difficulty getting a good night's sleep, and suffering from chronic pain all can make life difficult. It's also not uncommon to feel out of sorts emotionally and still not recognize—or admit—that something's wrong in your life.

About 15 to 20 percent of the American population is affected by some type of mental disorder, from the mild to the incapacitating, from the short-term to the persistent. While it's possible to learn how to prevent or reduce the effects of stress and anxiety, prevention isn't always possible for other maladies of the mind. Many forms of depression, as well as obsessive-compulsive disorder and schizophrenia, are biological in origin and often respond well to medication.

One common misconception is that mental and emotional illnesses strike because the victim lacks willpower or is morally weak. In fact, biochemical influences in the brain have increasingly been shown to be the precipitating factor in many disorders of mind, mood, and behavior.

All kinds of help and treatments are available for the stress and strain that gnaw at our mental and emotional well-being. In some cases, a good self-help book and the motivation to change your behavior may offer the right dose of insight and guidance. Millions of people find solace and practical ways to approach living through specialized self-help groups. For others, depression, sudden attacks of anxiety, disturbing thoughts, severe mood swings, or a compulsion to repeat an action hundreds of times are among the problems that signal a need for treatment by a mental health care professional.

Stress

Stress is a real part of life. For many of us—especially the frazzled—stress is having to juggle one demand after another and finding it harder to keep up.

Stress is really a term from the science of physics. By definition, stress describes what occurs when external pressure is applied to a solid object, such as a metal, resulting in a strain that produces fatigue in the metal. It makes sense to consider the origin of the term when talking about the stress that we experience.

Back in the 1940s, pioneering stress researcher Hans Selye called the stress phenomenon a response—"the nonspecific response of the body to any demand made on it." However vague this concept may sound, it remains the best working definition of stress. Stress is a lot like cholesterol—it can be good or bad. If it's an adverse and negative experience, it's distress. But if it's challenging in a constructive sense, then it's "eustress"—a Selye-coined term for positive stress.

Because stress is so subjective, what you find distressing may be someone else's cup of tea. For one person, it may be invigorating to work hard; for another, working hard is debilitating—even if each is doing the same job. This is partly because of the outside stressor that's introducing the stress and partly because of the individual reacting to it.

Distress may occur as a symptom of the frustrations of commuting, job pressures, family feuds, unemployment, money worries, or health concerns. Eustress, or beneficial stress, can arise from demands that make life interesting or more exciting, such as starting a new job, facing a deadline, getting married, retiring, or having a new baby.

The right amount of stress can gear you up to greater productivity, to find a hidden reservoir of strength or inspiration to finish a project on time, or to cope with an unexpected situation. More stress than we can handle often causes such physical symptoms as headaches, muscle tension, digestive upset, and sleeplessness.

Stress in any form triggers a "fight or flight" response in the body that prepares you to react quickly when faced with a challenge. The stress reaction causes a whole chain of events in all body systems. The brain stimulates the production of hormones that accelerate some body activities while slowing down others. For instance, the heart pumps faster and harder, blood pressure increases, the breathing rate increases, and blood flow to certain organs decreases so that more blood can travel to the muscles.

When the danger is over, your body returns to its previous state of inner harmony—unless you refuse to let go of your fears and apprehensions. Continually overreacting to stressors keeps you primed for fight or flight. The body never has a chance to repair itself. Too much stress appears to increase the risk of high blood pressure, heart disease, depression, gastrointestinal problems, headaches, muscle spasms, and fatigue.

Stress at Work

According to Public Health Service estimates, stress contributes to absenteeism, lost productivity, and company health care expenses by as much as $50 billion to $75 billion annually.

In 1990, scientists reported that a group of 215 healthy American men aged 30 to 60 working in high-strain jobs were three times more likely to develop high blood pressure than men in low-strain jobs. The men wore ambulatory blood pressure monitors that allowed the investigators to obtain frequent blood pressure readings during the workday. Those at higher risk of developing hypertension also experienced a thickening of part of the heart muscle.

Recent studies have shown that jobs that call for a high level of performance and offer a high degree of control give workers opportunities to learn new skills and to grow in their expertise. Rigid or passive job requirements, on the other hand, place low or no demands on skills, abilities, and decision making, so skills erode from lack of use.

The worst job strain is having high psychological pressure with little leeway to make decisions. This group of workers has a low sense of control over their work and may have the highest health risk for heart disease.

Most research on occupational health has been done on men. At this point, relatively few occupations have equal proportions of male and female workers. But the studies acknowledge that in general a woman's average level of decision latitude is markedly lower than a man's. Women also have a higher proportion of high-strain jobs.

A sense of control in your work is obviously important. If it's in short supply, a social support system can help take the edge off some of the negative aspects of high-strain jobs. Both male and female workers experience much less depression when they have the support of friends and family.

Managing Stress

The best way to handle stress effectively is to understand that stress isn't an alien force that assaults you or "happens" to you. Stress is what you do with what life serves up on the daily menu of events—or as Selye called it, your response.

Sorting out the sources of stress in your life is one way to get a handle on the problem. But recognizing stress isn't always easy. If you experience persistent fatigue, anxiety, and a loss of interest in work and life in general, it may be due to stress—or even depression—and is worth a visit to your family physician.

Every day, you win some and you lose some. To be an effective player, it helps to have a few good strategies.

- Learn the value of control. We know that to succeed we must struggle for some control over the course our lives will take. But we must also develop the art of handling the world within—that is, our response to those incidents and events that make up our life story. When life hands you a loss, instead of brooding use the experience as a learning opportunity.
- Set goals for yourself, especially in areas over which you have control. Spending time on a hobby or leisure activity, getting a college degree, going for additional job training, learning a new skill, or joining a club or community group can pay high dividends in satisfaction.
- Look at your life-style choices and see if they are working in your favor. Three factors that play a big role in stress management are minimal or no use of stimulants and intoxicants, such as nicotine, alcohol, and caffeine; a daily relaxation session that offers at least 20 minutes to recharge your mental and physical batteries; and regular physical activity.
- Incorporate some social involvement into your life. Isolation isn't conducive to good health.

A Louis Harris survey taken in 1985 reported that 69 percent of Americans undertook specific actions to control stress. The measures they cited were getting enough sleep, socializing regularly, participating in community groups, and physical activity. These respondents latched onto some good ways of adapting to contemporary life. If you haven't done anything for yourself yet, get started as quickly as possible. You can create your own stress management program or join a program.

There are no industry standards that govern stress-management programs. So it's up to you to determine whether a program is likely to match your expectations. Find out if it's really a stress-management course by asking which specific techniques are taught. Some programs actually teach assertiveness training, but call it stress management. Ask about the credentials of the instructors and how long they've been teaching stress-management. Talk to people who are currently enrolled in courses to see whether they're getting some real benefits from their investment of time and money. Most organized programs generally last from six to eight weeks.

Techniques commonly used to abate stress include relaxation therapy, meditation, deep-muscle relaxation, self-hypnosis, exercise, and behavior modification.

It's not unusual for a primary care physician or a mental health care provider to recommend a self-help book on relaxation. The reading prescription may be a supplemental part of the therapy, or the treatment itself. Many such books, or the techniques they offer, are now available in audio and video cassettes.

Anxiety

Anxiety is a vague sort of threatening feeling in which you anticipate that something unpleasant is about to happen. It's normal to experience some anxiety in certain situations—it may even serve you well. A student facing finals who is able to focus her attention on her studies or a rookie minor league player up at bat in the season opener both may perform better because of their anxiety. In both cases, the anxious feeling disappears when finals and the game are over.

When anxiety becomes persistent, you find yourself feeling apprehensive about things for no apparent reason—a state of mind sometimes called needless worry. The typical symptoms include nervousness, worrying, and feeling jittery. Mild anxiety is distinctly different from fear, which is a response to a stimulus that you can clearly identify.

Anxiety can appear in several forms. The classification system that psychiatrists use—the Diagnostic and Statistical Manual of Mental Disorders (DSM-III-R, for short)—lists the following anxiety disorders: generalized anxiety disorder, panic disorder (such as agoraphobia, or fear of public places), simple phobias, posttraumatic stress disorder, social phobia, and obsessive-compulsive disorder.

Generalized Anxiety Disorder

This is the least specific form of anxiety. Typically, the symptoms are excessive anxiety and worry that persists for at least six months in two or more of your life circumstances. This could mean worrying about how you're going to make ends meet when you're really financially well off, or perpetuating some other fear that is unrealistic. Children and adolescents who are preoccupied with how they perform academically, athletically, and socially also experience this type of anxiety. Certain medications can cause anxiety. Illicit drugs and withdrawal from alcohol also can provoke anxiety.

Physical symptoms often accompany generalized anxiety disorder. These include palpitations, diarrhea, sweating, urinary frequency, insomnia, fatigue, irritability, and feeling on edge. Mild to moderate depression frequently occurs with this disorder.

If your symptoms are troubling enough to send you to a doctor, your physician must first rule out a physical cause for the symptoms.

Drug therapy has been effectively used to relieve the physical symptoms of anxiety but doesn't resolve the underlying anxiety disorder. If the cause of the anxiety is apparent and of a type that can be expected to resolve within a reasonable period of time, such as losing a job or grieving over the death of a spouse, a short term of antianxiety medication can prove helpful. In other cases of anxiety, behavior therapy or psychotherapy may be prescribed.

Some people may have an increased risk of becoming psychologically dependent on certain antianxiety medications—especially drugs from the family of benzodiazepines. Some of these drugs include alprazolam (Xanax), diazepam (Valium), lorazepam (Ativan), and chlordiazepoxide (Librium). Although the benzodiazepines are highly effective in relieving anxiety, they yield the best results when they are prescribed sparingly and are used for short periods of time.

A newly introduced drug compound called buspirone (Buspar) appears to be as effective as the benzodiazepines in anxiety treatment—but without the sedating and muscle-relaxing side effects. Buspirone appears to have little potential for addiction. Among the common side effects of buspirone are headaches and dizziness.

Tricyclic antidepressants, especially imipramine (Tofranil), are also prescribed for generalized anxiety disorder.

Psychotherapy, behavior therapy, and relaxation therapy may also help you better deal with generalized anxiety.

Panic Disorder

Panic disorders are characterized by the spontaneous onset of intense feelings of dread, apprehension, or fear accompanied by a sense of doom. Physical symptoms also tend to occur, including difficulty breathing, rapid heartbeat, and feelings of tightness in the chest. Dizziness, nausea, sweating, a feeling of pins and needles, and hot flushes and chills also are likely. Typically, there is a fear of losing control, going crazy, or falling down and creating a scene. Collectively, these symptoms form a *panic attack*.

Some people experience a single episode of panic symptoms, while others find their attacks recurring weekly or monthly. Panic attacks can be disabling if you begin to associate the symptoms with the place where the attacks occurred. It's typical to suffer a panic attack in an elevator or in a crowded department store, or in a railway or airline terminal, experience a second or even third similar episode in the same setting, and then begin to avoid the scene of the attack.

Many a social person has turned reclusive after suffering repeated panic attacks. (This fear of being in a place or situation where a panic attack might occur is known as *agoraphobia*. This phobia often follows panic attacks.) Others have made multiple visits to hospital emergency rooms because their symptoms led them to believe (wrongly) they were having a heart attack.

Psychiatric researchers have found that the triggering factor in panic attacks can often be traced to a biochemical abnormality in the brain. Psychologists, on the other hand, say the attacks may result from environmental cues that set certain psychological and physiological processes in motion.

Many—but not all—people who suffer panic attacks have a dramatic response to drug therapy. The medications that psychiatrists prescribe to stop panic attacks are tricyclic antidepressants and monoamine oxidase (MAO) inhibitors—both of which are used to treat depression. Alprazolam (Xanax) is also effective. Behavioral therapy to modify the fear of being in the place where the panic attack occurred also may be used in conjunction with medication.

Simple Phobias

A simple *phobia* may be the most common psychiatric disorder in the general population. A phobia is a persistent fear that makes little sense to you but causes you to avoid the object or the situation that makes you feel anxious. The fear of heights (acrophobia) may rank number one among phobias. Virtually every persistent fear gets its own name, from fear of cats (ailurophobia) and fear of baldness (peladophobia) to fear of marriage (gamophobia). Agoraphobia, or fear of public places, is not considered a simple phobia.

A phobia may develop gradually or may be sudden in onset. For instance, you may develop a fear of small insects (acarophobia) if you find a bug or two in your salad. That could mark the sudden development of an irrational fear. A passenger who survives an airplane crash virtually unscathed while other passengers have died or suffered serious injuries is a prime candidate for developing a flying phobia (pterygophobia). More likely, this passenger may also suffer from posttraumatic stress disorder (see following).

Generally speaking, you don't need treatment for a simple phobia unless it disturbs you or limits your activity. A fear of heights may not be a problem if you live and work in a one-story building and like to vacation in the flatlands. But if you're a painter or a roofer, then your phobia is a problem. Similarly, if you fear flying but find that you can get around just as well by car, train, or on foot, you don't have to confront your fear. If your profession is sales representative and your work requires air travel, then you need to get treatment.

Phobias can be effectively treated with behavior therapy. The treatment focuses on a process of gradual desensitization until your anxiety eventually disappears.

Posttraumatic Stress Disorder

People who have been through an intensely traumatic experience may suffer from a group of symptoms called *posttraumatic stress disorder*. The triggering event could be experiencing or witnessing a plane crash, automobile accident, physical violence or death, or the sudden destruction of your home or property.

The major symptom of PTSD is a persistent mental and emotional rerun of the traumatic experience—especially through recurring memories and dreams about the event. Other symptoms include avoidance of any thoughts, feelings, or activities that bring up recollections of the trauma, leading to an overall feeling of numbness. Irritability, difficulty sleeping, inability to concentrate, and hypervigilance—an inability to let down your guard and relax—also mark PTSD.

Sometimes these symptoms may not appear until six months after the trauma, but usually they appear sooner. If the painful recurring dreams and thoughts don't quit within a month, then professional help is necessary. A psychiatrist can prescribe appropriate medication to relieve the anxiety or depression and encourage the PTSD victim to begin to talk about the problem in therapy.

Social Phobia

Social phobia is a distinct anxiety disorder marked by a persistent fear of situations in which other people may scrutinize your actions, which you fear will embarrass or humiliate you. These unreasonable fears encompass such activities as eating or speaking in public.

It has been estimated that 2 to 3 percent of the population suffers from social phobia. The fears that social phobics harbor turn them into near-recluses who may be afraid to date or make friends, to contribute ideas at work, or to go on for further education or training because they're afraid of what others will think of them.

The causes of social phobia could be a combination of heredity, learned behavior, psychological problems, and just plain shyness. In any case, help is now available. Psychiatrists have reported good results by prescribing certain antidepressant medications in combination with counseling.

The dose of medication must be carefully monitored because some of these psychopharmacologic drugs may become habit-forming. Ideally, a treatment program should begin behavior therapy immediately—either before or when drug therapy is started. This way, social phobics can learn and begin using practical strategies for dealing with their fears.

Performance anxiety is really a form of fear that strikes some people who have to speak before an audience. The symptoms are dry mouth, accelerated heart rate, sweaty palms, trembling, and a feeling of breathlessness.

If you experience severe performance anxiety, ask your doctor about prescribing a beta-blocker. Provided that you can tolerate this type of medication, it is effective in blocking anxiety reactions, especially for those people who perform on stage on rare occasions. It's best to give this medication a single trial run a few days before your speech—just to make sure that you don't develop any adverse reactions.

Obsessive-Compulsive Disorder

Obsessive-compulsive disorder (OCD), once considered a rare disorder, now is thought to be relatively common. An obsession is a repetitive idea or impulse that is so intrusive that a person has no control over it. A compulsion is a repetitive behavior or ritual, such as repeatedly counting or touching something to ward off an adverse event or to satisfy your obsession.

Instead of checking a door once to make sure that it's locked, an obsessive-compulsive checks hundreds of times. Or a food shopper may carefully choose a head of lettuce at the supermarket, but return to the same bin several times before settling on the "right" one. This shopper may spend a few hours in the store instead of the half-hour it would normally take to shop.

An estimated 4 million American adults and children have OCD. They try to live normal lives by keeping their disorder hidden and they may succeed, but eventually their education, careers, and intimate relationships suffer—or collapse—as a result.

In 1989, the FDA approved the use of the antidepressant drug clomipramine (Anafranil) for the treatment of obsessive-compulsive disorder. This drug works by altering the brain's uptake of serotonin, a neurotransmitter, a chemical in the brain that serves as a messenger.

Obsessive-compulsive behavior also has been found to respond to new techniques developed by behavioral therapists that gradually expose the victim to the situation that provokes the behavior. The idea is to get the person who is compulsive about washing, for instance, to touch dirt and agree not to wash his or her hands for a certain number of minutes, and eventually, for a longer period of time.

In most cases, behavior therapy and a regimen of drug treatment can produce effective results in reducing or preventing obsessive-compulsive rituals.

Depression

Depression is one of the most common and debilitating problems that beset people—both young and old. At any point in time, an estimated one out of five Americans are suffering from depression.

Depression occurs insidiously. Any number of things can bring on a depressed mood, but often there is no clear cause. Among the usual provocateurs are psychological, environmental, and biochemical factors.

An emotional loss, a disappointment, a feeling of powerlessness, and even your own brain chemistry are typical triggers of depression. It's possible to develop depression as a side effect of taking certain medications. Some people become depressed when there's less light in the day during the winter months—a phenomenon known as *seasonal affective disorder* (see page 139).

Recognizing a case of depression is difficult for patient and doctor alike. Most of us occasionally fall into a blue mood, but most such experiences are transitory. A good example is returning to work after spending a few weeks away on vacation. You can identify the source of your low mood, but soon you regroup and return to your normal level of functioning. If you do have inordinate difficulty getting back into the spirit of work, your depression may be a sign that your job is too stressful and you need to look for a new job—or learn how to manage stress better.

If you can't rule out a case of the blahs, you may be experiencing a true depression, which is characterized by the following signs and symptoms:

- depressed mood (or irritability in children and adolescents) that occurs almost daily and lasts all day
- withdrawal from people and a lack of interest in activities you used to find pleasurable
- weight changes (loss or gain) and a decrease or increase in appetite
- change in sleep patterns. Typically, there is insomnia and waking up early in the morning without being able to fall asleep again. Occasionally, a person may sleep an excessive amount and find it extremely difficult to wake up.
- declining interest in sexual activity and performance
- feeling fatigued and having a lack of energy
- difficulty concentrating on work, or even on simpler things, such as reading a book
- a sense of worthlessness
- hopelessness that sometimes leads to thoughts of suicide
- persistent sadness and frequent bouts of crying
- neglect of appearance, chores, work duties, or assignments
- inability to make a decision, even over something simple

When a bout of depression is mild or if there are clear extraneous factors contributing to it, supportive family members or friends may be able to help you through it. The human spirit allows us to rebound at varying speeds and in different stages from painful events or grief over an emotional loss. But when the suffering is so intense that it disrupts your life and you can't put your problems into perspective, then professional help is necessary.

Eighty percent of people with depression will respond to the proper treatment. Patients who are depressed do best when they are referred to a psychiatrist for evaluation. This includes a complete physical and psychological workup to rule out any hidden physical illness or a chronic problem involving a job, spouse, or child. If the diagnosis indicates that drug therapy would help, a psychiatrist can prescribe the proper medication and the right dosage level, along with counseling. A variety of therapies also are available, including psychotherapy and behavior therapy.

Drug Therapy

Since the 1950s, drug therapy has consisted of the traditional antidepressants: the tricyclics and the monoamine oxidase (MAO) inhibitors. In 1987, a new class of drugs called serotonin reuptake inhibitors—one of which is known by the generic name of fluoxetine (Prozac)—was introduced.

All of these drugs appear to work by interacting with neurotransmitters or their receptors at the ends of nerve cells in the brain. When the medications kick in, they produce electrochemical changes that help regulate mood.

Tricyclics. The tricyclics derive their name from the three rings that form their chemical structure. These drugs work by affecting the pathways of the neurotransmitters norepinephrine and serotonin. Studies have indicated that when tricyclic antidepressants are administered in appropriate doses, they are effective in nearly 70 percent of the patients to whom they are prescribed.

These drugs must be administered carefully in increasing doses until your doctor determines the appropriate amount for you. It usually takes four to six weeks, during which time the dose is adjusted, for them to become fully effective. During this time, your doctor monitors the level by taking blood tests.

Some of the tricyclics can have such side effects as drowsiness, dry mouth, constipation, blurred vision, accelerated heart rate, light-headedness, and in some cases, weight gain. The tricyclics include the first-generation drugs imipramine (Tofranil), amitriptyline (Elavil), and doxepin (Adapin), and the more recently developed nortriptyline (Aventyl), protriptyline (Vivactil), desipramine (Norpramin), and amoxapine (Asendin). The early generation of tricyclics seem to produce more dramatic side effects than the newer drugs.

Monoamine oxidase (MAO) inhibitors. MAO inhibitors are used when tricyclic antidepressants don't work or if a patient is highly sensitive to their effects. This class of drugs works by disrupting the passage of enzymes that break down chemical messengers in the brain to produce their results. MAO inhibitors evolved from the drug iproniazid, which produced a euphoric feeling in patients who were taking it for tuberculosis.

One problem with MAO inhibitors is that they carry the risk of producing a sudden increase in blood pressure—or hypertensive crisis—in people who eat certain foods that contain the amino acid tyramine. When a psychiatrist prescribes an MAO inhibitor, the drug comes with a list of forbidden foods and medications. Some of these items include aged cheese, pickles, yogurt with active cultures, red wine, beer, overly ripe bananas, cold and allergy pills, and certain antianxiety medications.

New-generation antidepressants. A medication called fluoxetine (Prozac), which gained FDA approval in 1987 as an antidepressant, is currently much in use. Indeed, some patients who responded poorly to other antidepressants report relief for the first time. Because fluoxetine takes effect in about three weeks and usually works with a standard dose level, blood monitoring is unnecessary.

The known side effects include headache, nausea, nervousness, and occasionally slight weight loss. But the long-term effects of fluoxetine remain unknown. Some physicians have reported more serious adverse reactions in a small number of patients, including agitation, tremors, mania, and a preoccupation with suicide.

Although fluoxetine has been approved for use only as a treatment for depression, it appears that the drug may also be useful in the treatment of some anxiety disorders.

Electroconvulsive Therapy (ECT)

When drug treatment fails to relieve depression, ECT, which involves producing a controlled seizure in the brain, is considered a safe and effective treatment.

Fear, misunderstanding, and controversy have surrounded ECT since it was first introduced in the late 1930s. However, the safety of the procedure has been much improved over the last 50 years. A patient accepted for ECT must now undergo a careful physical evaluation, especially if there is a history of high blood pressure or cardiovascular disease. Anesthesia, muscle relaxants, and oxygen are administered during the procedure.

Short-term memory loss is the major side effect of ECT. Most disruptions of memory resolve within six to nine months after treatment. A National Institute of Mental Health panel has estimated that less than one-half of 1 percent of all ECT recipients suffer severe memory loss.

A typical ECT regimen includes a series of six to nine treatments, with two days between sessions. ECT should be performed in a hospital by a qualified psychiatrist. If this kind of therapy is recommended, it's essential to get a second opinion. Find out how often the doctor administering the ECT has performed this kind of therapy.

Mania

The other side of the coin in mood disorders is *mania*, which is marked by an elevated or irritable mood and racing ideas and activity. Whereas a depressed person tends to feel negative and low in self-esteem, someone who is manic has an inflated self-image that may border on the grandiose. A person in the throes of mania experiences a heightened sense of power and increased energy that often can lead to behaviors with dangerous consequences. Some of the more recognizable behaviors are going on a shopping spree and spending thousands of dollars, promiscuity, and reckless driving.

Manic episodes that alternate with periods of depression are called *bipolar disorder*. When a person experiences only manic highs without depression, the condition is known as *unipolar mania*. *Cyclothymia* is a milder form of manic-depressive illness.

Treatment with lithium is very effective in controlling the mood swings of manic-depressive illness as well as the agitated and sometimes delusional behavior that accompanies mania.

Seasonal Affective Disorder

The amount of light in your life literally may lighten your mood and keep depression at bay. Just like clockwork, some people become depressed every year in the period from autumn until spring, the time of the year when there are fewer hours of daylight. Because this disordered mood coincides with the onset of certain seasons, it is appropriately named *seasonal affective disorder* (SAD).

But the effects of SAD apparently aren't limited to people with the winter blues. People who work night shifts or suffer from jet lag may also be subject to the depression, irritability, sluggishness, and anxiety that characterize SAD.

The human body operates according to an inner body clock that regulates sleep cycles, temperature, and the release of hormones—a pattern that scientists call our circadian clock. Because the body's natural cycle is 25 hours and a day offers only 24 hours, something gets lost in the shuffle.

Scientifically timed exposures to sunlight or the right kind of bright artificial light appears to be helpful in relieving some cases of seasonal affective disorder. The use of phototherapy for seasonal depression is a relatively new concept that requires a certain kind of light and a specific amount of exposure in order to be effective. For this reason, self-help with phototherapy is not recommended. If you decide to seek this kind of treatment, be certain that the therapist has sufficient experience in treating SAD. Much study remains to be done regarding the effectiveness of light therapy.

Sleep

We all need to sleep—more or less. Most people need seven to nine hours of sleep a night, while others seem to thrive on six hours or less. All too often, the sleep you get and the sleep you need are as different as night and day.

In 1990, the government appointed the National Commission on

Sleep Disorders Research to come up with a long-term plan for fostering sleep research and education, as well as ways to put the medical applications of research into public policy. It is expected that the commission's recommendations will be used to improve safety in scheduling in such job areas as transportation, industry, and nuclear power plants.

Among the apparent reasons for our national sleep deficit are increased social, job, and family pressures that cut into time we might have once used for sleep. Shift work, which requires adapting to permanent or alternating night shifts, often is accompanied by difficulty in falling asleep. Jet lag, or traveling across a number of time zones, can be discombobulating and wearing to travelers. Round-the-clock television may entice many people to stay up too late when they have to arise early the next morning.

Most of us feel miserable or out of synch after a night of sleeping poorly or not at all but manage to regroup as soon as we can catch up on sleep. When sleep deprivation is mild—for instance, one to one-and-a-half hours less than you're accustomed to sleeping—your productivity tends to dip and your thinking is less efficient. But chronic sleep deprivation can be dangerous because it can impair your judgment and lead to delayed reactions and to accidents.

Losing just one night's sleep can impair the spontaneity, flexibility, and originality that allow you to deal effectively with new and unexpected situations. British scientist James A. Horne of Loughborough University studied a group of 24 college students and found that when all were well rested, they had comparable scores on tests that measured creative thinking. On the second night of the experiment, half were allowed to sleep while the other half stayed up all night. When tests were given the following day, the sleep-deprived group scored one-third to two-thirds lower in various aspects of creative thinking.

Even when money was offered as a reward for producing higher scores to boost motivation, the sleep-deprived students still fared worse than their well-rested classmates.

When people lose one night's sleep, their ability to use familiar skills in unchallenging situations remains basically unaffected. As long as the job at hand holds their interest, they usually can pull through by increasing their concentration. But two nights of sleep loss results in an impaired ability to deal with a well-known situation—even if you have been trained to perform a certain way in that situation.

From young adulthood until sometime after age 60, the average night's sleep is about seven to eight hours long. But at some point during your 60s or 70s, the nature of sleep changes. Come nighttime, instead of having the continuous period of sleep you're accustomed to, it becomes normal to spend less time in deep sleep and to experience more frequent awakenings. This kind of fragmented sleep is often mistakenly called insomnia, but it's actually a changing sleep pattern that occurs in healthy adults.

However, in some older adults, a sleep disorder or depression may be at the root of a sleeping problem. Among the more common sleep disorders are interruptions of normal breathing called sleep apnea and an involuntary jerking of the leg, known as restless leg syndrome (see page 144).

Insomnia

Millions of Americans frequently complain of *insomnia,* or difficulty falling asleep or staying asleep. Everyone experiences an occasional night of restlessness or very little sleep.

Insomnia may be a transient symptom of the stress of a job change, an argument with a spouse, jet lag, or sleeping in a different place. When the anxiety disappears, so does the insomnia.

Short-term insomnia can result from stressful situations such as a job loss, the death of a friend or family member, or concern over unusual symptoms before a doctor's appointment. This type of insomnia usually resolves itself in a few weeks.

Persistent, or chronic, insomnia can linger for months or years. When insomnia is long-lasting, it may be the symptom of a psychiatric problem such as depression. Or it may stem from alcohol use, reliance on sleep medications, shift work, jet lag, or sleep disorders. Excessive intake of stimulants like caffeine, appetite suppressants, and certain medications can also cause insomnia.

The early recognition and treatment of a sleep disturbance such as insomnia may be valuable in preventing such mood disorders as depression. With this in mind, there are several steps you can take to increase your chances of getting a good night's sleep:

• Establish a regular schedule for going to sleep and waking up. Stick to your established wake-up time every day—on weekdays and weekends—even if you had an inadequate night's rest. Having a fixed schedule helps program your inner sleep/wake cycles and usually improves sleep.

• Don't drink coffee, tea, or soft drinks that contain caffeine within four hours of your scheduled bedtime. Some over-the-counter diet pills and decongestants may contain the stimulant phenylpropanolamine (PPA), which can interfere with sleep.

• Eat dinner at the same time every day and avoid going to bed on a full stomach—especially if you are bothered by the gastric reflux that accompanies heartburn. People who experience a backup of stomach acid into the esophagus also can raise the head of their beds, or use an additional pillow.

• Avoid alcohol after dinner. Alcohol may make you feel sleepy and help you fall asleep faster, but it can disrupt normal sleeping patterns. As a result, your sleep is likely to be lighter and choppy, punctuated by sudden wake-ups.

• Engage in regular physical activity to help improve your sleep. Exercise has its best effect on sleep when it is done in the late afternoon or early evening. Avoid exercising too close to bedtime because it can have the opposite effect—stimulation instead of relaxation.

• Take time out to relax in the evening before you go to bed. If you've got a full schedule on the next day, make a written list of your priorities. After your list is made, there's no reason to stay awake worrying about remembering everything.

• Eliminate any distractions that can disturb sleep—within your control. Dark window shades and eye coverings can help keep out light. Sometimes, the sound from an air conditioner or fan can help muffle external sounds.

• Keep the temperature of your bedroom comfortable. A room that is too hot or too cold doesn't help you fall asleep.

• Some people benefit from daytime naps, while others find that napping can adversely affect nighttime sleep. Many experts advise that you should avoid napping—unless you find it beneficial.

• If you're not sleepy at your regular bedtime, don't go to bed. On the same note, if you've been in bed for about 20 minutes and haven't been able to fall asleep, get out of bed and read, watch television, or listen to music until you feel sleepy.

Chronotherapy. When all else fails, another approach that may be effectively used to reset your inner clock is *chronotherapy,* or time therapy. If you can't fall asleep until the early hours of the morning—a sleep disturbance known as *delayed sleep phase syndrome*—chronotherapy can help advance your inner time cycle up to an earlier hour.

Chronotherapy calls for moving your bedtime forward three hours each day until you finally achieve a time that suits you. For instance, if you're used to falling asleep at 3:00 A.M., you would stay up until 6:00 A.M. on the first day and sleep your full seven to eight hours. The second day's bedtime would be pushed up three hours to 9:00 A.M. and you'd again sleep your usual amount. On the third day, noon would be your target sleeptime. From there, you'd progress to 3:00 P.M., then to 6:00 P.M., on to 9:00 P.M., and finally arrive at your desired turn-in time: midnight.

Chronotherapy is not a treatment that should be undertaken on your own without first consulting a sleep specialist. For this treatment to work, you need to have the right setting. This requires a quiet and dark area in which to sleep uninterrupted during the day and a stretch of about eight days in which to accomplish the change.

Some people prefer to check into a sleep laboratory when adjusting their inner clocks. Others can work with a specialist, but do it on their own if they have the motivation and a supportive family or friends who can offer encouragement, meals, and peace and quiet during the transitional sleeptimes.

Although it's possible to change your inner clock, once you're operating on your new time, you have to be diligent about getting up at the same time every morning. Otherwise, you risk falling back into your earlier middle-of-the-night sleep/wake routine.

Sleeping aids. A variety of sleep-inducing medications are frequently prescribed for insomnia, but these drugs are best used sparingly under a doctor's orders. When sleeping pills, or hypnotics, are used for a period of time, it can be relatively easy to develop a tolerance to these drugs and become dependent on them for sleep.

Many people turn to over-the-counter sleeping pills when they suffer from insomnia. The main ingredient in some of these products is an antihistamine derived from cold medications that makes their users drowsy. The drawback with these products is that not everyone reacts similarly to antihistamines: some people become stimulated instead of sleepy. Some more serious side effects are also possible: confusion, dizziness, disorientation, double vision, and a feeling of being very tired. Most of these side effects are more frequent or more pronounced in older people.

Having a nightcap may seem harmless because of the initial relaxing effect created by alcohol. But after you've been asleep awhile, a sort of small-scale withdrawal takes place and interferes with deep sleep. You may experience disturbing dreams or a night of unsettled sleep.

Sleep Disorders

Whereas insomnia or a disturbance of sleep rhythm can usually be treated by changing your behavior, *sleep disorders* are a far more serious concern. Among the more common are *sleep apnea* and *restless legs syndrome.*

Sleep apnea. A potentially dangerous condition, *sleep apnea* is characterized by a 10- to 60-second halt in breathing, loud snores, and gasping for air in order to take in breath. This cycle of breaks in your breathing can repeat itself several times and severely disrupt your sleep. If you suffer from sleep apnea, it's impossible to discover the problem yourself.

The usual signs of sleep apnea are daytime tiredness, irritability, and complaints of snoring from a sleep partner. Difficulty concentrating and depression are other typical symptoms. Men age 40 and over are more likely to be affected by sleep apnea, especially if they are overweight. This disorder not only causes annoying snoring, but the lack of oxygen during the halt in breathing could trigger cardiac arrhythmias or a heart attack.

If you feel extremely sleepy during the day and are more moody and restless than normal, see your doctor. When sleep apnea is suspected, your doctor will refer you to a sleep center for diagnosis and a determination of the cause of the disorder.

Treatment may call for medication, weight loss, or, as a last resort, surgery to allow for unobstructed breathing during sleep. Mechanical devices have been developed to allow continuous air to flow into the breathing passages during the night. One such device is a face mask that is attached by tube to a small air compressor. The constant delivery of air through the nose can prevent the airways from becoming obstructed.

Restless legs syndrome. Just as sleep begins, you may experience a strange creeping and crawling feeling deep inside your leg that eventually causes you to move the leg in a jerking or kicking motion. Mild pain and cramps may also occur in restless legs syndrome. These symptoms usually will force you to get up and walk around to get rid of the sensation. As a result, you may have a problem getting back to sleep.

The cause of restless legs syndrome isn't always clear. If your family doctor can't explain your disorder, you may be referred to a sleep specialist for diagnosis. Restless legs may stem from peripheral neuropathy, a neurological condition that often occurs with diabetes. In some cases, an iron deficiency is responsible for the disorder, or it may develop as a temporary problem of pregnancy.

It's possible to treat the iron deficiency, but when restless legs results from a diabetic neuropathy, it may not be reversible. Drugs used to treat epilepsy have been employed to suppress the syndrome, but most restless legs sufferers develop a tolerance to these drugs. Home remedies also may provide relief for mild cases. One such remedy is to keep the legs cold at night, while the variation is to keep the legs hot.

Sleep Clinics

When all else fails, you may be referred to a sleep clinic. Because a variety of factors often interact to produce chronic insomnia or sleep disorders, neurologists, psychiatrists, and pulmonary or cardiac specialists may be called in to evaluate your condition.

There are a variety of tests to measure your brain wave patterns, heart and breath rate, body movement, and the level of oxygen in your blood. Depending on the test results and the diagnosis, you may be invited to check in for a few nights' stay at a sleep clinic for therapy.

Sleep clinics are usually operated by medical schools or large teaching hospitals. If you are advised to enter a sleep clinic, check your health insurance policy to see if this kind of treatment is covered. For a list of accredited sleep disorder centers in the United States, write to the American Sleep Disorders Association, 604 Second Street S.W., Rochester, Minnesota 55902.

Chronic Pain

Millions of Americans suffer from *chronic pain*—a situation in which constant or intermittent pain becomes the focal point of a person's life. When persistent pain cannot be attributed to injury or a clear physical cause, it may be called *psychogenic pain*. The word *psychogenic* literally means "born in the psyche," but it's a term that is of little use in dealing with chronic pain.

The study of pain doesn't lend itself to a convenient and well-defined separation between mind and body as causal agent. Actually, psychogenic pain often springs, at least in part, from a biological basis. Similarly, physical pain is never without an emotional reaction.

Your response to pain and your ability to cope with it are shaped by your personality, your cultural and ethnic background, your early developmental experience, your present circumstances, daily stresses, whether you feel a sense of control over your life, and the illness itself.

Chronic pain disorder is usually diagnosed if:

- someone reacts to pain more intensely and for a longer time than the average person
- there is no clear physical cause to account for the pain, or for its continuance
- the complaint of pain or the social and occupational impairment exceeds what would be expected from that problem

Conventional treatments for pain—bed rest, drugs, surgery, and physical therapy—typically leave chronic pain patients no better off than they were before seeking help. Many also risk becoming addicted to narcotics or tranquilizers that are often prescribed for pain.

After exhausting the conventional therapies, many pain sufferers turn to alternative treatments such as acupuncture, nerve blocks, relaxation techniques, and biofeedback. Some of these treatments work for some people, and others don't. While they may be worth exploring, be sure to seek advice from your doctor. As a last resort, he or she may refer you to a specialized pain clinic.

Pain clinics are usually affiliated with universities or teaching hospitals. The goal of treatment isn't to make the pain disappear but to improve the quality of life by learning how to cope with the pain and return to living a normal life. A side effect of this advanced treatment often is some reduction of pain. In some cases, the major benefit of visiting a pain management center is freedom from dependence on narcotics and tranquilizers.

The evolving field of pain management hasn't yet established any standards of practice. There is an accrediting body for chronic pain clinics, called the Commission on Accreditation of Rehabilitation Facilities, but it recognizes only programs that are comprehensive in nature. These programs use a team approach involving physicians, psychiatrists or clinical psychologists, specialized nurses, and physical therapists.

Pain clinics can be expensive, but their services are often covered by insurance. Certain insurance plans may require preapproval. Some programs are for inpatients only; others accept outpatients.

Not all clinics are alike in their approach to therapy. A clinic that is directed by a psychiatrist may stress behavioral techniques, while a program run by a physiatrist is more likely to emphasize physical rehabilitation. Similarly, an anesthesiologist-directed clinic may opt for more use of nerve blocks. Before enrolling, find out which type of therapy the clinic emphasizes. Ideally, patients should learn pain-relieving techniques that they can use later at home on a day-to-day basis after completing the program.

Eating Disorders

Eating disorders such as *anorexia nervosa* and *bulimia* respond best to treatment when they are caught early. The problem with these disorders is that their victims rarely seek help on their own. By the time a parent, a friend, or a mate begins to suspect that something is wrong, an anorectic may have lost an excessive amount of weight or a bulimic may have suffered physical damage.

People with anorexia harbor an intense fear of weight gain and feel a continuing need to diet. Someone with bulimia consumes large amounts of food at one time—a phenomenon called binge eating—and follows up with a purge induced by vomiting or a laxative.

Young women and a smaller number of young men are most likely to be afflicted with eating disorders. The cause of these disorders remains unknown, but it is thought that they have a psychological origin. Researchers are also investigating the possibility of a biological cause.

Some signs of anorexia are a preoccupation with food accompanied by bizarre eating patterns, such as cutting food into tiny pieces, or moving it around on a plate, but never eating it. Excessive exercise—often to the point of near-exhaustion—becomes a compulsion among some anorectics. Oddly, family members may not notice this behavior until the victim becomes emaciated.

Bulimia may be more difficult to detect because its victims do their binge eating in private. Anorectics have a tendency to isolate themselves socially and to have little interest in sex. Bulimics, on the other hand, are usually outgoing and are more likely to be involved in relationships. Aside from affecting several aspects of health and appearance, bulimia is a serious threat to mental health.

If left untreated, eating disorders can persist for decades. Bulimia can produce serious health effects ranging from tears in the esophagus, rotten teeth from constant vomiting, chronic fatigue, and depression. It also causes the parotid glands around the jaw to swell, eventually making its victims take on the appearance of chipmunks. Anorexia can curtail the menstrual cycle in women, and in men cause diminished sexual interest.

An estimated 30 to 60 percent of anorectics eventually fall prey to the binge eating of bulimia. Both disorders are difficult to treat. In either case, there is a risk of relapse. Bulimics frequently respond to psychotherapy and behavioral therapy. Treatment with tricyclic antidepressants or antianxiety medications may be helpful in some cases. Many bulimics appear to find value in self-help groups that have been formed for eating disorders. With anorectics, the treatment emphasizes maintaining a reasonable weight.

In most cases, these disorders can be treated on an outpatient basis. Experts in eating disorders note that hospitalization is usually necessary when a victim's weight falls to 30 percent below normal. Other considerations for inpatient treatment include problems like severe depression, thoughts of suicide, or the physical symptoms of starvation.

Substance Abuse

Public health experts can't say for certain how many Americans are victims of alcohol and drug abuse and dependency, but estimates place the figure at well over 18 million for alcohol alone. A growing number of people—especially adolescents and young adults—use such drugs as cocaine, heroin, and marijuana for pleasure, but often with serious results.

Alcohol

About half of all American adults use alcohol, but consumption doesn't always indicate a problem. When drinking alcohol becomes a compulsion, however mild, then it's time to get help. Alcoholism is often called the disease of denial because, typically, alcoholics deny that their drinking is out of control. Although there is no single accepted definition of alcoholism and no definitive criteria that doctors can use to make a diagnosis of alcoholism, there are categories that substance abuse experts use to indicate various stages of this problem. Most of those who will eventually become alcoholics go through these stages over a period of time.

Problem drinking generally indicates a pattern of alcohol intake that disrupts work, health, social life, and family life. Often, it leads to problems at home, missed days of work, and running afoul of the law.

Alcohol abuse is characterized by regular daily consumption of large quantities of alcohol punctuated by occasional periods of abstinence. These episodes of sobriety are followed by heavy drinking sprees that may last for days, weeks, or months.

Alcohol dependency, or alcoholism, is the third stage of the disease. An alcoholic develops an increasing tolerance for larger and larger amounts of alcohol, leading to such medical complications as cirrhosis, hepatitis, gastrointestinal bleeding, and cardiomyopathy, a disease of the heart muscle. Neurological and psychiatric changes can occur in a state of alcohol dependency, including loss of control and personality changes.

By the time an alcoholic progresses to stage four, poor physical health and impaired thinking are readily apparent. The fourth phase is marked by a complete loss of control over alcohol. An alcoholic who doesn't seek help and rehabilitation during the final phase falls into greater deterioration and faces the risk of a premature death.

Scientists recently identified a gene that appears to be associated with a hereditary vulnerability to alcoholism. However, the team of researchers who reported their findings in *The Journal of the American Medical Association* explain that there is no single gene that is responsible for all forms of alcoholism. Heredity is thought to be one part of a larger picture of alcoholism that also encompasses physical, social, and cultural influences.

There are two types of alcoholism that run in families and seem to be affected by genes as well as by environment. *Male-inherited alcoholism,* which can affect the sons of alcoholic fathers early in life, is characterized by moderate to severe alcohol abuse. A more prevalent type of alcoholism called *milieu-limited alcoholism* is thought to be the result of environmental influences in the family setting.

In any case, having an alcoholic parent is considered the strongest risk factor for developing alcoholism yourself—whether you're male or female. An awareness of your family history for alcoholism can help you to control your own drinking so as to head off any potential problems.

It can be difficult for physicians to detect alcohol abuse in patients because people commonly report consuming smaller amounts than is true. But sharing your knowledge of a family history of alcoholism with your physician can give your doctor the opportunity to work with you to help prevent problems.

While some people with a genetic vulnerability to this disease go on to alcoholism, others who are similarly predisposed are so motivated to avoid the problem that they either shun alcohol altogether or use it judiciously.

If you find that you begin to need alcohol to get through the day, it's an early warning sign of a serious disease, and you should treat it as such. Since alcohol is, like nicotine and caffeine, a socially sanctioned drug, it is widely used for various reasons—especially to relieve tension or to induce a state of being that seems to give pleasure. But beware, for alcoholism has a way of creeping up on you.

Treating alcohol abuse. There are various ways to treat alcoholism, but there is no cure for the disease. The only effective way to stop the associated physical, mental, and social damage is to abstain from alcohol. As many as 30 percent of alcoholics undergo a spontaneous remission or natural recovery from their problem. It's also interesting that surveys of recovered alcoholics suggest that although treatment plays some role in recovery from alcoholism, the main stimulus to changing drinking behavior comes from social pressures.

Most alcoholism treatment programs combine a variety of methods. Some may focus on behavior therapies, with an emphasis on learning techniques to deal effectively with situations and emotions that produce stress or anxiety, including the challenge to stay sober. Others may offer a variety of psychological treatment, such as individual counseling, along with group, marital, and family therapy. In some programs, pharmacological treatment with disulfiram (Antabuse) is offered, usually in combination with psychotherapy.

Organized treatment programs such as Alcoholics Anonymous are considered a part of standard treatment. It's been reported that more than 60 percent of the alcoholics who complete an AA program remain abstinent afterward. Some experts question this figure, stressing the lack of proper scientific controls and follow-up to determine just how many abstainers suffered relapses.

There are AA groups in most cities around the country. To find one near you, look in your telephone book for Alcoholics Anonymous.

Pregnancy and Alcohol. Infants exposed to alcohol before birth have a higher risk of abnormalities and birth defects. For this reason, and because it is difficult to estimate exactly how much alcohol causes problems in the developing fetus, pregnant women should avoid consuming any alcohol at all. Even if some guidelines call for avoiding only excessive amounts of alcohol during pregnancy, it's best to practice *total* abstinence.

The federal government's new rules on health-warning labels on alcoholic beverages are now in effect. The message on the labels is important and should be followed by every woman concerned about the physical and mental health of her child.

Cocaine

An estimated 2.2 million Americans—or about one out of every 100—use cocaine once a week. Once a drug that only the rich, the artistic, and the offbeat used for pleasure, cocaine has hit the nation's streets with a vengeance in a cheaper, more affordable form called crack. Crack, which comes in solid form, is smoked in a pipe. It is highly addictive and can lead to a desperate cycle of crack addiction. Cocaine can also be inhaled or taken intravenously.

Because some people have used the inhaled form of cocaine without becoming addicted, it has been rationalized that it's possible to use cocaine safely. But as the number of users has increased, so has the number of cocaine-related emergency room visits, cocaine-related deaths, and admissions to treatment programs.

A crack high begins within six to eight seconds of inhaling the smoke, but lasts for only a few minutes. The effect of cocaine sniffed into the nasal passages is apparent within two to three minutes of inhaling the powder. Cocaine that is mainlined (injected) takes effect within 15 to 30 seconds.

Once the cocaine reaches the brain, it produces about 15 to 40 minutes of exhilaration, self-confidence, alertness, and heightened perceptions and sexual performance. Following the stimulation phase of cocaine, there is a period of sadness, restlessness, and irritability. These negative feelings can lead to depression and, commonly, the desire for another hit. Used repeatedly and in higher doses, the drug can lead to hyperactivity, impaired judgment, rambling speech, agitation, irregular sleep patterns, and aggressive or violent behavior.

Snorting cocaine or smoking crack regularly causes such local physical symptoms as sinus conditions, nasal sores, and other respiratory complications. Injecting cocaine, especially using shared needles, puts its users at high risk of AIDS and hepatitis. Other serious complications that can arise from cocaine use include stroke, heart attack, seizures, and irregular heartbeats. Among the possible psychiatric effects are anxiety attacks and mania.

When cocaine is used during pregnancy, it increases the risk of premature labor, spontaneous abortion, and complications at birth for the infant. Newborns who have been exposed to cocaine may have low birthweights and an increased risk of sudden infant death syndrome. Cocaine-exposed infants experience withdrawal symptoms such as seizures and extreme irritability. A large number of these children, as they grow older, have behavioral disorders that range from mild to severe.

Cocaine abusers may seek treatment when they develop a medical problem related to drug use or when they have an adverse reaction to a high dose of cocaine. An experience of craving for the drug during withdrawal also brings some users to doctors' offices.

Treatment is effective only when the patient has the motivation to change and to follow the treatment regimen. The first step is to stop using the drug. Once abstinence is accomplished, a variety of therapies are begun. Psychotherapy, individual counseling, or group therapy is used, along with membership in self-help support groups for recovering drug addicts such as Cocaine Anonymous or Narcotics Anonymous.

Heroin

Heroin is a derivative of the psychoactive—or mind-altering—substance morphine. It is a member of the opium family of drugs. An estimated 500,000 Americans are addicted to heroin, while about 2 million people use the drug on occasion.

Heroin is taken by direct injection into the bloodstream to produce a psychological high. Because it is administered intravenously, heroin use can be a major risk factor for AIDS among those who share needles.

The high from heroin is followed by such reactions as depression, loss of appetite, loss of interest in sex, constipation, drowsiness, and constricted pupils. Heroin addicts have a higher risk of mortality from drug overdose, suicide, and violence, as well as from infectious hepatitis, bacterial endocarditis, and respiratory failure.

Infants born to heroin users often suffer drug withdrawal symptoms and may be at a high risk for long-term psychological and behavioral problems.

Marijuana

Despite studies that have shown its regular use may cause more long-term health problems than previously thought, marijuana remains a heavily used recreational drug in America.

Because marijuana contains several psychoactive ingredients, it produces a variety of effects on the thoughts, feelings, moods, and perceptions of users. This substance, derived from the plant *Cannabis sativa,* may produce relaxation or euphoria, heightened sensations, depression, or paranoia. Along with these immediate reactions come some short-term side effects, notably reduced attention span and difficulty concentrating, apathy, and lethargy. Delayed reaction time in occasional users should preclude driving, as with alcohol.

The main active ingredient in marijuana is tetrahydrocannabinol, or

THC. After THC is inhaled from a marijuana cigarette, it enters the bloodstream, then the brain, fatty tissues, and reproductive organs. Chronic use of THC does reduce the production and motility of sperm, but this limited observation has not been related to decreased fertility. Chronic pot smokers may also be doing as much, if not more, harm to their lungs than tobacco smokers.

THC appears to linger in the body's fatty tissues. Habitual users of marijuana may develop a permanent accumulation of this substance, although the long-term effects of this remain unknown.

It is thought that when pot began its rise to popularity in the 1960s, it had a lower THC content. Today's marijuana bought on the street is apparently much more potent, possibly because growers have managed to produce a more powerful plant.

Marijuana long has been viewed as nonaddicting, but it's now recognized that users can develop a psychological dependence on the drug. Marijuana also remains in the body for a long period of time, so it can show up on drug tests weeks after ingestion.

Getting Help

If you have health insurance, you may find that your policy places a cap on mental health coverage. As health care enters the era of managed care and utilization review, the current trend among insurers is toward outpatient treatment and short-term therapy rather than traditional long-term treatment. This may not be bad if your problem is mild to moderate and doesn't require hospitalization.

A 1989 status report on the health care industry's impact on psychiatry by the American Psychiatric Association notes that many employers have redesigned aspects of their employee benefits. One such approach requires the employee who uses mental health services to pay a larger share of the costs. Another is to offer less coverage for high-cost inpatient treatment while increasing coverage for outpatient care.

Even if you don't have insurance, help is available through community mental health centers or clinics, family service agencies, and through some residency programs affiliated with large hospitals or medical schools.

There are many types of qualified therapists available. Your family doctor may be able to make a referral. If you have friends who recently underwent therapy, they may be able to recommend a qualified mental health professional. Otherwise, you can call the local branch of the American Psychiatric Association and ask for a list of board-certified psychiatrists in your area. Referrals are also available from such professional organizations as the American Psychological Association, the Association of Certified Social Workers, the American Association for Marriage and

Family Therapy, and the American Association of Pastoral Counselors.

If you live in a town with a medical school or teaching hospital, call and ask for the department of psychiatry or the department of social services and speak to someone who can make a referral. Many hospitals now have separate referral services that furnish the names of qualified specialists. Or you can call the regional office of various self-help groups near you for the name of an appropriate community or voluntary organization.

Therapy

Long before the development of chemical agents for the management of such disorders as depression, mania, and schizophrenia, all you could do was talk about your feelings, thoughts, and behavior. This time-honored approach remains the treatment of choice in many cases.

Psychotherapy, also called "talking therapy," is designed to make you feel better through support, understanding, and gaining a sense of direction or purpose. The goal of treatment is to share your experiences with the therapist in order to better understand your emotions and behavior and to come up with strategies to help make your life work better.

There are many different types of psychotherapy:

• *Psychoanalysis* is an intensive form of psychotherapy that stresses unconscious and unresolved conflicts from childhood. This long-term therapy uses a technique called *free association* in which you say whatever comes to mind while the analyst interprets these associations in order to give you insights into your behavior. Psychoanalysis requires frequent office visits and can be expensive.

• *Psychodynamic psychotherapy* is based on psychoanalytic techniques. Recently, there has been a shift in favor of the short form of psychodynamic therapy. Instead of the patient doing all of the talking, this kind of therapy encourages greater interaction between you and the therapist. On the average, short-term therapy requires 12 to 25 once-a-week visits. Because the therapy is goal-oriented in its approach, the intent is to come up with a more immediate solution to a single problem.

• *Cognitive therapy,* another form of short-term treatment, is designed to correct any negative thinking patterns that you may have about yourself. Your self-image and the way you see yourself are the raw materials you work with in cognitive therapy. Role playing, keeping a daily log of your thoughts, and homework assignments are used.

• *Behavioral therapy* is based on the principle of earning a reward for choosing a positive behavior over a negative behavior. For instance, eating to allay anxiety is a negative behavior if you're overweight and it makes you feel guilty and causes your self-esteem to slide. Behavioral therapy aims to dispel such negative thinking by retraining you to think about the positive instead.

• *Marriage and family therapy* is used to resolve conflicts within the family setting. This type of short-term counseling addresses problems relating to marriage, divorce, child rearing, sexuality, and child, spouse, or elder abuse. The underlying principle of this therapy is to find reasonable alternatives and solutions to problems as well as to learn ways to prevent recurrences of the conflict in the future. In some cases, the solution may simply be understanding that people have different personality styles and learning to make slight adjustments in your attitude and behavior.

Specialists

Several kinds of professionals, with different types of training, experience, and qualifications, can provide treatment and counseling for a wide range of mental and emotional needs.

All of the mental health practitioners listed here are considered psychotherapists. Because psychotherapy is not an area regulated by law, people with little or no training, or those who use questionable practices, can call themselves "therapists." Always ask about a professional's training, credentials, and areas of specialization so you can be sure that the psychotherapist you choose is legitimate.

Psychiatrists.   A psychiatrist is a physician, complete with a medical degree, and is the only mental health professional who can prescribe drugs. Most psychiatrists are board-certified by the American Board of Psychiatry and Neurology. All of them should bear a current license from the state in which their practice is located. Because of their medical and specialty training, psychiatrists can evaluate and diagnose the entire range of mental disorders. A psychiatrist is more likely to detect the physical signs that may be present as part of a psychological problem. Some psychiatrists, although medically qualified, may not specialize in the talk therapies. When this is the case, they will refer you to an appropriate and qualified therapist.

Psychoanalysts.   Psychoanalysts are psychiatrists or psychologists who have undergone the long-term therapy of psychoanalysis themselves and have devoted additional years of study to this area.

Psychologists.   Psychologists have academic doctoral degrees in several specialty areas relating to human behavior. While some strictly conduct research, others—known as clinical psychologists—undertake additional training so that they can treat patients. In most states, a psychologist in private or group practice must have successfully completed a Ph.D. program and passed an examination to earn a professional license. Many clinical psychologists perform psychotherapy.

Social workers. A psychiatric social worker has a master's degree in social work with some training in psychotherapy and usually continuing postgraduate education in psychotherapy. Because social workers are trained to help people deal with getting agency or governmental help for personal or family problems, they may take on only cases that call for short-term treatment. Social workers are highly skilled at steering their clients in the right direction—whether to a self-help group or to another therapist who can provide the appropriate therapy for a specific problem. Psychiatric social workers are certified by the states in which they practice.

Counselors. Clinical mental health counselors have master's degrees and must undergo a period of supervised training before treating patients. Some go on for further postgraduate studies, additional clinical training, and take an examination to qualify as a certified clinical mental health counselor. Some counselors limit their practice to guidance or vocational services, but today a greater number are qualified to do psychotherapy.

Marriage counselors and family therapists. Mental health professionals from a range of disciplines call themselves marriage counselors and family therapists. Among these are psychiatrists, psychologists, psychiatric social workers, and mental health counselors. They are either Ph.D.s or master's-prepared. Many marital and family therapists are members of the American Association for Marriage and Family Therapy, which requires specialized study and supervised clinical experience to gain membership.

Pastoral counselors. Pastoral counselors are ministers, priests, or rabbis who hold bachelor's or master's degrees in divinity and have usually taken additional training in counseling. Some pastoral counselors have pursued a master's- or doctoral-level curriculum in mental health and have qualified for certification by the American Association of Pastoral Counselors.

Psychiatric nurses. Registered nurses who have advanced academic degrees and specialized training with an emphasis on mental health are called psychiatric nurse-practitioners. This type of nurse-practitioner is often trained to do psychotherapy in a group practice, hospital, or clinic. A psychiatric nurse-practitioner should not be confused with a psychiatric nurse, who is a registered nurse who cares for mental health patients in hospitals.

6

Growing Older

Richard S. Rivlin, M.D.

After years of studying large groups of otherwise healthy people over 65, gerontologists report that the outlook for keeping your body and your mind healthy into old age is better than ever. Medical investigators still can't explain the mechanisms of the aging process, or why each one of us ages differently. But clues to successful aging are emerging.

We do know that the ability to age well involves the mind and spirit as well as the body. The genes you inherit are important, as is your life-style, attitude, environment, socioeconomic status, and sheer luck. Equally important is the feeling of being in control of your life. Having a social network—supportive spouse, family, friends, or neighbors—is also beneficial to your health.

Learning how to age successfully, then, is an acquired skill. It's a skill that we all have to acquire fairly early in life, too. Many good health habits begin in early adulthood, to be carried on right through our mature years. Let's take a look at what we can do to help prevent many diseases and premature aging before they occur.

Causes of Aging

Life expectancy has been on the upswing in America since the turn of the century. These gains are due to improvements in health care, nutrition, childhood immunization, housing, sanitation, and expanded social service programs.

Based on overall life expectancy figures, the U.S. Census Bureau projects that the over-65 population will total 39 million by the year 2010 and 66 million by 2030. There are gender differences: women have a greater life expectancy than men—with an advantage of more than seven years.

The maximum human life span appears to be about 110 years. Scientists do not know why each species has a set life span, nor do doctors know what causes the human body to age, but it's becoming clear that aging is a "mixture of multiple causes," according to one biologist. Several theories have been proposed that shed some light on the aging process.

Cellular theory. Your cells, apparently, can divide a limited number of times before they either stop making copies of themselves or start making imperfect copies that can result in cancer-causing mutations. Also, the older a cell population grows, the more frequently the DNA (hereditary material of a cell) makes mistakes that it cannot repair.

Genetic theory. You have a built-in genetic program that activates certain cells on a predetermined schedule. Based on this theory, your internal clock knows when it's time for growth (such as during youth and adolescence), when it's time for cells to be replaced at their normal rate, and when to slow down.

Since each person has a different genetic makeup, this theory may help to explain why certain physical changes associated with aging occur at a different rate in each person. Each family, then, has its own aging pattern and its own genetic susceptibility to certain diseases. Many questions still surround the role of your genes in normal aging, as well as how heredity figures in certain diseases that have a genetic component, such as Alzheimer's disease.

Free-radical theory. Under certain conditions, unstable molecules of oxygen in the cells can create potentially harmful waste products, called free radicals, which are formed as a byproduct of oxygen metabolism. One of these waste products that may accumulate in your tissues is a material called lipofuscin, which consists of pigment and chemicals from the cells. Lipofuscin is found mainly in the brain, and it is not certain whether its presence is dangerous or not.

Hormonal theory. Hormones control and influence many of your body's activities as well as your emotions, thought processes, and appearance. Your hormones direct your growth, development, and, possibly, aging.

In women, for instance, the hormone estrogen seems to offer protection against heart disease during the years before menopause. When the time is right, hormones deliver the message to tell the body to halt the menstrual cycle. This hormonal event, or menopause, results in low-ered estrogen levels that are associated with osteoporosis and an increased risk of cardiovascular disease in some women.

Immune system theory. Your immune system is strongest during youth and young adulthood. As you grow older, it takes longer to respond to infectious agents. With advancing age, the immune system may even begin to attack the body's own normal tissue as it does in rheumatoid arthritis or systemic lupus erythematosus, a disease of the connective tissue.

All of the above theories sound plausible, and have some scientific evidence to back them up. But a definitive theory of aging has yet to be found.

Aging begins at conception and continues all your life. Growing older eventually may bring some distressing physical changes, although aging is not synonymous with illness or disease. True, each organ system grad-ually slows down as you grow older. In some systems, such as the kidneys, the body naturally loses cells, while in other areas, your reaction time decreases, and you may not be able to adapt quite as quickly to demands for more power, speed, or stamina.

Some of these factors are beyond your control. For instance, your genes strongly determine when you'll get your first wrinkle and whether you'll become bald. But there are other important factors of aging over which you do have some influence. For example, constant exposure to sunlight results in aged-looking skin. Excessive noise can cause early hearing loss. Smoking, lack of exercise, and excessive alcohol intake can all contribute to premature aging.

Too, there's a tendency to blame aging for many chronic health problems when much of the fault really lies with faulty living habits. If we examine certain aspects of aging, it's possible to see that lack of awareness and careless living sow the seeds of many future illnesses.

Aging and the Skin

Your skin is a subtle recorder of time. It is at this superficial level that you first notice the most visible signs of aging. The skin's outer layer, or *epidermis,* is constructed of orderly, organized rows of cells in youth and young adulthood. The two layers of your skin and the subcutaneous layer of fatty tissue below house several structures and tiny organs, including blood vessels, hair follicles, sweat glands, oil-producing glands, and the proteins collagen and elastin.

With aging, these tissues undergo a change in the way they work and in the architecture of their cellular structure. For instance, as elastic fibers in the second layer of skin, or *dermis,* break down, they become brittle and can't snap back into place as readily. The result is saggy skin. A decrease in collagen, a protein that gives the skin and connective tissue its strength and firmness, reduces the skin's youthful flexibility.

Several other factors may influence the way your skin ages. People who get regular vigorous *exercise* seem to have more vibrant-looking skin than their sedentary counterparts. Exercise stimulates the skin, the underlying connective tissue, the blood vessels that nourish the skin, and the muscles below. The result often is tighter, healthier skin.

Proper *cleansing* improves the ability of oxygen to reach your pores. Regular use of a *moisturizer* can also help prevent your skin from becoming dry by keeping the skin's own moisture from evaporating. It's best to apply a moisturizer when your skin is still damp after cleansing your face, or after bathing.

Stop smoking. Smoking contributes to premature aging because it constricts the blood vessels and decreases the flow of oxygen to the skin. Heavy smokers may have significant premature wrinkling.

Exposure to the sun is the leading cause of premature aging of the skin. Although sunlight is a good source of vitamin D, dermatologists who study its cumulative effects call it a "notorious enemy" of good skin. Excessive exposure to sunlight can result in skin cancer, benign growths, blotching, uneven pigmentation, as well as coarse, yellowed, saggy, and deeply wrinkled skin. None of these sunshine-induced skin problems stems from the aging process itself. Fair-skinned people especially are susceptible to sun-induced damage. The darker your skin, the greater the supply of a pigment called melanin, which protects you against the sun's harmful ultraviolet rays.

The Sun and Your Skin

Preventing sun damage is your first line of defense in maintaining a healthy skin. The hidden danger in sunlight is the ultraviolet light that is invisible to the naked eye. Exposure to the short, high-energy rays of light called ultraviolet B (UVB) causes sunburn.

An isolated, accidental episode of sunburn is uncomfortable, but usually isn't harmful over the long term. The danger and the damage come from regular overexposure to sunlight over a period of years. Degenerative changes in the skin occur because the energy from the light triggers a reaction inside your cells that gradually breaks down chemical bonds and disorganizes the otherwise orderly rows of cells. Wrinkling, dryness, irregular pigmentation, and, increasingly, benign and malignant skin growths are the price of prolonged exposure to sunlight.

Severe sunburn is especially dangerous for young people. Children and adolescents who suffer several episodes of severe sunburn with blistering have a greater risk of developing the most deadly form of skin cancer, malignant melanoma, as adults. The incidence of this once-rare skin cancer now is on the rise.

Although in the past suntanned skin was widely perceived as a sign of health and vigor, this view is slowly changing for two reasons: an increasing awareness of the growing danger of skin cancer and a realization that protecting your skin from too much sun is a better long-term investment in skin care than is a tan.

There are several ways to protect your skin from cumulative sun damage. If you must spend time outdoors, avoid the midday sun—from 11:00 A.M. to 3:00 P.M.—when sunlight is strongest and most damaging to the skin.

Protect yourself against the sun's rays. Wear a hat, clothing with long sleeves, and long pants that fully cover your legs. Most important, apply a high-strength sunscreen to your skin *before* you venture out into the sun. A chemical in most sunscreens popularly known as PABA (para-aminobenzoic acid) is highly effective in screening out the sunburn, or ultraviolet B, rays. If you have a skin reaction to PABA, other preparations are available. Benzophenone compounds, which absorb both the sunburn and suntan rays, offer good protection. A sunscreen that contains cinnamate as an active ingredient may also be used in place of PABA.

Commercial sunscreens come with an *SPF,* or *sun protection factor,* a rating that ranges from a low of 2 to the high 30s. The SPF number approximates the time you can stay in the sun before your skin begins to burn. For instance, if you have very fair skin that burns easily and you use a sunscreen with an SPF of 15, you can tolerate 15 times more sun. In most sunny settings within the continental United States, a sunscreen with an SPF of 15 offers ample protection.

Regardless of your type of skin—fair, medium, or dark—it's essential to protect yourself. A sunscreen is most effective when applied to your skin 45 minutes to an hour before you go outdoors. If you go into the water or perspire heavily, it's prudent to reapply the sunscreen—even if the label says the product is waterproof.

Retin-A

In January 1988, dermatologists reported in *The Journal of the American Medical Association* that they were able to reverse some of the effects of sun-damaged skin by applying *tretinoin,* popularly known as *Retin-A.* This vitamin-A derivative, which has long been used in the treatment of acne, reduced the number of fine lines in most members of the group being studied. Other benefits included the fading of so-called age spots, or brown spots, and improved blood flow to the skin.

Researchers don't know exactly how Retin-A works against sun-damaged skin. The medication appears to make the skin look smoother, but it's not certain what kind of changes Retin-A produces in skin cells. Retin-A's long-term effects also remain unknown.

Adults who want to use Retin-A for its supposed antiaging effects must realize that the drug apparently is effective only with continuous use. Once you stop using it, the beneficial results disappear and the wrinkles may return.

Most people who use Retin-A experience such short-term side effects as skin inflammation and irritation. Because this preparation makes the skin highly sensitive to sunlight, anyone using Retin-A must wear a sunscreen when going outdoors.

Although the Food and Drug Administration has approved the use of Retin-A only for the treatment of acne, dermatologists can prescribe tretinoin for prematurely wrinkled skin. If you decide to try Retin-A, make sure you use it only under the supervision of a dermatologist.

Retin-A is a lower-dose formulation of the oral medication isotretinoin (Accutane), which was found to cause birth defects when taken during pregnancy. If you are pregnant, avoid using Retin-A.

The Hair

Graying of the hair is nothing more than a gradual slowdown in the pigment-producing cells in each hair follicle. The rate of change varies from person to person—you may notice your first gray hair as early as 20 or as late as your mid-80s. Heredity and hormones strongly influence baldness, thinning, and graying of the hair.

Both men and women experience *hair loss*. Men may notice some thinning beginning around age 30. Women generally don't experience hair loss until after menopause, when this hormonal shift leaves them with dwindling levels of estrogen. Recent childbirth, infection, certain medications, chemotherapy, and anemia may also produce temporary hair loss. Once the problem is resolved, normal hair growth usually resumes within a few months.

It's normal to lose up to 75 hairs a day as part of the hair replacement cycle. When baldness occurs, some hair follicles stop working and lost hairs are not replaced. Others may continue production, but instead of producing normal strands of hair yield a fine, nearly invisible hair called *vellus.*

Minoxidil

In 1988, the Food and Drug Administration approved the use of the prescription drug *minoxidil* (Rogaine) for the treatment of male pattern baldness. Before its approval as a hair restorer, minoxidil was used to treat high blood pressure, and the discovery of the drug's ability to grow hair was accidental. A large number of people using the medication for hypertension reported that they experienced new hair growth. Scientists reformulated the hypertension medication into a topical solution and found that twice-a-day applications to the scalp produced hair growth in some users after three or four months of use.

Minoxidil produces sparse hair growth on the top of the head, but not around the temples. After using the topical medication for eight months to a year, new hair growth tapers off. The catch is that you have to continue applying minoxidil in order to maintain the new growth. If you stop the applications, the new hair will fall out in three or four months.

Even so, the substance doesn't work in everyone. Those under 30, those who have been losing hair for less than five years, and those who have been balding only at the crown experience the best results. Those with receding hairlines seem to get no benefit from minoxidil. Studies are being conducted to determine whether it is effective in women.

When taken orally for hypertension, minoxidil can produce serious side effects in some people. When minoxidil solution is applied topically, your scalp and bloodstream absorb very little of the drug and it is considered safe for external use. The most common side effect of minoxidil is itching, which may result from its ingredients or may point to an allergic reaction to the substance. Researchers have not yet determined whether topical minoxidil has an adverse effect on users with cardiovascular problems. The long-term side effects of minoxidil aren't known yet.

Since new hair growth plateaus after you use minoxidil for about a year, the long-term benefit may be questionable for some users. A few studies have shown that some of the newly grown hair falls out after one year despite continuous use of minoxidil. These considerations, along with a cost of $50 to $85 for a one-month supply, lead to the conclusion that minoxidil may not be the ideal solution for every bald spot.

Although minoxidil may not produce the results most balding men would like to have, and may produce no permanent results at all in some users, it is the only product approved by the FDA for stimulating hair growth on the head. In 1989, the FDA banned the sale of nonprescription lotions and creams that claimed to grow hair or prevent baldness. The

FDA also noted that there is no evidence that products taken orally, such as vitamins or food supplements, can prevent or cure baldness.

Hair Transplants

Hair transplants are a popular although expensive way to fight baldness. You need a qualified, skilled surgeon to extract small sections of your scalp hair from the back and sides of your head and implant them into balding areas. Because only a limited number of hair sections can be transplanted at a time, it may take a year or two to complete a hair transplant.

The procedure is painful and carries the risk of infection, scarring, and postoperative bleeding. In addition, the cost for a series of hair transplant procedures over a period of a year or two can easily reach as high as $15,000. Although serious medical complications from hair transplants are relatively rare, dissatisfaction over the cosmetic results is more common. If you are considering a hair transplant, do some research first. Ask your doctor or a dermatologist for a referral to a reputable surgeon who is qualified to perform this kind of surgery. When you meet with the surgeon, ask to see "before-and-after" photographs of other patients' hair transplants, and inquire about the cost, efficacy, and safety of the procedure.

Our Changing Senses

Sight, hearing, taste, touch, and smell are acute when we are young. As we grow older, changes occur. When we strain our eyes to focus, move closer to hear a conversation, or find that we're adding extra flavorings or spices because our food seems to have lost its zing, we're adapting to subtle changes in our senses. The trick is to distinguish between the inevitable flattening of perception that normally occurs over years and those changes that signify illness, disease, or environmental injury.

Vision

Visual changes are fairly common by the time most people reach 40. It's fairly typical to notice a difference in the way your eyes focus when you're reading or doing close work. If you find that you're stretching your reading material in front of you or that you can't see clearly at a distance, you may have one of the two most common age-associated conditions to occur in the eyes.

Farsightedness, or *presbyopia*, commonly begins around age 40. The lens in the eye loses some elasticity and can't respond as well to changes in light patterns entering the eye when you shift your focus from far to near. In order to focus your eyes while reading, you may notice that you're holding the printed page farther away. Eyestrain is a common symptom of presbyopia. To correct this condition, your ophthalmologist will prescribe reading glasses.

Nearsightedness, or *myopia,* is an error of refraction that causes incoming rays of light to focus in front of the retina and produce a blurry image. (Incoming light should fall precisely on the retina. In presbyopia, the incoming light focuses behind the retina.) In myopia, it is distant objects that are unclear and difficult to focus. Prescription eyeglasses or contact lenses can correct myopia.

Your visual acuity remains fairly constant through your young adult years. But sometime between the ages of 40 and 50, you may notice a slight decline in your ability to see fine details. The pupil, a small opening that regulates the amount of light entering the eye, decreases in size. As a result, less light is available to stimulate the rod and cone cells of the retina in the back of the eyeball. These cells are responsible for perceiving light and color and sending this information to the brain via the optic nerve. When light levels are low, the loss of acuity makes it somewhat more difficult to see as sharply as before.

The 40s are a time to begin a program of routine vision checkups. Aside from catching any age-associated visual changes that may require eyeglasses, serious eye problems may begin quietly during mid-adulthood. Glaucoma, cataracts, macular degeneration, and diabetic retinopathy are the most common disorders that can rob you of your eyesight. These problems aren't as easily corrected as farsightedness or nearsightedness. But with regular checkups and good eye care, it may be possible to prevent or manage these serious eye problems. Although there is no consensus on how frequently vision screening should be performed in adults without symptoms, it is a good idea to get a visual acuity test at least every two to five years once you reach 40, and every two years after age 60.

Glaucoma. *Glaucoma,* a buildup of fluid pressure in the eye, follows an especially insidious course. In *chronic glaucoma,* there are no symptoms until irreversible damage has occurred. *Acute glaucoma* is characterized by sudden pain in the eyes, blurred vision, the appearance of haloes around lights, and headaches. Without immediate treatment of acute glaucoma, you risk permanent loss of vision.

Because glaucoma presents no signs or symptoms in its early stages, the only course of prevention is early diagnosis and treatment. If you have a family history of glaucoma, your risk of developing the disease may be higher. Blacks may face a much higher chance of suffering glaucoma, according to a study conducted by the Johns Hopkins School of Medicine. That the black population in the United States as well as in other countries has much higher rates of glaucoma than Caucasians supports the theory that genetic factors play a role.

To diagnose glaucoma, an ophthalmologist uses a device called a *tonometer* to measure the pressure in your eye. If the pressure is high and the doctor suspects glaucoma, another test, called *gonioscopy,* may be necessary to inspect the drainage system inside the eye chamber.

When glaucoma is detected in its early stages, your ophthalmologist will prescribe medicated eyedrops to control the condition before the increased pressure does damage. Two commonly prescribed drugs are pilocarpine (Pilocar) and epinephrine (Adrenalin), which reduce the internal pressure in the eye. Beta-blocker eyedrops may also be prescribed to reduce the production of fluid. When drug therapy doesn't produce results, laser surgery may be recommended to widen drainage passageways and relieve the internal pressure that way. Early drug or laser therapy can help prevent blindness from glaucoma.

If you are over 65, it is recommended that you seek periodic testing for glaucoma from an eye specialist every one to three years. Many primary care physicians have neither the training nor the equipment to test for acute glaucoma. Consult an eye specialist for acute glaucoma screening.

Cataracts. As you grow older, your eye's lens—a crystal-clear capsule at birth—may cloud up, at times to the point that it becomes opaque. As this process goes forward, you develop the progressively hazy vision that characterizes a *cataract.*

Although cataracts have long been considered an inevitable part of aging, it is possible to reduce the risk of cataract formation. Many cases of cataracts are hereditary, and others are a result of trauma to the eye, disease (especially diabetes), or a reaction to certain drugs. But there is some evidence now that people whose work brings them into contact with high levels of X-ray and microwave radiation may be at higher risk, though there is no current evidence that the level and type of radiation emitted from video display terminals produces cataracts. A study at Johns Hopkins University has also linked cigarette smoking with the formation of cataracts.

Excessive exposure to the ultraviolet light in sunshine has long been associated with cataracts. A study of Chesapeake Bay area residents whose work on the water involves constant exposure to sunlight seems to confirm this. The main culprit is the shorter-wavelength ultraviolet B radiation—the same kind of light that produces sunburn and can lead to skin cancer.

Because cataracts form slowly over a period of years, it's prudent to begin protecting your eyes from sunlight as early as possible. Wearing a hat with a brim that shades the eyes helps cut the exposure to ultraviolet light. Wearing sunglasses also protects your eyes.

The main symptom of a cataract is blurred or double vision and a sensitivity to glare. Surgery is the only treatment. During the surgical procedure, an eye surgeon removes your clouded lens. Eyeglasses, contact lenses, or an intraocular lens implant will then have to take over the job your surgically removed lens used to do. Intraocular lens implants (IOLs) are used in many elderly patients with great success. Despite the promising results of IOLs so far, we don't know how well these lenses will endure over long-term use.

Sunglasses

Not every pair of sunglasses offers the kind of ultraviolet radiation protection you need. A labeling system developed by the American Standards Institute offers consumers information on three categories of protective lenses. When buying nonprescription sunglasses, try to choose glasses that tell you the category of the lenses under this system.

- Cosmetic sunglasses are recommended for use around town. These lenses block at least 70 percent of UVB rays, 20 percent of UVA light, and 60 percent of visible light.
- General-purpose sunglasses are recommended for outdoor activities such as driving, boating, hiking, and flying. They cut out 95 percent of UVB radiation, about 60 percent of UVA sunlight, and 60 to 92 percent of visible light, depending on the darkness of the lens.
- Special-purpose sunglasses are recommended for use in bright sunshine, such as on beaches and ski slopes. These glasses block approximately 99 percent of UVB, 60 percent of UVA, and 97 percent of visible light.

Macular degeneration. A leading cause of vision loss in people over 50 is *macular degeneration*. For unknown reasons, the macula—or central part of the retina that is responsible for producing sharp central vision—loses cells. As this happens, you gradually lose your ability to see fine details, until you are left with a permanent blind spot in the center of your visual field. The disorder doesn't affect your side vision.

Macular degeneration has subtle symptoms that may vary from person to person. Straight lines tend to look wavy and distorted, words may look blurred, or you may notice an empty spot in the center of vision. Women tend to develop macular degeneration more often than men. If anyone in your family has macular degeneration, you may have a higher risk of developing the condition.

There are two forms of macular degeneration, but no cure for either one. In the more common type, the tissues of the macula thin out and there is no way to stop the deterioration. The other form of the disease involves the blood vessels behind the retina. If the problem is detected early, laser therapy may be effective in halting the destruction of this tiny part of the retina.

When laser treatment isn't possible, low-vision aids such as magnifying glasses, large-type books and newspapers, and other devices may be helpful.

The National Society to Prevent Blindness recommends that you regularly take a self-test for macular degeneration. Select an object with a straight line, such as a door frame or a few lines of type on a page. Cover one eye and see if the line is still straight, then repeat the test with the other eye. If the line appears bent, or you notice a blank spot, see an ophthalmologist.

Diabetic retinopathy.   One possible complication of diabetes is *diabetic retinopathy*—a condition that can cause loss of eyesight. Diabetes can weaken the blood vessels in the retina, causing them to break open and leak. After these vessels hemorrhage, scar tissue forms on the retina and some vision is lost.

You may notice a slight, gradual blurring of vision; this is an early warning sign of one form of diabetic retinopathy. The second form produces cloudy vision or a complete loss of sight. In some cases, there is the danger of a detached retina.

With early diagnosis and treatment, it is possible to stop the damage from leaking blood vessels. Laser therapy is effective in sealing these leaks, and in some cases a surgical procedure called a vitrectomy may be necessary.

The best way to prevent diabetic retinopathy is to control your diabetes. If you have diabetes, part of your regular care should be an annual examination by an ophthalmologist. If you have any signs of the disease, immediate treatment and careful monitoring can prevent loss of vision.

Detached retina.   Although a *detached retina* isn't a common condition, it occurs often enough in middle-aged and older adults. If you develop a detached retina and ignore it, you run the risk of impaired or lost vision.

Retinal detachment usually results from an injury to the eye, a blow to the head, or as an aftereffect of cataract surgery. It begins with a small tear in the retina, which allows fluid to seep into the area. The fluid pulls down on the retina until it falls down, like a curtain.

Symptoms include flashes of light, floating dark spots, and a partial loss of peripheral vision that appears like a dark shadow blocking the view from the side, top, or bottom of the affected eye. With immediate treatment, you have a better chance of retaining your vision.

Hearing

More than 8.8 percent of the American population has some form of hearing loss, according to the National Center for Health Statistics. Hearing loss may be hereditary in some families, or be the result of injury, infection, or occupational exposure. But increasingly, environmental noise is responsible for a growing incidence of hearing loss. Prolonged exposure to loud machines, motors, rock music, and a variety of modern environmental sounds takes its toll on your ability to hear.

For sound waves from the world outside to have any meaning for you, they must pass successfully through three compartments—the outer ear, the middle ear, and the inner ear—to your brain. The outer ear picks up sound waves and sends them through the auditory canal that leads to the eardrum. As the sound waves strike the membrane of the eardrum, the vibration sets off an amplification process within three tiny bones inside your middle ear. From there, the pulsating sound waves are transmitted to your inner ear, where about 30,000 highly sensitive hair cells convert the sound into nerve impulses for transmission to your brain.

If the sound is loud and persistent, it can cause irreversible damage to the hair cells. The level of noise, measured in units of energy called decibels, is rising in the environment and so is the incidence of hearing impairment in early and middle adulthood.

Hearing loss.   There are three different types of *hearing loss,* but most is directly related to the gradual erosion and deterioration of the hair cells.

Conductive hearing loss occurs when sound waves can't travel from the outside to the inner ear, usually because ear wax or an infection blocks the way (see Chapter 7). If infection is present, medication can be prescribed. In some cases, hearing loss may be due to otosclerosis (see Chapter 7). Surgery is often successful in correcting this condition.

Presbycusis, or age-related hearing loss, is common. The first signs of this form of nerve deafness may appear as early as the 30s, although they may not be noticeable for several years. In presbycusis, your ability to hear high-frequency sounds declines and it becomes difficult to distinguish certain sounds used in speech. There is no cure for presbycusis, but hearing can be improved by wearing a hearing aid.

People who find it hard to hear often resist seeking treatment. If you have trouble hearing, do not assume it is part of the aging process. Many types of hearing loss can be treated, and others can be corrected through the use of hearing aids.

The symptoms of hearing loss include difficulty distinguishing words, the perception that others mumble and slur their speech, an inability to hear a faucet dripping or musical high notes, and constant background noise in your ears.

If you notice any changes, consult a physician whose medical specialty is the ear (an otologist) or the ear, nose, and throat (an otolaryngologist). If necessary, the physician may refer you to an audiologist for more detailed hearing tests. The test results may be helpful in deciding whether you would benefit from a hearing aid and which type would be best for your particular needs.

Find an audiologist who is up-to-date. Many people with hearing loss are discouraged because they remember the lack of success their parents may have had with old-fashioned hearing aids, most of which were simple amplifiers that made every sound louder. The result was that turning them up to hear conversation better caused such a din that distinguishing what was being said was often more difficult with the aid than without it. Some newer equipment uses tiny computers that identify for amplification only those frequencies in which you have lost hearing. Others match received sounds to a voice imprint, and amplify only those sound patterns it recognizes as speech.

Another problem in finding the proper aid has to do with vanity. Though people are no longer embarrassed to wear eyeglasses, they want their hearing aids to be as tiny and inconspicuous as possible. This caused the industry to make the aids smaller and smaller, instead of making them better and better. If it turns out that your problem can best be corrected by a behind-the-ear model, or even by one with a shirt pocket control, make sure the cosmetic factors remain secondary to the functional factors.

The Gums and Teeth

Losing teeth is not a natural part of aging. The full set of 32 teeth that you develop by age 20 is designed to last a lifetime. Although dentures and dental implants are available for people who lose their teeth, the most practical way to keep your own teeth is to practice prevention.

Good dental care is relatively simple but requires diligence. It calls for brushing your teeth after eating meals and snacks and flossing at least once a day. Drinking fluoridated water helps protect the teeth from decay, as do certain fluoride mouth rinses and toothpastes. Eating a healthy diet helps strengthen the teeth. Finally, making regular visits to your dentist for a cleaning and checkup should be part of your program to fight tooth loss.

Your teeth are essential to the health of your oral environment, to the enjoyment of food, and to the joy of a smile. Good teeth solidly ensconced in healthy gums allow you to chew your food properly as the first step of digestion. Chewing helps to exercise your jawbone and also stimulates the production of saliva, which has a natural ability to cleanse the mouth.

When you eat sugary foods without cleaning your teeth afterward, the bacteria in your mouth soon begin to produce an acid that attacks the tooth enamel. This acid saps calcium and phosphate from the teeth and the process of tooth decay begins. Both children and adults tend to have healthier teeth when fluoride is used to fight tooth decay.

Plaque and periodontal disease. *Plaque* is an invisible bacterial film that forms constantly on your teeth, even during sleep. If you don't remove plaque from just below the gumline and in between the teeth at least once every 24 hours, it calcifies into a hard substance called tartar, or dental calculus.

The plaque you allow to accumulate attracts more plaque. Worse, it pushes the gum margin (gingiva) away from the tooth and allows bacteria to collect and thrive, until the area becomes inflamed. When this occurs, you have *gingivitis*. As bacteria and debris build up, they release toxic substances that work their way down the side of the tooth to the underlying bone. Eventually, the bone erodes, and the teeth become loose and may even fall out.

About 80 percent of American adults have some form of periodontal disease, according to the National Institute of Dental Research of the National Institutes of Health. Gum disease is so prevalent that it has replaced tooth decay as the top cause of tooth loss. Because it does its damage insidiously, you may not suspect that anything is wrong until your teeth feel loose in their sockets.

Although plaque is the main cause of gum disease, other factors may have a role. These include malocclusion, better known as a "bad bite"; clenching or grinding the teeth; poorly fitting crowns or leaky fillings; tobacco; medical conditions such as diabetes and blood disorders; pregnancy; lack of fluoride; and diet.

Treating gum disease. Treatment of gum disease varies with the severity of the problem. Your dentist may recommend a professional cleaning treatment known as *deep scaling* to scrape away dental calculus and any deep pockets of infection. Deep scaling combined with *root planing*, which removes diseased gum tissue adjacent to the tooth, encourages the growth of healthy gum tissue. Scaling, along with a judicious program of brushing and flossing at home, is effective in many cases. If infection is too deep or widespread, surgery may be recommended.

Treating advanced periodontal disease can be a long and costly ordeal. Prevention is a simpler and cheaper route:

- Brush and floss daily.
- Use disclosing tablets or solutions as recommended to pinpoint

areas of heavy plaque that may require more thorough cleaning.
- Visit your dentist at least twice a year for a professional cleaning. If you tend to build excess plaque or are occasionally neglectful, more frequent professional cleanings may be in order.
- Improve your brushing techniques. An ideal time for a refresher is during your twice-yearly cleanings. The type of bristles, the way you hold the brush, the motion and pressure of the brush, and the length of the cleaning all make a difference in whether you're doing a good job. Ask your dentist or hygienist if you're using the right methods. Surprisingly, many adults still don't know how to brush their teeth.

Enamel. Although the enamel on your teeth is the hardest substance in the body, even the healthiest teeth lose a small amount of enamel during each decade of adulthood. Your teeth also tend to discolor. Certain foods—especially coffee, tea, and red wine—react with plaque to stain the teeth. Smoking also causes the teeth to turn yellow.

As you grow older, a substance directly below the enamel, called dentin, may become translucent and make your teeth look a little darker. Beneath the dentin is the dental pulp, where nerves and blood vessels are located. Beginning in your 20s, the pulp slowly begins to lose cells, blood supply, and sensitivity. Eventually, the reduced blood flow to the area leaves an older tooth more susceptible to infection.

If infection occurs, and your dentist says extraction is the only solution, you may need to find another dentist for a second opinion. Review your options carefully.

A tooth endangered by infected pulp can be saved. Dentists trained in endodontics remove the diseased soft tissue, nerves, and blood vessels, sterilize the pulp chamber and root canal, and fill the passage with a material that prevents further infection. When root-canal therapy is complete, a crown is necessary to fully restore the tooth.

Replacing teeth. If you're like most people, you've lost one or more teeth to decay, periodontal disease, or an accident. For some reason, a missing tooth is considered important when the gap is in the front of the mouth, but insignificant when it's on the side or back. Either way, a missing tooth can change the appearance of your face and if it isn't replaced, the loss throws the rest of your teeth out of alignment.

Sometimes teeth are so beyond repair that they need to be extracted. Replacement may be with a bridge, which relies on your remaining, natural teeth for support, or dentures, which take the place of your natural teeth. Dental implants may be recommended in cases where dentures don't work.

In a *dental implant,* artificial teeth are attached to your jawbone in a surgical procedure. Although new surgical techniques and materials have improved the outlook for dental implants, their long-term success has not yet been demonstrated. Also, implant procedures can be expensive. Among the possible complications of implants are bone infection and nerve damage in the lips and jaw. If you are considering dental implants, a dentist experienced in performing this procedure can tell you if you are a good candidate.

Orthodontics. Braces aren't just for kids anymore. When your own teeth are so crooked or crowded that you have a bad bite or are self-conscious about your smile, you may decide to join the estimated 15 percent of adults from 20 to 60 who wear braces. (Note that in some cases, braces cannot produce straight teeth.) When discussing brace treatment with an orthodontist, the first question to ask is how much money and time you'll have to invest. Find out how this specialist intends to solve your problem, what kind of result to expect, whether any of your teeth will need to be extracted, and which type of bracing appliance will be used.

The Bones, Muscles, and Joints

Over time, the stature and contours of our bodies change. Your scale may register the same weight at age 50 as it did when you were 25, but the distribution of those pounds is different.

You stand tallest in your mid-20s, when the backbone has finished growing. The intervertebral disks that form a cushion between each bone, or vertebra, of the spine account for nearly a quarter of your backbone's length. As you grow older, these disks begin to dry out, causing the vertebrae to collapse and move closer together. Eventually everyone shrinks a little in height.

By age 35, men and women achieve their peak bone mass. Soon, the body's natural removal of some bone cells begins. In women, the bone loss process accelerates after menopause because the levels of the bone-protecting hormone estrogen drop off. This process, called *osteoporosis,* is a disease once thought to be an inevitable part of aging.

Osteoporosis

We all lose bone as we grow older, but in osteoporosis, a progressively disabling disorder, the bones become so light and porous that any kind of movement can cause a fracture.

An estimated 15 million to 20 million American adults over 45, most of them women, are affected by osteoporosis. Because this disorder quietly robs the skeleton of calcium over a period of decades, many of its victims aren't aware that there's a problem until they suffer a fracture.

Although there are treatments to halt further bone loss in newly diagnosed cases, it's impossible to restore the bone that has already been lost. The only chance of beating osteoporosis is in preventing it.

Confusion and controversy surround the prevention and treatment of osteoporosis. Among the commonly prescribed preventive measures are adequate calcium intake, exercise, and estrogen replacement therapy. But because each woman's risk profile differs, the prescription isn't the same for everyone. While a combined program of calcium consumption and exercise may be effective for some women at high risk, others might want to discuss the pros and cons of estrogen therapy with their doctors.

Risk factors.   To determine your risk profile for osteoporosis, you need to consider a number of factors, from your ancestry and family history to your life-style. Although it can't be said with certainty who will get the disease, there is well-established evidence that helps identify those most at risk.

- *Sex.* Women are at greater risk than men of developing osteoporosis, for two reasons: first, their bone mass is about one-third less dense than that of men; and second, from early adulthood to the later years, men lose 17 percent of their spongy porous bone while women lose 29 percent.
- *Age.* About 25 percent of all women over 60 have spinal compression fractures that cause the characteristic stooped posture of osteoporosis. Nearly one-third of the women who reach 90 suffer a hip fracture.
- *Race.* Black women have heavier and thicker bones and, accordingly, a lower risk of osteoporosis. Caucasian and Asian women have a much higher risk of age-related bone loss.
- *Body build.* Small-boned women are especially susceptible to osteoporosis.
- *Weight.* Underweight women are more prone to osteoporosis than heavier women, who tend to have more of the bone-protecting hormone estrogen.
- *Early menopause.* Surgical removal of the ovaries or an early cessation of menstruation cuts off the supply of the hormone estrogen, which has a protective effect on bone.
- *Prolonged use of cortisone drugs.* These hormones can have an adverse effect on bone-forming cells and help cause the breakdown of bone tissue.
- *Inactivity.* A sedentary life-style and long periods of immobility, such as being confined to bed while recovering from an illness, cause rapid bone loss.
- *Smoking.* Cigarette smoking appears to bring on an earlier menopause than your genes had planned. The earlier the menopause, the greater the bone loss.

• *Alcohol.* Heavy use of alcohol depresses bone formation by its effect on bone-building cells called osteoblasts.

• *Calcium.* An adequate calcium intake before menopause, through the diet or through calcium supplements, can help strengthen the bones. Calcium is also used in conjunction with other treatments to prevent bone loss during and after menopause.

• *Diet.* Certain substances in some foods encourage calcium loss. These include excess protein consumption and phosphates in soft drinks. When the diet is high in sodium, the kidneys have to excrete more calcium.

Other risk factors may influence the development of osteoporosis, but the evidence remains too sketchy to draw any conclusions at this time. Drinking fluoridated water is thought by some to build bone; consuming too much caffeine and taking certain diuretics may turn out to speed loss.

Calcium. The bones and teeth hold most of your body's calcium. The small amount that circulates in the bloodstream is necessary for conducting electrical impulses in the nerves, contracting muscles, and coagulating blood. When calcium levels in the bloodstream are low, the body taps your bones for calcium. Occasional withdrawals aren't harmful, but extended periods of calcium depletion cause the gradual thinning of bone.

A number of hormones influence the creation of new bone tissue and the destruction of older bone. As long as these hormones stay in balance, and you consume enough calcium in your daily diet, the drain on the bones should be minimal.

The U.S. Food and Drug Administration's Recommended Daily Allowance for calcium is 800 milligrams. However, a panel of scientists assembled by the National Institutes of Health for consensus conferences on osteoporosis recommended that postmenopausal women at high risk of developing osteoporosis should take 1,500 milligrams of calcium a day. The NIH panel recommends that other adults should consume 1,000 milligrams daily.

Calcium is an essential nutrient and diet is the best source of this mineral. Dairy products such as skim milk, yogurt, low-fat cheese, and ice cream, and other foods such as broccoli and canned salmon and sardines, are excellent natural sources of calcium. Occasionally, people develop an adverse reaction to milk, or a lactose intolerance, as they get older. If you find that you develop unpleasant symptoms such as gas and bloating after drinking milk, try lactase-added milk.

Some studies have shown that calcium supplements after menopause have only a marginal effect in slowing bone loss. But even though the benefit may be small, it's worth the effort if you can slow the loss of bone to any degree.

Exercise.   Increased physical activity of the "weight-bearing" kind can help increase bone mass. Light to moderate exercise that puts stress on the weight-bearing bones—the spinal column, hips, and the long bones of the legs—is beneficial to building strong bones. Weight-bearing exercise includes walking, jogging, aerobics, bicycling, dancing, rope jumping, and stair climbing.

A word of caution: most young adults and men and women in their 30s and 40s who are in good health can tolerate a moderate amount of high-intensity exercise and build bone mass. But women over 65 who already have been diagnosed as having osteoporosis may damage their fragile bones if they suddenly decide to begin exercising. Consult your physician about an exercise program that's right for your age and physical condition.

Screening for osteoporosis.   To date, there are no established guidelines for the routine radiological detection of osteoporosis. Nevertheless, many clinics offer such detection services to women—especially those in the 45-to-70 age group. One such test uses a technique called *single-photon absorptiometry,* or SPA, which measures bone in the forearm. This test, however, cannot assess the risk of fracture in the spine and hip—the major areas where osteoporosis occurs.

Two tests do offer a high degree of accuracy, but are very expensive. They are *dual-photon absorptiometry* (DPA) and *quantitated computerized tomography,* or CT scanning.

Most medical authorities do not recommend routine radiologic screening for people who have no symptoms.

Treatment.   Three drugs have been approved by the Food and Drug Administration for the treatment of osteoporosis: calcium, estrogen, and calcitonin—a hormone that blocks bone loss. Sodium fluoride therapy has been the subject of much study as a possible way to increase bone density; some clinical trials have shown that although fluoride may increase bone mass, the bone is not strong enough to withstand fractures.

A new treatment with the drug etidronate (Didronel) appears to strengthen brittle bones in the spine and reduce the incidence of new spinal fractures. A study published in 1990 in *The New England Journal of Medicine* reported that postmenopausal women who were given a regimen of etidronate and calcium for two years increased the density of their spinal bone by about 5 percent. These women also suffered half as many painful vertebral fractures as the untreated group.

Etidronate apparently works by slowing the breakdown of bone tissue—a process called resorption—and sets the stage for new bone to form in its place. As we age, more bone is broken down than rebuilt. The etidronate-calcium combination, which is given in separate cycles, seems to help restore the balance of the bone-building activity. Etidronate is available in pill form, so it is easy to administer.

Although etidronate has not yet gained FDA approval for the treatment of osteoporosis, the drug is used to treat Paget's disease, another bone condition. No major adverse side effects were reported in the women who took etidronate for two years; only 5 to 6 percent of the participants reported experiencing nausea and diarrhea. Scientists don't know whether there are any long-term side effects. Doctors have yet to determine the effectiveness of etidronate when compared with hormone replacement therapy or calcitonin treatment.

Men with osteoporosis generally do not need hormonal replacement therapy. However, some men with low testosterone levels may require sex steroid replacement. Calcium supplements with vitamin D may also be prescribed.

Hormone replacement therapy. Estrogen, with its proven ability to preserve bone in women prior to menopause, also has a protective effect when it is given to postmenopausal women at high risk for osteoporosis.

As effective as estrogen therapy may be against osteoporosis, the very mention of the therapy tends to evoke concern and confusion among women. As a result, many women who have been advised by their physicians to follow an estrogen replacement program don't comply with the doctor's orders because they fear developing cancer or unpleasant side effects.

Estrogen therapy is recommended for women who are at increased risk for osteoporosis—as long as the women do not have a history of vaginal bleeding, liver disease, cancer, or thromboembolic disorders (blood clots). Because there are so many uncertainties in patients' minds surrounding hormonal replacement therapy, you should ask for information on the risks and consequences of osteoporotic fractures, the risks and benefits of hormonal therapy, and alternative approaches to osteoporosis prevention.

When you ask about the benefits and risks of estrogen therapy, these are some of the key issues to consider:

- *Benefits* A halt in bone loss and a reduction in fractures; elimination of hot flashes; restored flexibility, secretions, and lubrication in the vaginal tissues, which tend to atrophy during menopause; and, possibly, a lower risk of heart disease.
- *Risk* The question of an increased risk of uterine cancer or breast cancer, depending on the form of estrogen replacement being used.

Hormonal therapy was once administered only in pill form but has since become available in a skin patch that is worn on the abdomen, where it delivers estrogen transdermally directly into the bloodstream. It has not yet been determined that the skin patch delivery system is as effective as the oral route.

A 1989 Swedish study captured wide attention when it suggested that long-term estrogen therapy can increase the risk of breast cancer, especially when estrogen plus progestin is used. However, other studies suggest that an estrogen-progestin regimen can reduce the breast cancer risk.

In the face of so much uncertainty, it may be difficult to decide if you should begin hormonal replacement therapy. With your doctor's guidance and your careful consideration of the benefits and risks, you should be able to make an informed decision that's right for you.

The Muscles

No two people have exactly the same amount of body fat and *lean body mass,* a term that covers the nonfat part of you and includes muscles, organs, connective tissue, bone, and water.

When you're physically inactive, you lose lean body tissue. In its place comes fat. Muscle strength and flexibility also decline. Inactivity robs your body of energy and strength and may accelerate aging. Anyone who's ever been sidelined for a long period of bed rest as a result of illness or an accident may recall how difficult it was to resume an active life after the prolonged inactivity. A few weeks of doing nothing can make the body feel decades older.

It had long been thought that losing muscle mass was an irreversible function of aging. But medical scientists at the Tufts University Human Nutrition Research Center of Aging demonstrated that men and women in their 60s, 70s, and 80s were able to reverse the muscle mass loss process and increase the size of their muscles after undertaking a weight-training regimen geared to their age group.

Unused muscles tend to waste away. Between ages 30 and 80, the body loses about 30 percent of its muscle mass. But if you keep your muscles active, they will show less of a change over the years.

Exercise and aging. Research into exercise physiology has shown that regular exercise can recharge your strength and flexibility, keep your body firm and fit, and boost your self-esteem. Several studies suggest that physical activity may be beneficial to your heart and blood vessels, lungs, muscles, and metabolism. Regular exercise also appears to help prevent constipation, which in turn may help protect against colon cancer.

Scientists don't know why exercise reduces the risk of death from heart disease and cancer. In a study released late in 1989, more than 13,000 men and women were followed for eight years to measure fitness by performance on a treadmill. After making adjustments for age, the researchers found that as the exercisers' fitness levels rose, their longevity increased. The most dramatic health gains were recorded by the least fit men and women who moved from the sedentary group to the next level of fitness out of five possible groups.

Exercise is a powerful prescription that many doctors recommend in the prevention and control of several diseases, from adult-onset diabetes and high blood pressure to osteoporosis and heart attack. If you don't exercise regularly now, but would like to begin a program, be sure to clear it with your doctor first.

The Heart and Lungs

Your heart is a strong muscular pump that can stay healthy if it is not allowed to deteriorate or become diseased. During an average lifetime of 70 years, your heart will beat more than 2.5 billion times.

Your maximum heart rate—the heart's ability to beat faster with exercise—declines progressively with age. Cardiac output, or the amount of blood the heart pumps with each beat, begins to decline as early as age 20. With each succeeding year, there is about a 1 percent decline in cardiac output. Yet studies suggest that with regular exercise, cardiac output can remain relatively constant.

Blood pressure levels often increase with age. Although nearly half of American men and women who reach their mid-70s develop hypertension, some people consistently register the ideal blood pressure reading of 120/80 even in old age. When hypertension is mild, doctors often try to control the condition without medication. This prescription includes weight loss if necessary, dietary modification, lowering alcohol intake, and regular exercise.

Preventing heart disease. *Arteriosclerosis,* or hardening of the arteries, is directly related to aging and affects nearly everyone to some degree. It occurs when the blood vessels lose their elasticity between the 20s and 60s.

Under the general heading of arteriosclerosis comes another form of this disorder, called *atherosclerosis,* a progressive disease of the arteries. Fat, cholesterol, and other substances accumulate inside the artery walls and reduce the flow of blood through the vessels. Although atherosclerosis is a major cause of heart disease, it is not a natural part of aging.

Men have a higher risk of heart attack until women begin catching up to them in their mid-50s, when the protection of estrogen is lost following menopause. Researchers suspect that the beneficial effect of estrogen is due in part to its role in raising the level of so-called good (high-density lipoprotein) cholesterol in the bloodstream. The hormone also appears to help the blood vessels retain their elasticity.

Better breathing. Your lungs achieve their VO_2 *max* or maximum oxygen uptake around age 20. (Your VO_2 max is your ability to inhale oxygen while you're working hard at physical labor, exercising, or climbing stairs.) An inactive person can expect VO_2 max to decline to two-thirds of capacity by age 60.

Although your VO_2 max drops with age, a number of studies have shown that physically active people can slow the decline. Many middle-aged and older adults who undertook regular exercise programs recorded VO_2 max levels comparable to sedentary people 10 and 20 years younger.

Digestion

After about age 40, your stomach gradually begins to secrete less gastric acid and may feel sluggish at times. As a result, it may become more difficult for your body to absorb nutrients. For instance, the intestine is less able to absorb calcium as you grow older.

Peristalsis, the muscular action that propels food along the digestive tract, slowly decreases with age, and food takes longer to move through the system. A common complaint of growing older is *constipation,* a problem that results from decreased muscle tone and motility in the large intestine. For occasional constipation, you may find relief by increasing the amount of fiber, or roughage, in your daily diet, including whole-grain cereals and breads, fresh fruits, and vegetables. Persistent constipation calls for a full medical evaluation.

Heartburn, a problem more likely to bother those over 40, occurs when stomach acid moves up toward the esophagus and causes irritation, pain, or burning. You may be able to avoid distress by taking a few simple measures, such as not eating too close to bedtime.

It's also possible to develop an adverse reaction to milk as you grow older. After years of drinking milk, you may find that you cannot digest milk or its products—a condition known as *lactose intolerance.* The problem stems from a reduced intestinal production of *lactase,* the enzyme that's responsible for breaking down *lactose,* the sugar in milk. If you have a lactose intolerance but still would like to drink milk, you can buy lactase-added milk, which contains specially added enzymes.

Metabolism

Rats placed on a restricted low-calorie diet live about 50 percent longer than average. Most scientists strongly suspect that if such an experiment were possible in humans, the results would be the same.

Your metabolism slows down gradually after age 20, and it takes longer to burn off the food you have eaten. It's been estimated that the number of calories we need drops off 2 to 5 percent each decade after age 30. To avoid becoming a storage depot for fat, there are two choices: cut calories from your diet or burn off more calories through exercise.

The Immune System

An entire theory of aging centers on the immune system. It appears that with aging, the body gradually loses its "biological memory" and has a harder time recognizing viruses and other hostile microorganisms it successfully drove away in the past.

Occasionally, the aging immune system mistakes its own proteins or tissues for *antigens,* or foreign invaders, and begins attacking its own tissue in a process called *autoimmune disease.* This process appears to be linked to an age-related decrease in *antibodies,* substances that fight disease-causing microorganisms. Rheumatoid arthritis, lupus erythematosus, myasthenia gravis, and possibly multiple sclerosis are examples of autoimmune disorders.

The risk of developing cancer is greater as you grow older for several reasons, including age-related immunological changes, life-style factors such as cigarette smoking, and exposure to toxic materials. Immunologists believe that the immune system readily distinguishes normal cells from cancer cells and immediately destroys any abnormal cells that enter the body. This theory of immune surveillance holds true as long as the body is healthy and the immune system is working properly. By practicing good health habits, and avoiding cigarettes, unnecessary radiation, and hazardous chemical substances in the environment, you can hold down the risk of developing certain forms of cancer as you grow older.

Hormones

More than 100 hormones regulate the functions of the human body. Collectively known as the endocrine system, these glands produce several changes as you grow older—from slowing down the body's metabolism to triggering menopause in women.

Many hormonal functions change with aging. One change involves the body's balance of salt and water, which affects your blood pressure. Others include the level of sugar in your blood, your reaction to stress, and your sex drive.

Your metabolism, the way your body uses fuel, is under the control of the thyroid gland. As the thyroid undergoes changes in size and structure with aging, your metabolism slows. The most common result of a slower metabolism is weight gain from burning fewer calories than you consume. To counter this hormonal change, eat less and exercise more.

Human Growth Hormone

The search for the ever-elusive fountain of youth took yet another turn when scientists reported that experimental treatment with human growth hormone seemed to mitigate some effects of aging. A study published in 1990 in *The New England Journal of Medicine* reported that a group of 21 healthy men who received a genetically engineered version of the hormone for six months had physical improvements in their skin and an increase in muscle tissue similar to that of men 10 to 20 years younger.

The men, who ranged in age from 61 to 81, were healthy but had low production of human growth hormone. For six months, 12 of the men received injections of the hormone three times a month. Nine other participants received no treatment at all. At the end of the treatment period, the results among those who got the drug were very striking.

Lean body tissue, which includes muscle mass, increased by 8.8 percent, fatty tissue declined by 14.4 percent, and skin thickness increased by 7.1 percent. These percentages are comparable to those found in younger men. A slight increase in the density of bones in the spinal column was also reported.

During childhood, the pituitary gland produces this hormone so that normal growth can occur. The adult body still secretes the hormone, but production begins to taper off around age 30. As growth hormone gradually declines, there is a loss of muscle tissue and the accumulation of fatty tissue. Some people continue to produce adequate levels of growth hormone as they grow older, while others have a deficiency of this substance.

Although human growth hormone has been used to treat children deficient in the hormone, researchers don't know the implications of treatment in older adults. Stronger muscles, tighter skin, and, possibly, stronger bones are among the benefits of the therapy; but health risks from taking an excessive amount of the hormone may be cause for greater concern.

Many scientists hail the results as "exciting," but they also note that the findings remain preliminary and should not be considered a panacea to prevent normal aging. However alluring human growth hormone injections may sound to those who would like to undo some of the traces of time, it's clear that the findings are preliminary and allow no meaningful conclusion at this time.

Among the short-term side effects are a slight increase in blood pressure. The possible long-term effects remain unknown. If growth hormone is given in excess, it has the potential to affect the body adversely, possibly leading to arthritis, diabetes, enlargement of the face and hands, heart failure, and cancer.

Scientists don't know how long the effects of the hormone injections can be expected to last. And a treatment regimen modeled after the one used in the study is estimated to cost close to $14,000 a year. For reasons of cost alone, this kind of therapy isn't accessible to many people.

Although the interest and demand for growth hormone may be great, only older adults with a measurable deficit of the hormone would be eligible for treatment. Some scientists believe that encouraging a low-fat diet and exercise among older adults is just as beneficial in helping to build muscle mass.

Diabetes

Adult-onset *type II diabetes* is a common hormonal disorder that occurs as people get older, but most frequently in those who are inactive or obese. Blood glucose levels rise with age and, for unknown reasons, the body becomes resistant to insulin. When this happens, it leads to a situation in which blood levels of glucose increase, causing damage to the blood vessels. You may be able to help prevent or control type II diabetes by getting regular physical exercise and maintaining your normal weight.

Sex hormones

Sexual desire (libido) is influenced by hormones, beginning with the pituitary gland in the brain. This gland stimulates the release of other hormones until finally a woman's ovaries release a great deal of estrogen and a man's testes release testosterone. Men and women both produce the same sex hormones—although in different amounts. The level of sex hormones gradually decreases with age in both sexes. Arousal may take a little longer as you grow older, but otherwise, a fall in hormone production should not halt normal sexual function.

The Nervous System and the Brain

An average person is endowed with about 100 billion brain cells. Between 10 billion and 15 billion of these are *neurons,* or nerve cells, and the rest glial cells that support the work of the neurons. Between young adulthood and old age, large numbers of brain cells die off as a normal part of aging.

Unlike other cells in the body, cells in the brain and nervous system don't replace themselves. When nerve cells are damaged—from drug and alcohol abuse, disease, accidents, and aging—they are lost forever.

Although nerve cells die, the communication links between cells, called *dendrites,* do not. These branchlike projections tend to shrink with age but remarkably also appear to have a reserve capacity to grow—apparently to compensate for damage when the brain suffers an injury. Some scientists studying the aging brain have suggested that dendrites continue to grow in response to intellectual challenge and mental exercise regardless of age.

Losing brain cells doesn't necessarily mean you are losing intelligence. Many of the disappearing cells are in those parts of the brain that govern vision, sleep, and even anxiety. For example, by the time men and women reach 60, they often find themselves sleeping fewer hours each night. It is also known that some areas of the brain show relatively little decline in cell population. One such area is the hypothalamus, which regulates the release of hormones into your body.

Because the brain takes longer to process information and to signal the spinal cord to initiate action, your reaction time to various stimuli tends to increase as you grow older. For instance, a tennis ball speeding across the court is harder to return, or getting your foot from the gas pedal to the brake of your car may take a fraction of a second longer. Chemical messengers called *neurotransmitters,* found at the end of nerve cell branches, are essential for keeping electrical signals moving through the nervous system; some decline with age while others remain stable.

Studies of people from their 50s up have shown that those who exercise regularly—at least three times a week—can improve their reaction time as well as their muscle strength. Aerobic exercise seems to yield the greatest benefit. In some studies, the participants also experienced improved memory and perception.

It's natural for memory to decline a little with age. Memory lapses—such as temporarily forgetting someone's name, forgetting to do something, or misplacing your keys—are benign occurrences. Although some people begin worrying about memory loss in their 40s and 50s, you may not notice any memory lapses until much later.

Senility is not a normal part of aging. If you have serious memory loss, an inability to concentrate, and feel confused, consult a physician. These symptoms, which can be caused by medication, alcohol, depression, or distraction, are too often presumed to be signs of the degenerative brain disorder commonly known as *Alzheimer's disease.*

Alzheimer's Disease

When people are asked what they fear most about aging, the answer is almost always the same: *Alzheimer's disease.* Since the fastest-growing segment of the population is the elderly, projections by the National Institute on Aging for the future are disturbing. Estimates for the year 2050 place the nation's Alzheimer's victims around 14 million.

Alzheimer's disease was first described in 1906 by the German neurologist after whom it is named. But it wasn't until the 1970s, when medical scientists realized that the problem wasn't rare, that major research efforts were focused on the disorder. Today, scores of scientists are searching for clues to the cause, cure, and prevention of Alzheimer's disease.

In an Alzheimer's brain, there is a degeneration of nerve cells in areas of brain tissue that are responsible for memory. An affected nerve cell loses its ability to secrete the neurotransmitter acetylcholine, which is a chemical that carries messages between certain nerve cells in the brain. Major research efforts are focused on finding an effective drug to slow down or halt the breakdown of acetylcholine in the brain and possibly stem the loss of memory. The greater the reduction of acetylcholine, the higher the mortality of brain cells.

The reason that brain cells die is unknown. Among the possible causes are genetic links, slow-acting viruses, and environmental toxins—especially aluminum.

Since it was first reported in the 1970s that deposits of aluminum were found in some Alzheimer's brains during autopsy, many people have been afraid to use aluminum cookware. But aluminum is found in more than your pots and pans. It's ubiquitous—the metal is present in the soil, drinking water, food, air, antacids, and antiperspirants. In any event, at this time there is no persuasive evidence convicting aluminum as a causative factor in Alzheimer's disease.

Diagnosis. Although there still aren't any clear answers, research and increased awareness have helped doctors more readily distinguish between benign forgetfulness, potentially reversible disorders, and Alzheimer's disease.

While Alzheimer's disease claims the greatest attention as the most common form of *senile dementia,* there actually are more than 50 causes of dementia—many of which can be reversed with treatment after the underlying disorder is corrected. They include:

• Multi-infarct dementia, which consists of many small strokes, none of which are physically disabling.

• Long-term use of certain prescription and over-the-counter drugs, singly or in combination, can produce toxic conditions in the body that lead to mental confusion and loss of memory.

• Depression may produce such symptoms as apathy, withdrawal, difficulty in sleeping and in making decisions which may be misdiagnosed as Alzheimer's. Drugs and psychotherapy may be helpful in treating depression.

• Brain disease caused by metabolic changes can cause confusion, changes in behavior, errors in thinking, and impaired consciousness. Among the many disorders that can produce these symptoms are chronic alcoholism, liver failure, vitamin B_{12} deficiency, diabetes, kidney failure, and malnutrition.

• Hypothyroidism—a disorder in which the thyroid gland produces inadequate amounts of thyroid hormones—may cause the body's physical and mental activities to decline.

It is paradoxical that many people in the early stages of Alzheimer's disease are not diagnosed, whereas others with correctable conditions are mistakenly labeled as irreversibly demented. There is no standardized test yet available to make a definite diagnosis of Alzheimer's disease.

Until there are answers, it's a waste of time to brood in advance over a disease that may not affect you. Instead, if you think you are growing forgetful, you can try some positive mind games, such as *mnemonics,* techniques that help improve the memory—such as making written lists, writing down important points, and underlining items or dates so that they stand out when you scan your notebook or calendar. Add a little structure to your life by keeping your keys, glasses, bills, and other items in a certain place. And create mental pictures of things you want to remember. For instance, if you park your car in a large lot and note that you're in section E, associate the letter E with something that will help you retrieve your car later—such as E for "easy to remember."

Assessing Your Health Risks

By the year 2002, nearly one-third of the American population will be 55 or older. If you're among this group, it may be time to assess your health risk factors as well as your social and psychological risk factors.

In a classic study of nearly 7,000 adults in Alameda County, California, conducted in 1965, epidemiologists identified seven healthy habits that appeared to have a positive effect on longevity. The researchers found that men of 45 who regularly followed six or seven of these habits gained more than 11 years in life expectancy. For women, the gain was seven years.

Here's the list of health practices that formed the centerpiece of the study. How many are a part of your life-style?

1. Do you smoke?
2. Do you drink more than a moderate amount of alcohol?
3. Do you eat breakfast regularly?
4. Do you snack a lot between meals?
5. Are you able to maintain a normal weight for your height?
6. Do you sleep seven to eight hours a night?
7. Do you get moderate exercise on a regular basis?

"No" answers to nos. 1, 2, and 4 and "yes" to nos. 3, 5, 6, and 7 have been correlated with good health. The habit of eating breakfast regularly has come under some criticism, but researchers have found that participants who ate a breakfast every morning and snacked only rarely reported better physical health than those who skipped the first meal of the day. Moderate amounts of regular exercise are important, as is enough sleep. Cigarette smoking, drinking too much alcohol, and becoming overweight are especially detrimental to good health.

7

Common Health Complaints

Peter A. Gross, M.D.

If you suffer an ache, a fever, nausea, or a sudden immobilizing pain, you must rely on your own judgment in deciding what to do. Will the condition resolve on its own, with self-care, or do you need to see a doctor?

This section provides general guidelines for dealing with most common and a few not-so-common and serious health complaints. Special attention is given to the cause, symptoms, treatment, and, when applicable, the prevention of each problem.

This information should be used for reference only. It is *not* a substitute for diagnosis and treatment by your physician.

Gastrointestinal Complaints

Almost everyone suffers an occasional bout of heartburn, nausea, vomiting, and diarrhea. These common gastrointestinal complaints often tend to be self-limiting, but there are instances when a digestive problem calls for prompt medical attention.

Gastritis

Gastritis, or an inflammation of the mucus lining of the stomach, can result from drinking too much coffee or alcohol, consuming foods that cause an allergic reaction, infection, and as a side effect of aspirin, ibuprofen, and certain prescription drugs.

Symptoms often include pain, nausea, loss of appetite, and vomiting. In most cases, the discomfort lasts for one or two days and then disappears. No treatment is usually necessary, although over-the-counter antacids may provide some relief, as does avoidance of coffee, strong tea, and alcohol. Eating small meals consisting of bland foods (as opposed to heavy and spicy foods) is also recommended, at least until all symptoms have disappeared.

Indigestion

The discomfort that can occur after eating is often described as *indigestion* or *dyspepsia*. Symptoms may include a dull feeling or a gnawing discomfort in the chest or upper abdomen, abdominal pain, bloating, nausea, and gas.

While indigestion usually is attributed to eating particular foods or beverages, or eating too heavily or too quickly, there may be other causes, including anxiety and stress. Although chronic indigestion is a recurrent problem for some people, in most cases it is a benign disorder and with time will disappear on its own. However, if the symptoms become severe and persistent, a more serious condition, such as an ulcer, gallbladder disease, or even stomach cancer, may be the cause.

If you suffer from chronic digestive disorders and your doctor is unable to diagnose a physical cause, you may be able to find relief by modifying your diet, stopping smoking, and reducing the stress in your life. Avoid using aspirin or ibuprofen—they may cause bleeding in the stomach. Use acetaminophen (Tylenol) instead. Over-the-counter antacids may also help relieve your symptoms.

Excess Gas

Your digestive tract produces a certain amount of gas as part of its normal daily activity. You can't prevent the formation of gas, but it is possible to reduce the amount of gas that may cause you discomfort or embarrassment.

Gas in the intestinal tract comes from two major sources:

- *air* that some people tend to swallow as they eat and talk
- *the colon,* where undigested parts of food, such as sugars and carbohydrates, are acted upon by bacteria that normally inhabit the large bowel. As the bacteria come into contact with the intestinal contents, fermentation occurs and odor-causing gases such as carbon dioxide, methane, and hydrogen sulphide are produced

Belching and burping usually result from swallowing air. Eating too fast, talking while eating, chewing gum, and smoking may contribute to air swallowing. Chronic, or repeated, belching only encourages gulping more air and aggravates the problem.

Abdominal bloating, or an uncomfortable buildup of gas, often may be caused by disorders of the intestinal tract, including irritable bowel syndrome, or by diet. *Flatulence,* or the frequent passing of gas from the rectum, is caused mostly by the consumption of carbohydrates that are not completely digested by the time they reach the lower intestinal tract. These undigested foods pass on to the colon, where they are acted on by bacteria.

Gas-forming foods in your diet, including beans, cabbage, broccoli, brussels sprouts, cauliflower, and eggplant, can also cause excess gas. An intolerance to the lactose in milk can result in abdominal bloating and gas as well. Other possible causes may include a sensitivity to a certain food, an overgrowth of bacteria in the small intestine, or, rarely, partial blockages of the intestine.

Ulcers

An *ulcer* occurs when a small portion of the lining of the stomach or the duodenum becomes eroded and inflamed. This raw area causes a burning or gnawing pain. The exact cause of an ulcer (which usually measures between the size of a dime and a half-dollar piece) is not known. However, several factors play a role in ulcer formation, including an excess amount of the stomach's digestive enzyme pepsin and hydrochloric acid, as well as decreased ability of the mucus layer to resist ulceration.

Ulcer pain and symptoms vary with each person. You may experience pain when your stomach is empty or immediately after you eat; the most common time is between one to three hours after eating. Pain may last from a short period of time to a few hours. Appetite loss, weight loss, and occasional vomiting can occur. When discomfort and stomach pain last more than two weeks and the usual antacids fail to relieve your symptoms, consult a physician as soon as possible.

Treatment may include eliminating irritating foods from the diet, including coffee and tea, and taking medications such as cimetidine (Tagamet) and ranitidine (Zantac) to decrease the amount of acid produced in the stomach.

Heartburn

When digestive juices from the stomach flow back upward into the esophagus and produce pain and burning (esophageal reflux), the discomfort is called *heartburn*. A related condition that may contribute to heartburn in some people is *hiatal hernia,* in which part or all of the upper stomach bulges upward through a weakened opening (hiatus) in the diaphragm. The reduced muscle tone of the circular diaphragm may allow the acid contents of the stomach to reverse direction and travel up instead of down.

The symptoms of heartburn can range from mild discomfort to painful burning in the throat or chest. (Often, the pain may be mistaken for a heart attack. See Chapter 3.) Antacids can temporarily relieve the symptoms.

You can reduce the frequency and severity of heartburn by following these steps:

- Eat small, frequent meals instead of large meals.
- Don't eat snacks or meals too close to bedtime.
- Avoid acidic foods—especially citrus juices and tomato products.
- Avoid alcohol and cigarettes, because both can increase stomach acid production and cause heartburn.
- Raise the head of your bed about four inches to reduce reflux while you are sleeping.
- Don't wear tight-fitting clothing around the waist; it can be uncomfortable and increase abdominal pressure.
- If you are overweight, losing excess pounds may lower abdominal pressure and reduce heartburn.

Women commonly experience heartburn during pregnancy.

Vomiting

Vomiting is a symptom of many disorders. It may be a response to a number of stimuli: gastritis caused by a viral agent or bacterium, food poisoning, motion sickness, alcohol, medications, or emotional distress. Women can experience nausea and vomiting during pregnancy, especially during the first three months.

If the cause of vomiting is a virus, or excess food and drink, the condition usually is self-limiting and not a matter of serious concern. Prolonged nausea and vomiting may indicate disorders in other parts of the body than the stomach, including appendicitis, cancer, intestinal obstruction, kidney disease, liver disease, or a brain tumor or head injury. If vomiting recurs often or is accompanied by severe abdominal pain, or contains red blood or dark brown granules that look like coffee grounds, consult a physician immediately.

Diarrhea

Diarrhea, or bowel movements that are very frequent and very loose, is a mechanism the body uses to protect itself. By quickly sweeping out any infectious or noxious agent, the intestinal tract can return to its regular job of absorbing nutrients and fluids.

Acute diarrhea is usually triggered by infectious agents like viruses or bacteria. These agents are commonly acquired by ingesting contaminated food or water and through person-to-person contact with someone who is infected. In most cases, this intestinal upset produces liquid stools, often with mucus. Although an acute episode of diarrhea causes discomfort, it usually resolves itself within a few days.

Traveler's diarrhea, or turista, may occur when you travel to other parts of the world, especially to countries where you may not have resistance to local microorganisms in the food and water. The symptoms include nausea, abdominal cramps, bloating, vomiting, low-grade fever, malaise, and an urgent need to evacuate your bowels. Most cases of traveler's diarrhea stem from contact with toxin-producing *E. coli* bacteria.

You can prevent traveler's diarrhea by avoiding such foods as raw vegetables, raw seafood, raw meat, and unpeeled fruit when you travel. Shun tap water, ice made from tap water, and unpasteurized milk and dairy products. Beware of food sold by street vendors, no matter how tempting.

If you suffer from acute diarrhea, it is essential that you replace the fluids lost by your intestines in order to avoid dehydration. Diluted fruit juices, soft drinks, clear broth, and in the case of traveler's diarrhea, bottled water from a known source, help to replenish lost fluids. Avoid milk and dairy products. Eating salted crackers also helps restore the body's mineral balance. Bismuth subsalicylate (Pepto-Bismol) also may provide some relief from your symptoms. If you take this product, use it only as directed. (Children especially should avoid consuming large quantities of bismuth subsalicylate.)

Severe forms of diarrheal disease that produce dehydration, fever, diarrhea that persists for more than one week, or blood in the stools requires a doctor's care.

Constipation

Constipation is a temporary or persistent difficulty in moving your bowels. *Temporary constipation* may occur if your regular diet or routine is disrupted. *Chronic constipation* may be due to poor diet, dehydration, stress, certain medications, or the pressure of other activities that allow you to ignore your body's call.

When you feel the urge to evacuate your bowels, you must respond within a limited amount of time or the sensation disappears for variable amounts of time. If you keep ignoring the call, the fecal matter remains in the colon, allowing the intestinal tract to absorb more and more water from the usually soft fecal contents. As a result, the stools become harder and more difficult to expel and the constipation can become persistent and chronic.

Regularity is an individual matter. For some people, it is normal to have a daily bowel movement or perhaps even two or three a day. For others, bowel movements three times a week are normal. With a mild case of constipation, nature usually takes its course and the body gets back to regular functioning after a few days. A mild laxative might help relieve temporary constipation, but laxatives in general should be used with caution.

Repeated use of laxatives may irritate the intestinal lining and also may weaken the bowel's muscle tone. Instead, increase the amount of fiber in your diet by eating more whole grains, fruits, and vegetables. (You may suffer from excess gas and indigestion if your system isn't accustomed to fiber. To avoid discomfort, increase your fiber intake gradually.) Because fiber retains water, it makes the stool bulkier, softer, and easier to pass. Regular exercise is also helpful in stimulating the bowels.

If these measures fail to relieve your constipation within a few weeks, consult your physician.

Irritable Bowel Syndrome

Irritable bowel syndrome, or IBS, is a common disorder that affects millions of Americans. IBS, also called spastic colon, is often characterized by episodes of diarrhea that alternate with constipation, and may include such symptoms as abdominal cramps, nausea, and excess gas.

While many people who are diagnosed with IBS can trace this disorder to stress and emotional upsets, the condition may be caused by overactive nerves that control the intestines. Many IBS sufferers have an intestinal nervous system that is overly sensitive to stimuli, such as certain foods or stress. An intolerance to milk products (lactose intolerance) may also produce similar gastrointestinal symptoms.

To treat IBS, a doctor first must rule out serious disease and then work to help you identify any foods or situations that may trigger your symptoms. Behavior modification may also be recommended to help reduce stress.

Inflammatory Bowel Disease

The term *inflammatory bowel disease* (IBD) covers two separate but serious inflammatory diseases: Crohn's disease, or regional ileitis, and ulcerative colitis. *Ileitis* is an inflammation of the ileum, the lower part of the small intestine. *Colitis* is an inflammation of the large intestine or the colon.

IBD affects people of all ages, but typically occurs during adolescence and early adulthood. The attacks may be sudden or gradual in their onset. The symptoms may be continuous, or they may subside only to flare up every few months or years.

The symptoms of the two diseases are slightly different. Crohn's disease is characterized by pain in the right side of the abdomen, a slight fever, cramps, and diarrhea. The inflammation produced by Crohn's disease commonly affects the ileum, or last part of the small bowel, but may affect any part of the gastrointestinal tract.

Ulcerative colitis typically begins by inflaming the lining of the rectum. It tends to produce pain in the lower left side of the abdomen, and is accompanied by diarrhea, weight loss, and rectal bleeding. If the disease remains confined to the rectum, you have a milder form of ulcerative colitis, called ulcerative proctitis.

In addition to causing intestinal distress, IBD may precipitate conditions elsewhere in the body, including the eye, the skin, the joints, and the liver.

The cause of IBD is unknown, but it often is hereditary. If your IBD is chronic, the treatment will include dietary modification, behavior modification to reduce stress, and medication.

Diverticulosis

When areas of the colon wall weaken, little pouches called diverticuli may form and cause *diverticulosis,* a condition that usually causes no symptoms. If these sacs become inflamed or infected, the condition is known as *diverticulitis.* Abdominal pain and fever often accompany a case of diverticulitis. Sometimes these pockets become inflamed and form an abscess. If diverticulitis is left untreated, the infection can perforate the intestinal wall and cause peritonitis, an inflammation of the abdominal cavity lining.

Very mild cases may be treated with a liquid diet and antibiotics. More severe cases of diverticulitis require hospitalization in order to administer intravenous feeding and antibiotics. A severe attack of diverticulitis increases the risk of a future episode.

It may be possible to prevent diverticulosis by eating a diet high in fiber, including fresh fruits, vegetables, and whole grains.

Hemorrhoids

More than half of all American adults over 50 have had *hemorrhoids* at some time during their lives. When blood vessels in the anal canal and rectum are subject to repeated pressure, the vessels may swell and bulge to create hemorrhoids. These dilated blood vessels may be internal or external. Internal hemorrhoids don't always produce symptoms, although occasionally they may bleed, itch, and protrude down toward the anus.

Constipation is considered the chief cause of hemorrhoids. However, frequent bowel movements also can cause hemorrhoids. The increased abdominal pressure that is common during pregnancy and in obesity can also contribute to their formation.

While internal hemorrhoids are covered with a mucus membrane that has no nerve endings to sense pain, external hemorrhoids occur in a highly sensitive area and can produce severe pain, especially if a hemorrhoid develops a blood clot. Sitz baths (sitting in a tub of warm water), pain relievers, and stool softeners may help to relieve symptoms. Self-treatment with over-the-counter remedies may provide lubrication as well as relief for irritation, although none of these products can actually shrink hemorrhoids, as is sometimes claimed.

Medical treatment for internal hemorrhoids that bleed persistently and protrude include injection techniques, rubber band ligation, and photocoagulation, a method that uses infrared light or a laser to burn the tissue.

To help prevent hemorrhoids, increase your daily intake of dietary fiber to minimize the likelihood of the constipation that causes increased anal pressure. If you are subject to hemorrhoids, you can help control any itching or irritation in the area by practicing good hygiene and keeping the external skin around the anus clean and dry.

Parasites

Many parasites are endemic to the United States. Among the sources of parasites are household pets, contaminated food, water, and soil, and even sexual partners. When a parasite enters your body, the symptoms may range from a feeling of vague discomfort to abdominal cramps and chronic diarrhea.

One of the most common parasites in the United States is *Giardia lamblia,* a protozoan that can be transmitted through a water-borne infection or from person to person.

Symptoms of giardiasis can include diarrhea, nausea, abdominal cramps, flatulence, and fatigue. Campers and travelers are the most likely groups to be affected by giardia, although entire communities have become ill after drinking giardia-infested water. To reduce your risk of ingesting the parasite, never drink untreated water from an unknown source. A crystal-clear mountain stream far from civilization may contain microscopic giardia cysts from animal droppings. Boiling such water for at least 10 minutes can help destroy the parasite.

In areas where there is poor sanitation, amoebal organisms (*Entamoeba histolytica*) may be spread through fecally contaminated food, water, or soil. Sexual activity, especially among male homosexuals, also may lead to the transmission of amebiasis.

The symptoms include diarrhea accompanied by cramps and, in some cases, bloody stools. If left untreated, the organism may persist for a few weeks and then quiet down, only to settle in the liver, where it can form abscesses. Therapy depends on the severity of the illness and on the anatomic location of the disease—that is, whether the infection is inside or outside of the intestine.

The parasite *Toxoplasmosis gondii* commonly infects birds and small mammals. Humans may develop the parasitic disease *toxoplasmosis* when they come into contact with infected cat feces or eat undercooked meat.

Symptoms often resemble those of infectious mononucleosis: low-grade fever, fatigue, and swollen glands. The disease usually is self-limiting and the symptoms tend to subside over a period of several weeks. If the infection becomes chronic, it can be severely debilitating, though.

Pregnant women must be especially vigilant about contracting toxoplasmosis because the parasite can infect the fetus and cause birth defects that may lead to blindness and mental retardation. If you are pregnant, avoid eating raw or undercooked meat. If you have a cat, ask someone else to change the pet's litter box until after your infant is born.

The infectious disease *cryptosporidiosis* is believed to be acquired through direct contact with infected animals or humans, as well as through infected food and water.

Symptoms include watery diarrhea, upper abdominal cramps, flatulence, and weight loss. Travelers and healthy people who acquire cryptosporidiosis can expect the infection to last from 10 days to two weeks.

The disease is usually self-limiting. Although drugs are being tested for use against cryptosporidiosis, there is no effective therapy at this time.

If you consume raw or undercooked pork, you risk the chance of a *trichinosis* infection, if the eggs from the roundworm *Trichinella spiralis* are present in the meat.

Some people with trichinosis show no symptoms. But when the infection is severe, diarrhea and abdominal discomfort may appear within a day or two. After about a week of incubation, the intestinal symptoms disappear to be replaced by fever, muscle aches, fatigue, headache, swelling around the eyes, and a rash. If the worms are not expelled from the body, they can bore into the heart, lungs, or nervous system, sometimes with fatal complications.

Mild cases require rest and analgesics. Depending on the severity of the infection, the drug thiabendazole (Mintezol) or cortisone may be prescribed.

Several types of *tapeworms* can invade the human body. The most common are found in fish, beef, and pork that is eaten raw or is inadequately cooked.

Sometimes there are no symptoms or just mild discomfort. However, depending on the tapeworm, there may be anemia, gas pains, diarrhea, weight loss, and fever. A number of medications are available to treat this condition.

Gallbladder Problems

The gallbladder is a small pear-shaped organ that aids in the digestion of fats by storing bile, a substance produced by the nearby liver. When called for by the body, this stored bile is released into the small intestine. Among the components of bile are cholesterol, bile salts, and bilirubin, a bile pigment from hemoglobin released by the breakdown of old blood cells. If an imbalance in these substances occurs, tiny solid particles may form and develop into one or several gallstones; some are made up almost entirely of cholesterol, while others are formed from calcium or bile pigments.

People with gallstones may have no symptoms at all, or only minor, transient symptoms. However, if a gallstone slips into its drain pipe—the cystic duct—and blocks that duct, it can cause an inflammation of the entire gallbladder, a condition called *cholecystitis*. On occasion, cholecystitis is caused not by the blockage of the cystic duct but by infection, but either way it can produce pain in the upper right abdominal area, often accompanied by nausea and vomiting. This pain, which may be referred to the back, near or between the shoulder blades, can become intense and last from a half hour to several hours. In addition, fever and chills can develop and in some cases jaundice may occur (a yellowing of the skin). If you have already been diagnosed as having gallstones and experience any combination of these symptoms, call your doctor immediately. Contrary to popular belief, indigestion, flatulence, belching, and intolerance to fatty foods are *not* signs of gallbladder disease.

Doctors often recommend the removal of the gallbladder. In 1989, cholecystectomy, the surgical removal of the gallbladder, was the third most frequently performed operation in the nation. However, there are alternative treatments, including medications that slowly dissolve cholesterol gallstones. Doctors can also remove gallstones by snaring and extracting them by means of little baskets attached to special instruments. Recently *laparoscopic* cholecystectomy has been introduced. This procedure enables patients to go home after a day or two instead of the five to seven days in the hospital that is required after the usual operation. *Gallstone lithotripsy* remains experimental. This is a procedure that uses shock waves to fragment the stones into particles the size of sand grains, which are easily passed through the duct. This new therapy has not yet gained approval from the Food and Drug Administration.

Several factors are associated with the formation of gallstones. One is diet; eating a low-fat, high-fiber diet may help prevent gallstones. Age is another. Women are more likely to develop gallstones than men, especially during the period from adolescence to the completion of menopause.

Hepatitis

Hepatitis is an inflammation of the liver, most often caused by exposure to one of the hepatitis viruses, although alcohol, drugs, or infectious agents can also play a role. Depending on the form of the virus to which you were exposed, the severity of the illness may range from mild inflammation to serious liver damage.

Hepatitis A, or infectious hepatitis, is transmitted by fecal contamination of food and water, as well as through direct physical contact with someone actively infected. You may be infected with the hepatitis A virus for two to six weeks before any symptoms occur. In most cases, its symptoms are fairly mild and similar to the flu syndrome: nausea, abdominal discomfort, weakness, and loss of appetite. The urine may take on a brownish tinge and the stools become very light in color. Jaundice may occur. Some of those infected may have no symptoms.

Hepatitis A is usually self-limiting. Most people fully recover from hepatitis A and do not become carriers of the disease, but they cannot be blood donors. Bed rest has not been shown to be helpful. Avoid alcohol to prevent damage to the weakened liver.

If you are traveling to a country where infectious hepatitis is prevalent, you many want to consider receiving injections of gamma globulin, antibodies that prevent or reduce the severity of illness if you do become exposed.

Hepatitis B, or serum hepatitis, a more serious disease, is spread mainly by direct contact with infected blood. Transfusions, inoculation with a dirty hypodermic needle, and sexual contact are some of the ways you can get this disease. An infected pregnant woman can pass it to her fetus. The virus is present in all bodily fluids of an infected person, including saliva, tears, semen, and menstrual fluid.

The incubation period for hepatitis B may be much longer: about four weeks to six months. Symptoms are similar to those for hepatitis A, though they tend to be more severe. However, even with this serious disease, some victims may have vague symptoms or none at all. Of those infected, most recover completely. You should note that an estimated 10 percent become carriers of hepatitis B, and many go on to develop chronic liver disease; complications of untreated hepatitis B may lead to liver cancer or chronic liver disease, such as the scarring of cirrhosis or chronic hepatitis.

To make a diagnosis, your doctor will do blood tests. If the test shows the virus or antibodies to the virus, your doctor will recommend rest, a low-fat, high-carbohydrate diet, and small amounts of fluids at frequent intervals. Alcohol must be avoided.

Although no drug regimen exists to treat those already infected, a vaccine will help prevent hepatitis B in people with healthy immune systems. It is recommended for people at high risk: health care workers, sexually active homosexual men, patients who receive transfusions of blood, such as hemophiliacs, intravenous drug users, people receiving hemodialysis treatments, and household members or sexual partners of those who are hepatitis B carriers.

At least two other hepatitis viruses exist. They are grouped together and called *non-A/non-B hepatitis* viruses and involve a variety of symptoms and transmission methods similar to those of hepatitis A and B.

Many people who become infected with these strains develop acute hepatitis and recover, whereas others carry the virus but show no symptoms. Non-A/non-B hepatitis can cause chronic liver problems, including cirrhosis and liver failure.

These non-A/non-B viruses have been so elusive that until recently there was no way to detect their presence in donated blood. A test is now available to detect one of these strains, hepatitis D, and in 1990, a new test developed to screen blood for hepatitis C, which is also transmitted through blood transfusions, was approved by the Food and Drug Administration.

Cirrhosis

When *cirrhosis* occurs, liver cells are damaged or destroyed. As scar tissue forms, the original architecture of the organ is changed, preventing the liver from performing its work.

While excessive alcohol consumption is a frequent cause of cirrhosis, the disease may also occur as a result of hepatitis, chronic heart failure, or chronic obstruction of the common bile duct. Certain drugs and chemicals may also be toxic to the liver and result in cell damage.

Among the signs and symptoms of cirrhosis are enlargement of the liver, jaundiced skin, accumulation of fluid in the abdominal area called *ascites,* nausea, loss of appetite, and the development of small spidery networks of blood vessels on the face, arms, and trunk.

Depending on the cause of cirrhosis, it may be possible to halt the progress of the disease. For instance, if it is alcohol that has damaged the liver, the progress of the disease may be arrested by abstention from alcohol.

Appendicitis

Your appendix is a fingerlike projection at the beginning of your large intestine in the lower right abdomen. We become aware of it only if it becomes infected, then swollen and inflamed, a condition called *appendicitis.* Symptoms may include pain that starts suddenly in the center of the abdomen and spreads to the lower right side. Loss of appetite and nausea may be accompanied by vomiting.

Other conditions produce sudden pain similar to that of appendicitis, and making a diagnosis can be difficult. But it can be vital. Once a diagnosis of appendicitis is made, or strongly suspected, the matter becomes a medical emergency. Treatment is emergency surgical removal of the appendix. Failure to seek treatment creates the serious risk that the infected appendix will rupture, spilling into the abdomen the contents of the intestine, along with bacteria, causing *peritonitis,* a dangerous inflammation of the membrane that lines the abdominal cavity.

Cancer of the Esophagus

When cancer occurs in the esophagus, the rapidly multiplying cancerous cells may narrow your gullet and make swallowing difficult—a condition known as *dysphagia.* If you develop a problem swallowing solid foods, consult your doctor. To diagnose esophageal cancer, your doctor will order an X ray that requires you to drink a preparation made of barium. Further testing includes an examination of the esophagus with a flexible scope, and the removal of a small piece of tissue for biopsy.

Early diagnosis improves the survival rate of esophageal cancer. If the tumor is located in the lower third of the esophagus and has not spread to other parts of the body, surgical removal usually is the recommended treatment, followed by radiotherapy. If surgery cannot be performed, radiotherapy treatments may be prescribed.

Esophageal cancer is uncommon in the United States. If you smoke, you are five times more likely than a nonsmoker to develop cancer of the esophagus. Alcohol also has been associated with esophageal cancer.

Cancer of the Stomach

Although an estimated 23,000 new cases of stomach cancer occur each year, gastric cancer is on the decline in the United States. Diet may play a major role in this form of cancer, but there is no conclusive proof. Having an ulcer on the lining of the stomach doesn't mean that cancerous changes will follow.

Stomach cancer often has no symptoms. As the tumor grows, it may produce symptoms in its later stage, including ulcerlike pain, feeling full after eating a small amount of food, loss of appetite, bloating, difficulty swallowing, vomiting, and weight loss.

Diagnosis includes barium X rays, examination of the stomach with a flexible endoscope, and a tissue biopsy. If the cancer cells are confined to one area of the stomach, surgery is recommended and chemotherapy may also be added. If the tumor is very extensive, surgery may not be performed and only chemotherapy may be administered.

Because the cause of gastric cancer remains unknown, it is difficult to recommend a specific course of prevention. A low-fat, high-fiber diet is believed to have a major role in the prevention of cancer.

Polyps

Polyps are abnormal growths in the mucosal lining of the large intestine. There are various kinds of polyps; some are benign, others may be the precursors of colorectal cancer. Although the presence of polyps is not always apparent, signs to watch out for include blood in the stool and, rarely, watery diarrhea.

If your doctor suspects polyps, diagnosis is usually made via barium enema and colonoscopy examination. Polyps are removed with a specially equipped colonoscope and examined for the presence of abnormal cells. If a polyp is suspected to be an *adenoma,* a biopsy is taken. Depending on the diagnosis, the adenoma may be removed via colonoscopy, or surgery may be required. Following removal, periodic checkups are necessary to look for recurrences or for any changes in the intestinal wall.

Cancer of the Colon and Rectum

The second most common form of cancer in the United States is colon and rectal cancer. Scientific studies suggest that the environment in which you live and work and the diet you eat may have a strong influence on your risk of developing colon and rectal cancer.

The risk of developing colorectal cancer increases slightly at age 40 in men and women, but its incidence is much higher after age 50. Some people may have a higher risk profile, for these reasons: a family history of colorectal cancer or any form of cancer; a family history of developing polyps in the mucosal lining of the large intestine; a personal history of endometrial, ovarian, or breast cancer; and ulcerative colitis.

When cancer cells invade the colon, the main symptoms are a change in bowel movements and habits, bleeding, slowly developing anemia, and, occasionally, pain. Diagnosis is by the same techniques used for polyps—barium enema, a colonoscopy (sigmoidoscopy), and biopsy.

Treatment is surgical removal of the affected part of the colon and rectum. The need for a colostomy, or permanent opening in the abdominal wall from the bowel, depends on the location of the tumor and the extent of the disease. Radiation therapy and chemotherapy may be required as part of follow-up care.

To help prevent colon and rectal cancer, everyone over 40 should discuss the risks, benefits, and costs of screening tests for fecal occult blood and sigmoidoscopy with their regular physician. Increasing dietary fiber and reducing fatty foods may help you reduce your risk of cancer.

If you are over 40 and one of your first-degree relatives (i.e., mother, grandmother, aunt) has colorectal cancer or if you have had endometrial, ovarian, or breast cancer, it is recommended that you have a fecal occult blood test once a year and a sigmoidoscopy every three to five years. If you have a family history of colon polyps or any form of cancer, earlier and more frequent screening for colon and rectal cancer is recommended.

Urinary System

Your kidneys clean your blood at the rate of more than a quart every 10 minutes, filtering out wastes for removal in the form of urine. Depending on the amount of liquid you consume, and how well they're working, your kidneys may expel from less than one quart to more than six quarts a day through the urinary tract.

Urinary Tract Infections

When infectious agents—especially bacteria—gain entry to the urinary tract, these microorganisms can upset the ecology of this normally sterile area and cause a *urinary tract infection,* or *UTI.* Depending on how far the bacteria travel, a UTI may occur without symptoms and clear up on its own, or it can give you more acute symptoms that require medication. UTIs are a common problem for women because the anatomical architecture of the area allows relatively easy access to bacterial invaders. The last exit of your urinary tract is the *urethra,* through which urine leaves the body. Women have much shorter urethras than men— about 1.5 inches compared to 8 or 9 inches—and a greater risk of UTIs. If bacteria enter the urethral tube, infection can spread into the bladder, move up through two narrow canals called the ureters, and settle into your kidneys.

The bacterium responsible for most UTIs is *E. coli,* which is a normal inhabitant of your intestinal tract. When *E. coli* bacteria from a bowel movement travel the short distance from the anal opening to the nearby urethral or vaginal opening in women, infection is likely. Also associated with UTIs are sexual intercourse, pregnancy, and diabetes.

The most common infections are urethritis, cystitis, asymptomatic bacteriuria, and pyelonephritis.

Urethritis is an inflammation of the urethral tube, which carries urine from the bladder for excretion. This condition is very common in both men and women. The symptoms include a frequent urge to urinate although you void only a small amount. There may be a burning sensation while urinating and possibly blood in your urine, which may have a strong odor. There may also be a watery discharge. Chronic urethritis in men may be due to infection with the chlamydia microorganism (see Chapter 4).

Cystitis is a bacterial infection that settles into the bladder. Its symptoms include pain and burning while you urinate and a frequent urge to empty your bladder although you produce very little urine. Another condition, called "honeymoon cystitis," is not cystitis at all. It occurs in about half of all women who had no previous sexual intercourse; the painful urination may be due to irritation, although infection may be the cause of the problem.

Asymptomatic bacteriuria occurs when you have a significant amount of bacteria in your urine, yet show no symptoms of infection. It is a common problem among young and teenaged girls. Routine testing is recommended for asymptomatic bacteriuria using dipstick urinalysis in the following groups: preschool children, people 60 and over, pregnant women, and diabetics.

Pyelonephritis is a kidney infection that is most often caused by bacteria that migrate up the urinary tract from the bladder to your kidneys, though occasionally the bacteria are carried to your kidneys by the bloodstream. Symptoms include pain in the back slightly above your waist, chills and fever, and nausea and vomiting. You may also have painful, burning, and frequent urination.

Whereas some UTIs are so mild that they may resolve on their own, others require medical attention. If you suspect that you have a UTI, see your doctor. Diagnosis includes a sample of urine for laboratory analysis.

If your urine culture indicates a UTI, your doctor will prescribe antibiotics, the most commonly effective treatment. There's a special note of importance here: although medication may relieve your symptoms within a few days, you run the risk of a recurring problem with UTIs if you don't take the *full dosage* of your antibiotics for as long as prescribed.

To help prevent UTIs, practice some good habits: women should always wipe from the front to the back after a bowel movement. Keep the anal area clean and dry—as part of your regular hygiene and especially before sexual activity. Drink lots of liquids—especially water—to help flush bacteria out of your urinary tract. Urinate when your bladder sends the message; if you wait too long, you may be inviting bacteria to grow.

Before engaging in sexual activity, empty your bladder. After sex, try to urinate again to help clear out any bacteria that may have entered your urinary tract. If you've had recurring UTIs and your doctor thinks that the infection is related to sexual activity, you may be advised to use prophylactic antibiotics before or after sex. Other measures you may want to take include wearing cotton underwear and avoiding irritating soaps and hygiene sprays.

Kidney Stones

Each year, well over 300,000—for some reason, more men than women—Americans suffer the pain of *kidney stones,* or renal calculi.

Kidney stones begin to form usually during the 20s and 30s when a microscopic fragment in the urine crystallizes. Gradually, this fragment attracts more undissolved substances and after a period of time, a stone develops. Calcium is one of the most common ingredients of kidney stones, often in combination with other substances. Sometimes, a metabolic abnormality can result in calcium kidney stones, or uric acid stones. Urinary tract infections may also encourage the growth of a kidney stone. Occasionally, stones form for no discernible reason. Some kidney stones may produce no symptoms, while others may pass through the urinary tract in sandlike fragments and cause little pain or, if there's an obstruction, produce severe symptoms.

A common symptom of kidney stones is severe pain, called renal colic, that starts as stabbing pain in one side of the back. As the stone travels through the urinary tract, from kidney to bladder to urethra, the site of the colicky pain shifts to the new location of the stone, until you pass the stone. You may also have blood-streaked urine. If infection is present, other symptoms are likely to occur, such as fever and painful and frequent urination.

Treatment of kidney stones begins with drinking a large amount of liquid (three to four quarts) every day—especially water. This helps dilute your urine and keeps it from becoming too concentrated. When a stone that causes pain or blocks the flow of urine doesn't pass through your urinary system on its own, you'll need further treatment to remove the stone.

Sometimes, medication is used to help discourage stone formation.

Thiazide diuretics may be effective against calcium stones because these drugs increase the amount of urine you excrete and lower its calcium content. Uric acid stones may respond to allopurinol (Lopurin), a medication used to treat gout. D-penicillamine may be used for some cystine (an amino acid) stones.

When these methods fail to eliminate your kidney stone, several innovative techniques can offer relief. *Lithotripsy,* or shock-wave treatment, is highly effective in pulverizing some kidney stones into fragments about as large as sand grains. *Percutaneous stone extraction,* which is done through a needle-sized hole in the skin, uses a radiologically guided instrument to locate the stone and pull it out. If the stone's diameter makes removal difficult, doctors can fire an ultrasound probe to smash it. *Laser therapy* is the newest and simplest nonsurgical treatment for kidney stones—especially those that have reached the lower ureter. If you have a very large stone or an infection, surgery may be recommended, though today such surgery is not common.

Once a stone is removed, your doctor will analyze its chemical composition. After identifying the causative chemical, you will be given a treatment plan to help prevent the development of new stones.

If you've had one kidney stone, you have a strong chance of forming another. Still, you may be able to prevent a recurrence by following a few preventive measures. Your doctor may prescribe some medications to discourage stone development. Drink as much fluid as possible. Specific dietary restrictions depend on the type of stones you form.

Incontinence

A fairly common but rarely discussed problem, one that is a source of much dread and embarrassment, is *urinary incontinence,* or an involuntary releasing of urine from the bladder.

Incontinence is not a disease but a symptom of some other condition that often can be treated and cured. In many cases, it is a temporary problem caused by a local infection of the urinary tract or the use of certain medications. Some women whose pelvic floor muscles are weakened from childbirth suffer incontinence. Men with prostate disorders may have problems with it. If you frequently ignore your body's command to urinate, there is a risk that over a period of time, muscles will weaken and you will develop the problem. Some diseases, such as diabetes, multiple sclerosis, depression, and even prolonged constipation, can result in incontinence.

There are several different types of incontinence. *Stress incontinence* results from weakened tissues around the bladder. A cough, sneeze, laugh, running, or lifting something can result in the release of a small amount of urine.

Urge incontinence is a powerful, uncontrollable, and usually un-expected urge to urinate that results in wetting yourself a little before you can make it to the toilet. *Overflow incontinence* occurs when you dribble a small amount of urine because your bladder is full to the point of overflowing. A condition called *irritable bladder,* in which your bladder contracts uncontrollably, bears a close resemblance to urge incontinence.

Depending on the cause of the problem, doctors use several non-surgical therapies to treat incontinence. If your pelvic floor muscles are weak, exercises can be prescribed to help strengthen the area around the bladder and urethra. "Bladder retraining" emphasizes timed trips to the restroom and muscle-strengthening exercises for the lower urinary tract. Biofeedback is another technique that uses pressure measurement devices in combination with specially prescribed exercises.

When none of these methods work, surgery may be recommended to reposition the bladder neck or to correct an obstruction that blocks the flow of urine. Urologic surgeons can even replace the sphincter, or control muscle at the bottom of the bladder, to prevent the involuntary release of urine.

Prostate Disorders

The prostate gland is a part of the male reproductive system. Because this gland surrounds a portion of the urethra, the tube that carries semen as well as urine from the body, its very location often affects the urinary tract as a man grows older.

The prostate, located just below the bladder in the lower abdomen, is about the size of a walnut. It secretes prostatic fluid that helps sperm to flourish and flow freely during ejaculation.

Your prostate gland may become enlarged at some time during your adult life for various reasons, such as an infection called *prostatitis,* a common but often harmless condition called *benign prostatic hypertro-phy,* or as a result of *prostate cancer.*

Prostatitis.   *Prostatitis* is an inflammation of the prostate gland that may result from an invasion of bacteria, although sometimes its cause is unknown.

Acute prostatitis develops suddenly with such symptoms as fever, chills, pain in the lower back and the perineal area between the anus and penis. Urination may be difficult and painful.

Chronic bacterial prostatitis, one of the most common causes of persistent urinary tract infections in men, begins with milder, although annoying symptoms that tend to linger. This problem brings burning, painful, and frequent urination. You also may suffer pain in the lower back and in different parts of the genital area. The infection will be treated with antibiotics.

Chronic nonbacterial prostatitis is the most common type of prostatitis. It is usually more difficult to treat because its cause is unknown. Some antibiotics have been effective in relieving symptoms. Some doctors recommend massage, sitz baths, or anti-inflammatory medications.

Benign prostatic hypertrophy (enlarged prostate). At puberty, the prostate gland begins to grow, until it weighs just under one ounce by age 20. For unknown reasons, it continues to increase in size until by the time many men reach 40, they have signs of an enlarged prostate. By age 50 and over, between half to three-quarters of all men experience symptoms of *benign prostatic hypertrophy* (BPH), or an enlarged prostate.

When the prostate increases in size, it can compress the urethra and obstruct the free flow of urine. Typical symptoms include difficulty in starting the flow of urine, a weak stream, frequent voiding of small amounts of urine, and dribbling urine after you thought you had emptied your bladder. In rare cases, it may be impossible to urinate at all—a condition that can lead to acute kidney failure if left untreated.

Although this disorder is usually not dangerous in itself, it can create other more serious problems. It can cause cystitis or, if an enlarged prostate impedes the flow of urine, it can lead to a kidney infection. Or, it may result in the accumulation of urine in your bladder until it overflows involuntarily, causing incontinence.

Once prostatitis is ruled out, the only treatment to correct an enlarged prostate is a commonly performed surgical procedure called a transurethral resection, or prostatectomy. Doctors insert a thin, flexible tube with a fiberoptic lens into the penis and locate the area of enlarged tissue. They then send a delicate cutting instrument through the tube to clear away part of the gland.

A transurethral resection normally doesn't interfere with sexual ability. In a small number of cases, incontinence may follow a prostatectomy.

Prostate cancer. More men suffer from an enlarged prostate than from *prostate cancer*. At the same time, prostate cancer is the second most common cancer to plague American men and a major cause of death; each year, about 96,000 new cases are reported.

Because the risk of prostate cancer increases with age—beginning around age 50—and because early detection improves the chance of a cure, rectal examinations should be a part of your routine physical checkup. In most rectal examinations, the doctor inserts a gloved finger in the rectum to check the nearby prostate gland for any abnormal changes. A newer test employs an ultrasound probe to examine the prostate tissue. If cancer is suspected, a biopsy is taken.

When this type of cancer is detected in its early stages, the disease is usually confined to the prostate gland. Treatment is either through removing the entire gland and the adjacent lymph nodes or through radiation therapy. Both approaches offer cures as well as their own possible complications, such as painful urination, incontinence, and impotence. Discuss the benefits and risks of each treatment with your doctor before making a decision.

Endocrine System

Your endocrine system controls your body by deploying hormones—which operate as chemical messengers—into the bloodstream to deliver those hormones to your cells. Hormones team up with your nervous system to help keep your metabolism—or the rate at which the cells burn fuel—working efficiently. Occasionally, an endocrine gland may produce too much or too little of a hormone and upset the balance. The most common endocrine disorder is diabetes, followed by thyroid disease.

Diabetes Mellitus

Diabetes mellitus, commonly known as *diabetes,* affects about 11 million Americans. In diabetes, your body can't control the amount of sugar (glucose) in your blood for one of three reasons: either there isn't enough insulin being produced by the pancreas, the cells fail to respond to insulin (insulin resistance), or a combination of those two.

Normally, your pancreas continuously produces small amounts of insulin, with increased production of this hormone after you eat. As soon as your body converts carbohydrates into glucose, insulin makes it possible for the cells to tap into this most basic source of fuel necessary for energy. When insulin is in short supply, your cells can't access the glucose they need and the unused glucose stays in your bloodstream. After several years, there may be damage to tissues, organs, and nerves throughout your body. Severe complications or even death may occur if diabetes isn't properly managed.

Diabetes that goes undiagnosed or is poorly controlled can make you more vulnerable to blood vessel damage, kidney failure, stroke, blindness, and the nerve damage of peripheral neuropathy (see page 233).

There are two major types of diabetes, although some people with the disease don't belong in either category.

Type I insulin-dependent diabetes typically begins during childhood, adolescence, or young adulthood. This type is also called juvenile-onset diabetes. However, in some cases younger people may develop the maturity-onset form of the disease—type II diabetes—and some older adults may get type I diabetes. In type I diabetes, the insulin-manufacturing cells inside the pancreas (the islets of Langerhans) produce very little or no insulin. The cause of type I diabetes is unknown, although heredity, viral infections, and autoimmune disorders that prompt the body to attack its own insulin-producing cells all may play a role. About 10 percent of all diabetics in the country have type I diabetes.

Type II noninsulin-dependent diabetes usually occurs after age 40. About 90 percent of all people with diabetes have this form of the disease, in which the pancreas still produces insulin, sometimes in higher than normal amounts, but for some reason the cells can't effectively use it to burn carbohydrates. Some people may have a higher risk of developing type II diabetes, especially native Americans, blacks, Hispanics, and older Americans (more often women than men). The major risk factors include obesity (being 20 percent or more overweight) and a family history of diabetes. Unlike type I diabetes, in which symptoms start abruptly, type II diabetes is much more subtle and may have no symptoms. An estimated 5 million people have type II diabetes but don't know it.

Some women may develop *gestational diabetes* during their pregnancies. This temporary condition increases the risk of bearing an abnormally large infant, having a premature delivery, and *preeclampsia,* a condition marked by fluid retention during the advanced stages of pregnancy. Gestational diabetes also may put the mother at risk for the later development of type II diabetes. Pregnant women are routinely tested for glucose intolerance between the 24th and 28th weeks of pregnancy. If screening tests confirm the presence of diabetes, preventive care may be able to reduce the risk of a complicated delivery.

All these forms of diabetes can share common symptoms. They include frequent urination, excessive thirst, fatigue, increased appetite, vaginal infections or itching in the genital area, and a lower resistance to infection. Other symptoms are blurred vision, tingling in the hands and feet, and impotence in men. Weight loss may accompany type I diabetes, whereas weight gain is typical for type II diabetes.

If you have any of these symptoms, see your doctor about the possibility that you may have diabetes. Diagnosis includes taking a blood sample to measure the amount of glucose in your blood. If your blood glucose level isn't high but there is glucose in your urine, diabetes is still a possibility. In this case, you will need to return for an oral glucose tolerance test to confirm the diagnosis. This involves drinking a certain amount of glucose followed by blood samples to determine whether your blood sugar levels are too high.

If you are diagnosed as having diabetes, you can expect to live a relatively healthy and productive life as long as you take responsibility for controlling your disease. Good control of blood sugars may avoid some of the complications. Depending on the type of diabetes you have, your doctor will prescribe the appropriate treatment.

Type I diabetes requires daily insulin injections, a well-planned diet, and carefully timed meals and snacks. The treatment varies depending on your life-style and your health. For instance, regular physical exercise may yield the benefit of a reduced daily dose of insulin. Illness or stress may require increased amounts of insulin.

Insulin must be taken exactly as directed according to a carefully coordinated plan. While this medication can't cure diabetes, it can effectively control it. Missed injections or infections can cause the buildup of acidic substances called ketones in the blood. When the ketone level becomes dangerously high, it causes a condition known as diabetic ketoacidosis that can lead to coma. Apathy, thirst, nausea, and vomiting usually precede the loss of consciousness. Diabetic ketoacidosis requires treatment in a hospital.

A common problem that may result from taking insulin is a sudden lowering of blood sugar—called hypoglycemia—which may make you feel faint, sweaty, shaky, anxious, and produce the sensation of pins and needles around your mouth. If this happens, eat something sweet immediately. Ignoring hypoglycemia can result in loss of consciousness. Coma—or prolonged unconsciousness—is a medical emergency.

Type II diabetes usually can be treated successfully by controlling your diet (both the type and the amount of food you eat), losing excess weight, and exercising. When dietary control doesn't work, oral hypoglycemic agents may be prescribed. A small number of people with this kind of diabetes may need to take insulin.

There is strong evidence that it may be possible to prevent type II diabetes and its complications. Overweight people have about a three times higher incidence of type II diabetes than do normal-weight individuals, according to a 1985 National Institutes of Health panel. An excess of fat increases your body's resistance to the action of insulin. The aging process may also have a role in making your cells insulin-resistant. Weight reduction appears to be effective in reversing the abnormal changes that occur in type II diabetes. Exercise also has long been advocated as a part of the treatment for diabetes.

Dietary therapy is a key factor in diabetes management, according to the 1988 Surgeon General's Report on Nutrition and Health. Reducing dietary fat and simple sugars and emphasizing complex carbohydrates and fiber may be able to help restore a more normal balance of glucose and insulin in your bloodstream. Because most doctors are not trained in nutrition, many will refer you to a registered dietitian or certified nutritionist, who can create an appropriate diet for you.

If you have diabetes, you can remain healthy with self-discipline and self-monitoring of your blood sugar. Along with sticking to your diet regimen, exercising, and carefully following your medication schedule, you'll need to practice excellent hygiene. Keep your skin clean and pay special attention to your feet. An ingrown toenail, a small blister, or a cut could progress into a serious infection. Use caution with alcohol. And don't smoke—nicotine can constrict your blood vessels and increase the symptoms of poor circulation in your feet.

You can learn how to test your own blood sugar by using a blood-glucose-test kit. This allows you to monitor your treatment plan on a day-to-day basis.

Hypoglycemia

Hypoglycemia, or low blood sugar, is sometimes seen in diabetes, but it is usually indicative of some other disorder. Hypoglycemia is commonly—but mistakenly—thought to be associated with eating large amounts of sugary foods.

Symptoms such as fatigue, insomnia, weakness, dizziness, and many other common problems often have been attributed to hypoglycemia. In fact, the true symptoms of hypoglycemia are sweating, trembling, anxiety, and irritability accompanied by a documented recording of low blood sugar.

If you are a diabetic who takes insulin, you may experience a hypoglycemic reaction when you take too much insulin, stray from your meal plans, or exercise too vigorously.

Fasting hypoglycemia may occur in otherwise healthy people who miss one or two meals and then drink alcohol on an empty stomach. Other causes include reactions to certain medications, tumors of the insulin-producing cells in the pancreas, liver and kidney disease, hormonal disorders, and autoimmune abnormalities of the body's receiving sites—called receptors—for insulin.

Functional or *reactive hypoglycemia* is associated with symptoms that occur after meals. A leading cause of this type of hypoglycemia is previous stomach surgery; a disorder called the "dumping syndrome," in which fluids move too rapidly through the stomach, may result. In some cases, the cause is unknown.

To make a diagnosis, your doctor will need a description of your symptoms and some blood samples to analyze your glucose levels. Oral glucose tolerance tests are rarely helpful in diagnosing hypoglycemia because the results tend to be highly variable and even healthy people without symptoms can achieve hypoglycemic blood levels.

Treatment of fasting hypoglycemia involves correcting the underlying problem that is causing the condition. The reactive form of the disorder often responds to adjusting your diet and mealtimes. Instead of three meals a day, eating six smaller meals can help maintain your blood sugar levels. A diet that emphasizes fiber and complex carbohydrates with moderate amounts of protein may help slow down the absorption of glucose. Avoid simple carbohydrates that contain sugar except as an antidote to a hypoglycemic reaction.

If you have diabetes, you should know the signs of a hypoglycemic reaction and how to deal with it yourself. Always carry hard candy, sugar cubes, or glucose tablets to take at the first sign of a hypoglycemic attack.

Thyroid Disease

The thyroid gland rests with its two winglike lobes perched against the windpipe in the bottom part of your neck. From this command post, it produces thyroid hormone which helps regulate important aspects of your body's metabolism and helps determine how fast you burn up calories. Occasionally, your thyroid gland may produce too much or too little of the hormone and result in *thyroid disease.*

An overactive thyroid gland causes a condition called *hyperthyroidism,* which accelerates your metabolic rate. An underactive thyroid gland results in *hypothyroidism,* or a slowing down of many of your body processes.

Women have a higher incidence of thyroid disease. Older adults may have vague symptoms such as forgetfulness that actually stems from reduced thyroid production. Thyroid disorders often go unrecognized, are dismissed as part of aging, or are misdiagnosed as some other condition.

A possible cause of thyroid disease is an autoimmune disorder in which the antibodies that are supposed to protect you from infection attack your thyroid tissues instead. A condition called Graves' disease can overstimulate the thyroid gland, while another disorder, Hashimoto's disease, is a common cause of reduced thyroid function.

Hyperthyroidism may cause several signs and symptoms. Among these are restlessness, irritability, mood swings, difficulty sleeping, intolerance to heat, moist skin, tremors, shortness of breath, and muscle weakness. Irregular heartbeats, more frequent bowel movements, weight loss accompanied by increased appetite, and protruding eyes are other key symptoms.

The symptoms of *hypothyroidism* are pretty much the opposite. They include lethargy and tiredness, weight gain despite a decreased appetite, intolerance to cold, dry skin, difficulty with memory, swelling of the hands, feet, and face, muscle cramps, and constipation. The voice also may begin to sound husky. Women often experience heavier menstrual periods.

There is also a form of transient hyperthyroidism that is essentially self-limiting. *Subacute thyroiditis,* or subacute granulomatous thyroiditis, occurs fairly commonly between the ages of 30 and 60—usually more often in women. The cause of this condition is not known. Symptoms include enlargement of the thyroid gland, fever, chills, and malaise. There may be pain in the neck or ear or difficulty swallowing. Treatment may call for a mild analgesic such as aspirin. Prednisone may also be prescribed.

To make a diagnosis, your doctor will first examine your thyroid gland to check for signs of enlargement. A sample of blood will be taken for laboratory analysis of your thyroid function.

If you have a thyroid hormone deficiency, your doctor will prescribe a thyroid replacement supplement. After medication is begun, your doctor will periodically retest your thyroid function to adjust the level of your thyroid supplement.

Treatment for an excess of thyroid hormone (hyperthyroidism) may be done in two stages. The first line of treatment is antithyroid medication that suppresses thyroid hormone, such as propylthiouracil (marketed under its generic name) and methimazole (Tapazole). In many cases, drug therapy can relieve the symptoms and bring about a remission of the disease. Unfortunately, hyperthyroidism recurs in over 50 percent of patients after the drug is discontinued.

When medication is ineffective, radioactive iodine given by mouth is often used. The radioiodine is absorbed by the thyroid cells and destroys part of the gland. Surgery may be required in resistant cases or in people with very large thyroid glands. One concern with the surgical and radioiodine treatments is that the patient may develop hypothyroidism. If this occurs, thyroid replacement medications must be taken for life.

Postpartum thyroiditis, a painless form of the disease, can also cause transient hyperthyroidism and hypothyroidism. This disorder usually occurs within the first six months after delivery.

Bones, Muscles, and Joints

It's our bones, muscles, and joints that keep us in motion. Yet just being in motion—walking, working, exercising—can invite such common maladies as muscle cramps, joint pain, a bruised bone, stiffness, or back pain. Even getting too much bed rest can cause problems.

Many of these minor aches and pains disappear on their own or respond to self-treatment. It's important to be able to recognize the difference between a self-limiting problem and an injury that may get very much worse without medical treatment. Severe or persistent pain, swelling or limited ability to move a joint, and numbness should tell you that the injury requires a doctor's attention. How severe? How persistent? In some cases, it comes down to a judgment call.

When you stretch or partially tear a muscle or tendon by overexercising or overworking it, the injury is called a *strain*. A "pulled muscle" is just a muscle strain. Tiny tears appear in the muscle or tendon fibers and cause pain, swelling, and tenderness. Of the hundreds of muscles in your body, you are most likely to strain those in your upper arm, thigh, and back. Usually, a strained muscle can continue to be used, although the muscle may not work very efficiently and attempting to use it may be painful. A severely strained or ruptured muscle, which can be stiff, extremely painful, and severely swollen, requires treatment by a doctor.

A *sprain* is a stretch or partial tear in one of your ligaments, those tough cords of tissue that hold together bones, cartilage, and other tissues. A sprain may produce skin discoloration, and if the injury is severe, the joint may also look misshapen. Depending on the severity of a sprain, you may not be able to place any weight on the injured joint. If you have severe and persistent pain, seek medical care. Only by examining the joint—in some cases only by taking X rays—can a doctor distinguish between a serious sprain and a fracture. Sprains are usually treated by immobilizing the joint, usually by wrapping the area with a supportive bandage. If you have a fracture or chipped bone, a cast may be necessary.

Mild strains and sprains often respond to self-treatment. Remember the *RICE* rule: *R* for rest, *I* for ice, *C* for compression, and *E* for elevation. Rest the injured area. Apply ice to help reduce swelling and pain. Ice, which is effective only during the first 24 hours following an injury, works best when applied at regular intervals in an icepack or wrapped in a towel. After this 24-hour time period, apply moist heat at regular intervals to assist with the healing process. Compressing the area may help support the injured soft tissue. If you use an elastic bandage or strap the area with tape, make it snug but not too tight. Finally, elevate the injured area so that fluid can drain away from the area instead of collecting and causing swelling.

If you have suffered what you think is a mild injury, consider the first 24 hours afterwards as an official observation period. If the area feels and looks worse, consult your physician.

Dislocations

A bone popping out of its socket in a joint—usually at the shoulder, finger, elbow, knee, or hip—is called a *dislocation*. The affected joint stops working, becomes very painful and swollen, and may be discolored. Most often, the dislocation is caused by some injury to the area, but it is possible to experience spontaneous dislocations of the shoulder or jaw.

If you dislocate a joint, never attempt to reposition the injured area yourself. Seek medical attention. If the joint is partially dislocated, a doctor can manipulate it back into place. A sling may be applied to minimize strain on the healing joint. After a period of rest, normal range of motion gradually returns.

When the dislocation is serious or accompanied by a fracture, repositioning of the joint may have to be done under general anesthesia. When damage is extensive, the joint may have to be immobilized to allow healing to take place.

Fractures

A *fracture,* or break in a bone, may be caused by a variety of injuries—a fall, an automobile accident, a sports mishap, and even the physical stress of running.

Doctors have created categories of fractures. A simple fracture involves very little damage to the surrounding tissues. A compound fracture involves significant damage to the skin and tissues. The affected area may look deformed; in some cases a part of the broken bone protrudes through the skin. In a comminuted fracture, there are shattered pieces of bone around the break. When a child breaks a bone, the injury is often called a greenstick fracture because the elasticity of young bone gives it a tendency to bend and break incompletely.

Runners whose feet and leg bones constantly pound the ground occasionally suffer a partial fracture—also called a stress fracture—a hairline crack in a bone that often doesn't show on X rays until several weeks after the injury. If you have a stress fracture, rest is the only treatment that promotes healing.

Symptoms of a broken bone usually include severe pain that gets worse when you try to move the area, and swelling. Bruising may occur either at the time of injury or later. An injury that you mistake for a bad sprain may turn out to be a fracture.

If it seems that someone with you has broken a bone, seek medical attention at once. While you are waiting for help, keep these first-aid tips in mind:

• Placing wrapped ice on the injured area may help reduce swelling and pain.
• Don't try to move anyone whose back may be injured; even the slightest movement could result in permanent neurological damage.
• If the fracture is severe, don't give the injured person anything to eat or drink; doctors may need to administer general anesthesia to realign the broken bone.
• If the injured area is bleeding, apply a clean cloth to the area and apply direct pressure.

If you do suffer a fractured bone, here is what you can expect. After the diagnosis is confirmed with X rays, a simple fracture is treated by realigning the bone back—a process known as closed reduction. Guided by X rays and his or her tactile sense, a doctor will set or reposition the broken bone.

Open reduction is a surgical procedure that is usually done under general anesthesia. The skin and tissue surrounding the fracture are opened to allow full view of the fractured area. Besides repositioning the broken bone, the doctor may install a plate or pin to promote stability around the fracture.

Compound fractures that break the skin run a high risk of introducing a bone infection called *osteomyelitis*, as bacteria gain easy access through broken skin around the protruding bone. If left untreated or improperly treated, osteomyelitis can result in serious and possibly permanent bone damage.

Though doctors often immobilize a repositioned bone with a soft cast of one kind or another, most now encourage limited exercise as soon as possible as part of the treatment for fractures. Be sure to ask just which exercises you can do to help keep the muscles in the injured area from wasting away and your joints from becoming stiff.

Fractured bones heal at different rates. Age is one factor: children's bones heal more rapidly than adults. Another factor is the location of the affected bone. A long bone in your arm or leg surrounded by muscle usually heals faster than a fracture in a joint, such as a broken hip.

Muscle Cramps

When the fibers in a muscle suddenly contract or go into spasm, it causes what is commonly known as a *muscle cramp*. Taking exercise to a point that a muscle is overly fatigued often causes cramping, as does staying in a position that constricts the movement of a muscle for a long time. Most cramps produce intense pain but disappear within a few minutes. To help relax the cramped muscle and relieve the pain, gently massage the area. Be careful not to stretch the painful area too far; remember that the cramped muscle is resisting being extended and can be damaged if you engage it in a tug of war.

Tendon Injuries

Tendinitis, an inflammation of the tendons in a certain area, comes about through overuse of those tendons. Tendons are bands of tissue that link some muscles with bone. Tiny tears appear, and if the area is subject to continued use, the inflamed tendons become painful and tender. The shoulders and heels are most often affected. Rest is the first line of treatment. An analgesic may help relieve the pain. After a period of rest, gentle stretching may help prevent stiffness. If the pain persists after rest or gets worse, see your doctor.

Epicondylitis is the inflammation of the muscles around the elbow. It is usually twisting motions of the wrist that put the strain on the elbow muscles. The varieties of epicondylitis are identified by the sports in which they are most often found. When the pain occurs on the outer side of the elbow, it is called *tennis elbow*. When it occurs on the inner side, it is called *golfer's elbow*. But you don't have to be an athlete to suffer this ailment. If you work with carpentry tools, do a lot of yard work, especially raking, or play other sports—including baseball, bowling, and cross-country skiing—you may find youself being told you have tennis elbow or golfer's elbow without ever having played the sport. Rest may relieve the pain, but if it persists, consult a doctor.

When the casing around some tendons, especially those in the hands—becomes inflamed, we call it *tenosynovitis*. Repetitive motion such as typing or working on an assembly line may increase the risk of tenosynovitis. Other possible causes are infection and rheumatoid arthritis. When an affected finger stays bent in a rigid position, as if you had just pulled a trigger, this condition is also known as "trigger finger." Symptoms include pain and swelling, which usually go away with rest. But even after healing takes place, the area may remain tightened up, with movement difficult. If you have severe and recurring pain, see your doctor.

Back Pain

Back pain is one of America's most common afflictions. It has been estimated that most of us will suffer a backache severe enough to disable us at least once during our lifetimes. Here is one affliction where your age is not against you; studies indicate that people under 45 are sidelined by back complaints more frequently than older people.

There are many causes of back pain. Among them are physical stress, poor posture, a fall, a sudden strain, arthritis, a herniated disk, infection, osteoporosis, and benign and malignant tumors.

Most back pain occurs in the lumbar region, or lower back. Muscle strains, sprains, and spasms may produce pain and stiffness that limit your ability to get around. Rest, analgesics, and moist heat applications usually help relieve the pain. Very often, whether you seek medical help or not, low back pain improves on its own over a period of several weeks.

When your back injury produces severe pain, especially when the pain cannot be relieved by changing position, call your doctor and explain your symptoms. Prolonged numbness or tingling in an arm or leg, pain that radiates down an arm or leg, weakness in a muscle of the arm or leg, and pain in your back while resting may indicate that medical treatment is necessary.

Diagnosis requires a physical examination and a medical history to help determine the circumstances surrounding your symptoms. Your doctor will test your reflexes and check for muscle weakness. If your back pain came after a fall or an accident, or if your doctor suspects that a slipped disk is causing the problem, he or she may want to order X rays, a CT scan (computerized tomography) or an MRI (magnetic resonance imaging). Blood tests may also be necessary if infection, a metabolic problem, or a tumor is suspected.

As part of the treatment for back pain, many orthopedic specialists now recommend special daily exercises to strengthen the lumbar and abdominal muscles and to improve posture. Rest is an important part of the early stages of treatment, but getting too much rest may weaken your muscles at a time when they need to be strengthened.

If you have poor posture, or work in a job that requires repeated lifting, or if you must spend several hours a day driving a car or truck, you have a higher risk of low-back injury. Once you have a history of back pain you are at greater risk no matter your job. So, try to avoid that first injury.

To help prevent back injuries and relieve chronic low-back pain, it is recommended that you maintain your ideal weight and practice back-conditioning exercises. You might want to think about going to a back school. Back schools teach you how to sit, stand, sleep, and lift, with an emphasis on preventing injury. Some employers sponsor such schools for their workers; many hospitals and YMCAs all around the country conduct them. Fees vary. If your doctor recommends a back school your health insurance may pick up part or all of the cost.

You may prefer to begin your own exercise program to strengthen your back. People who exercise regularly may have a lower incidence of back pain. But before you start, be sure to get clearance from your doctor, as you should before beginning any exercise program.

Herniated Disk

The bones in your spine (vertebrae) are stacked on top of one another to form a column. Separating each vertebra is a cushion of pliable cartilage on the outside and a gelatinous material inside. Injury, wear and tear, poor posture, and aging may cause the gel inside to seep through the tough cartilage exterior and press on a nerve. When this happens, the condition is called a *herniated disk,* commonly referred to as a slipped disk.

Symptoms include pain in the affected part of your spinal column—most commonly the cervical, or neck, area or the lumbar region of your lower back. You may feel a dull ache in your neck or back, as well as stiffness. There may be numbness or tingling in an arm. Pain may start in the hip and typically shoots down the back of one leg, indicating *sciatica*.

If you have these symptoms, consult a doctor. The diagnosis includes a physical examination and a history to help establish the cause of your pain. In some cases, the physician may recommend diagnostic imaging tests (X rays, computerized tomography, or magnetic resonance imaging) to rule out other possible causes of your pain.

Treatment usually includes bed rest, anti-inflammatory drugs, and muscle relaxants. If the herniated disk is in the cervical spine, the neck area, a cervical collar may relieve and lessen the pain. In severe cases that affect the lower back, traction may be helpful. If the gelatinous inner material continues to protrude, surgery may be recommended. A small number of medical centers have successfully treated ruptured disks with injections of the enzyme chymopapain (Chymodiactin), which shrinks the damaged disk. A major risk with chymopapain is that in some patients it may produce anaphylactic shock, a life-threatening condition. Its use remains controversial.

To help protect your back from chronic pain and injury, practice good posture. Avoid becoming overweight because the additional weight places a great deal of stress on your back as well as distorting your posture. If you have rounded shoulders, you may be able to correct this condition with special exercises. In some cases, a brace may be helpful. Get regular physical exercise to help improve the strength and endurance of your back muscles.

Spondylosis

Degenerative changes in the disks between the vertebral bones in your back may cause your spinal column to become stiff and less flexible. This condition is known as *spondylosis,* or degenerative arthritis. Wear and tear and the loss of elasticity that come with aging are the usual causes of this condition.

When spondylosis is mild, there may be no symptoms. If a vertebral bone becomes flattened as a result of spondylosis, it may produce a small bony ridge or spur that presses on a nerve located near the spinal cord. If the pain is severe, surgery may be recommended to remove the ridge of bone.

Diagnosis includes a physical examination and X rays or diagnostic imaging to get a clear picture of the painful area. Sometimes there may be numbness or weakness in a limb, which disappears following treatment, only to recur. Conservative management, with rest and possibly traction, usually works. When neurological symptoms persist, surgery may be necessary.

Arthritis

If you have aching and painful joints, your problem may be nothing more than a temporary inflammation of a ligament, tendon, or one of the small sacs around the joints called bursae. But very often, joint pain is caused by one of the more than 100 forms of *arthritis*. This inflammatory joint disease causes pain that ranges from mild to severe and, depending on the type of arthritis, may even be crippling. Arthritis damages cartilage as well as other tissues and eventually may destroy the affected joint.

Among the more common forms of arthritis are *osteoarthritis, rheumatoid arthritis, gout, ankylosing spondylitis,* and *infectious arthritis.* Arthritis also may occur as the result of an injury, or as a complication of another disease, such as systemic lupus erythematosus, Lyme disease, psoriasis, ulcerative colitis, sickle cell anemia, or diabetes.

Early treatment of arthritis usually yields the best results, so seek medical attention when you notice the first symptoms of the disease, and you'll have a better chance of controlling arthritis. Although there is no cure for arthritis, there are a number of measures your doctor can recommend to help relieve your symptoms and possibly delay the progress of the disease.

Osteoarthritis

The most common cause of joint pain is *osteoarthritis,* also known as degenerative joint disease. This is a noninflammatory condition in which small breaks develop in the cartilage pads at the ends of bones where joints form. As the cartilage buffer deteriorates, the unprotected bone ends may grate together. Or a small ridge of bone may form in the joint.

Many factors play a role in degenerative joint disease, including constant use of the joint, repeated injury, normal aging, excess weight, and even your genes.

Joints in weight-bearing areas are most vulnerable to osteoarthritis— the hips, knees, feet, and spine. The finger joints, mainly the knuckles nearest the fingernails, are also frequently involved. If one of your legs is a little bit longer than the other, the joints in your knee, hip, or foot are subject to special wear and tear and may begin to deteriorate.

Symptoms usually include pain and stiffness when you exercise the joint. The pain normally goes away after resting for less than 30 minutes.

If you experience a great deal of joint pain, see your doctor, who will examine the affected joints. X rays and blood tests may be used to rule out the various forms of inflammatory arthritis, and you may be left with a diagnosis of degenerative joint disease.

Treatment includes pain relievers, such as aspirin or ibuprofen. Because these analgesics can cause gastrointestinal side effects in some people, it is important that you follow the instructions on the label, and that you report any stomach discomfort to your doctor. Because obesity is a common aggravating factor when osteoarthritis affects the hips and knees, weight loss is usually necessary for overweight patients. Ask your doctor which forms of exercise best suit your needs. Avoid any activity that causes pain.

Rheumatoid Arthritis

This disease produces inflammation of the synovium—the thin membrane lining the joint—and eventually may lead to damage of the surrounding tissues. But unlike osteoarthritis, which affects the major weight-bearing joints, *rheumatoid arthritis* can attack connective tissue and certain other organs throughout the body, as well as joints.

Although the cause of rheumatoid arthritis remains unknown, many researchers believe that it may follow infection with a viral agent or be due to an abnormality in the body's immune response. The disease can begin at any age. Adults usually develop rheumatoid arthritis during midlife or earlier. Children suffer from the juvenile forms of the disease, but with the proper treatment and care, most arthritic children have an excellent chance of getting through the painful early years without lasting damage to their joints.

Symptoms of rheumatoid arthritis differ from person to person. Early signs often include fatigue, weakness, and general aching in the muscles and bones. Later, you may notice that certain joints in the hands, wrists, elbows, and shoulders are painful, tender, swollen, and red. There is usually stiffness after sleeping or sitting several hours. The joint may feel more flexible after you move around a little. Although the symptoms most commonly develop over an extended period of time, about one of every five new patients experiences a sudden onset of the disease.

If you develop any of these symptoms, see your doctor. Because inflammatory joint pain may be a symptom of several disorders, your doctor must rule out several diseases before making a diagnosis of rheumatoid arthritis. Doing so may require a series of tests over several visits. However, with prompt and proper treatment, it is possible to get relief for your pain and to help minimize the damage from inflammation that now threatens to occur in your joints.

Treatment includes rest, regular exercise, and the use of aspirin or other nonsteroidal anti-inflammatory drugs to control inflammation. For severe cases, more powerful drugs may be used. These include the antimalarial drug chloroquine (Aralen), injections with gold salts, corticosteroids, penicillamine (Cuprimine), and methotrexate (Folex, Mexate) a drug used to destroy cancer cells. Certain joints can also be treated surgically.

As discouraging as a diagnosis of rheumatoid arthritis can be, it is important that you follow the instructions you receive. By sticking with your treatment program, you are likely to see a definite lessening of your symptoms. Patience, persistence, and a positive attitude go a long way in coping with rheumatoid arthritis. Your symptoms may go into remission only to flare up some other time—or they may disappear. But your best long-range hope is to stay with your program.

Gout

Gout is a form of arthritis that is often caused by a disorder of the body's metabolism. When your body produces more of the waste product uric acid than it can excrete through the kidneys, the leftover uric acid can form tiny crystals in the joints—classically, the big toe—where they form deposits. Other susceptible joints are the ankle, foot, finger, wrist, knee, and elbow areas. When the urate crystals form in the joint, they cause inflammation, making the joint feel painful, swollen, tender, hot, and red. The skin around the joint may look shiny.

There is a hereditary tendency toward developing gout, though the buildup of uric acid in the bloodstream can be the result of many other factors, including overweight, high alcohol intake, a high-protein diet, infection, or disease. Middle-aged men make up most of the gout population. When gout does afflict women, the onset is usually after menopause.

If you have an attack of gout, see your physician. Diagnosis includes an examination of the affected joint and your skin for external deposits of uric acid salts.

Although there is no cure for gout, it is one form of arthritis that is usually easy to control with treatment. Among the effective medications that can help prevent future acute attacks are colchicine (Colabid), nonsteroidal anti-inflammatory agents, and allopurinol (Lopurin).

Gout differs from other arthritic diseases in that it is characterized by acute attacks that are extremely painful but episodic. If you are in an early stage of the disease, you may go a year or more without experiencing another attack. But that doesn't mean the disease has gone away; high levels of uric acid in the blood can still be doing damage to your kidneys. Indeed, gout also differs from most other arthritic diseases in that the treatment regimen for the periods between the acute attacks usually differs from the regimen during an acute attack.

Untreated gout may lead to irreversible kidney disease or high blood pressure, as well as joint damage. Although one person may start at higher risk of developing gout than another, the disorder may affect anyone. You can hold down the risk by avoiding foods that are high in purines, such as liver, by getting rid of excess weight under a doctor's supervision, and by consuming alcohol in moderation.

Ankylosing Spondylitis

Chronic inflammation of the joints of the lower spine and the sacroiliac joints eventually may cause the affected bones in the spinal column and the pelvis to fuse together. Left untreated, the bones keep meshing together until the spine permanently locks into a bent-over position. This disease is called *ankylosing spondylitis*.

The cause of this progressively debilitating disease isn't known, but there is a strong genetic link to what's called the HLA-B27 antigen. Young men, usually whites under 40, are most vulnerable. The symptoms usually include aching in the lower back and morning stiffness that improves with exercise. The aching may resemble a mild discomfort easily dismissed as back strain. Early on, the symptoms may flare up, disappear, and return again. Your eyes may feel achy, watery, and look bloodshot. Other symptoms include fatigue, mild fever, loss of appetite, and weight loss.

If you have what seems to be a constellation of several of these symptoms, see your doctor. Early diagnosis and treatment emphasize keeping the spine flexible, strengthening the back muscles, and practicing good posture. Your doctor can prescribe special exercises or may refer you to a physical therapist to help you work toward preventing your back from becoming permanently deformed.

Infectious Arthritis

When bacteria, viruses, or fungi enter your bloodstream they may cause *infectious arthritis*. Here is one joint disease that can usually be cured, rather than just managed, provided you get prompt diagnosis and treatment.

Bacterial arthritis may be caused by staphylococcus or streptococcus organisms and, in certain settings, the gonococcus bacterium, which also causes gonorrhea. Healthy adolescents and young adults who are sexually active are at high risk for *gonococcal arthritis*. If you experience joint pain, see a doctor. Antibiotics are effective in clearing up the infection.

Lyme arthritis may occur after contracting Lyme disease from the bite of an infected tick. Certain ticks carry a coil-shaped bacterium called a spirochete, which may produce a circular rash that spreads outward from the point of the bite. If you don't notice the tick bite and don't develop a rash, a few days to a month may pass before you develop flu-like symptoms—fatigue, lethargy, fever and chills, and generalized aching. Pain may occur in a few joints, subside, and then flare up in different joints. In the later stages, the heart, nerves, and joints may become involved. Arthritis caused by Lyme disease is painful and may affect several joints. The attacks may persist for several years.

Early diagnosis and treatment of Lyme disease can help prevent the progression of the major complications of the infection, including arthritis. Antibiotics are prescribed to destroy the bacteria. Drug therapy is most effective when given early in the course of the disease. Even with early detection and treatment, the symptoms may persist for a period of time.

To help prevent Lyme disease, avoid tick-infested areas. If you must walk through tall grass and brush, wear long pants and tuck them into your socks. Select light-colored clothing so that if any of these speck-sized insects cling to the fabric you will have a better chance of seeing and removing them. Apply an insect repellant with DEET to your skin and clothing before venturing into fields or woodlands (do a patch test first to make sure you are not allergic). After your outing, check your skin carefully for ticks. If you have pets that go outdoors, brush them daily. A flea and tick collar also helps protect household pets against ticks.

Viral arthritis may develop as a result of infection with hepatitis B, infectious mononucleosis, German measles (rubella), and parvovirus B19, a newly identified virus. Fever, rash, and enlarged lymph nodes are often the first signs of infection. Joint pain may last a few days to a few weeks and usually resolves on its own when the infection disappears. Aspirin is usually prescribed for the inflammation.

Fungal arthritis is often linked with certain environmental conditions. The two most common fungal agents are coccidioidomycosis and histoplasmosis, which enter the body when you inhale fungal spores. Coccidioidomycosis is found in the southwestern United States and Mexico. Histoplasmosis is a problem in some parts of the northern and central United States and in some South American regions. Treatment is with antifungal drugs.

Bursitis

When pressure or injury irritates the bursa, a small fluid-filled sac that provides padding around a joint, an inflammation called *bursitis* may result. Pain and swelling are the main symptoms of bursitis, which affects the kneecap, elbow, shoulder, and hip.

Diagnosis includes a medical history, physical examination, possibly X rays, and bursa aspiration with a needle. When the diagnosis is confirmed, treatment may include rest, aspirin or nonsteroidal anti-inflammatory drugs to control the inflammation, and specially prescribed exercise to maintain range of motion in the joint. For severe pain and inflammation, your doctor may give you a local injection with a steroid medication. If infection is present, antibiotics will be prescribed.

There is a chance that bursitis may recur in the same joint. To help prevent future attacks, your doctor may advise you to eliminate or decrease the activity that led to your first episode of bursitis. If you have been given a prescribed program of exercise after you recover, follow it. By exercising the area regularly, you can help strengthen the surrounding muscles.

Bunions

A *bunion* is a swollen area at the base of the toe that causes pain and makes your foot look distorted. If you wear shoes that are too short, too narrow, or too pointy you may create a lot of pressure in the area. As the poorly fitting shoe forces your big toe to bend in toward the other toes, your foot responds by forming an inflamed protrusion (a bump) to help reduce this pressure.

There appears to be an inherited tendency toward bunions in some people. Women have a greater incidence of bunions than men. The main symptoms are pressure, pain, and the unattractive bony knob that forms on the foot. Treatment ranges from wearing wider shoes and using protective padding to surgery for more severe cases.

The Head and Nerves

Your brain and spinal cord are the main components of your central nervous system. Different sets of nerves that allow you to sense your surroundings, to move your muscles, and to continue the automatic operation of your heart, lungs, and intestines make up your peripheral nervous system. Your nerves constantly send messages to each other, but occasionally the messages get mixed or halted and produce neurological symptoms. A headache, dizziness, numbness in a limb, or pins and needles in your hands or feet may bother you occasionally and have little significance—or they may be a warning that something is wrong.

Headaches

Almost everyone suffers a *headache* from time to time. It's not uncommon that the pain of a severe headache may propel you to a doctor's office, wondering if you have a brain tumor. Yet in most cases, headache pain doesn't signify a serious illness, and you may be able to find relief by taking aspirin or acetaminophen.

There are several kinds of headaches, but tension headaches and migraine headaches are the most common. Other problems can cause headache symptoms: a diseased or sensitive tooth, ear infections, eye-strain or glaucoma, allergies, and certain diseases. Stress, sitting in the same posture too long, and irregular eating and sleeping patterns also may invite a headache.

Tension headaches affect more people than any other kind of head-ache. Symptoms include steady pain, usually in the front and back of the head and in both temples. After starting off as dull pain, the headache eventually feels like a tight band encircling your head. The muscles at the back of your neck may also feel tense. Often these headaches return every day, usually in the afternoon or evening.

Treatment of tension headaches should emphasize rest and relaxa-tion. Lying down for a while or taking a hot bath or shower may help ease your tension. Relief from tension headaches often comes from iden-tifying the cause of your stress and changing the situation or your be-havior to eliminate the problem.

Migraine headache, the other major type of headache, affects ap-proximately one-fourth of American adults. During a migraine attack, the blood vessels that lead to the brain are believed to contract—or go into spasm—and then swell, causing pain and often other symptoms. Because migraine headaches involve the blood vessels, doctors call them vascular headaches.

These debilitating headaches have a tendency to run in families. Migraine often begins in childhood—not as headaches, but as episodes of unexplained stomach pain. For largely unexplained reasons, women are more vulnerable to migraine than men, possibly because of shifts of hormones during the menstrual cycle.

Stimulating factors—weekends, holidays, and vacations—may set off a migraine in people who find it hard to relax. Foods, especially red wine and other forms of alcohol, chocolate, aged cheese, caffeine, nuts, and occasionally the seasoning MSG (monosodium glutamate) may cause headaches. Bright sunlight and getting too much sleep are also implicated as are certain medications—including estrogens and oral contraceptives.

Migraine headaches are divided into *common migraines* and *classic migraines.* In common migraines symptoms may include severe, recurring pain, weakness or nausea, and sensitivity to bright light.

Classic migraine provides its own warning signs—bright, flashing lights in the field of vision, a temporary blind spot, a feeling of pins and needles in the hands or face, difficulty speaking, and numbness on one side of your body. These preattack symptoms (the *aura*) generally precede the headache by about half an hour. These same symptoms also suggest a TIA (transient ischemic attack), or ministroke, so unless you have a history of classic migraines in which these signs have preceded your headache, do not rule out that they may be foretelling a more serious illness.

Typically, you can expect a migraine headache to last from a few hours to one day, although the time frame varies and may be longer. Relief often comes with rest in a darkened room.

Treatment often begins with prevention. By giving your medical history and describing what leads to your migraine attacks, you can help your doctor pinpoint the source of your migraine. Once this is identified, you'll need to avoid that triggering factor. Identifying the cause may take some detective work on your part, such as keeping a diary of what you eat, drink, or do that leads to a migraine attack.

For severe migraines that occur at least once a week, your doctor may prescribe medication to help prevent them. Among the drugs used to treat migraine are beta-blockers, especially propranolol (Inderal); calcium channel blockers; methysergide (Sansert); and the antidepressant drug amitriptyline (Elavil). Ergot preparations also may be prescribed.

Cluster headaches are a form of migraine that are so named because they occur in clusters—appearing once to several times a day with clocklike precision. Medical scientists have yet to determine what causes cluster headaches, or why they affect men more often than women.

Symptoms begin with piercing pain around the nostril or behind the eye that spreads into the forehead. The headache may cause a runny nose and watery eyes. Each attack may last from a half hour to two hours. After several weeks, the cluster headaches often disappear—sometimes for months or years. If you are having an episode of cluster headaches, try to avoid alcohol because it may encourage an attack. The treatment of cluster headaches may include oxygen inhalation, ergot, methysergide (Sansert), prednisone (Deltasone), or lithium.

If you have severe recurring headaches that don't respond to over-the-counter pain relievers, consult your doctor. After hearing your symptoms and taking a detailed medical history, your doctor should be able to make a diagnosis.

Some headaches may signal serious trouble and require prompt medical attention. Here are some symptoms that should not be ignored:

- sudden severe pain in someone who rarely gets headaches
- a headache accompanied by a stiff neck, fever, or sensitivity to light, especially if the headache becomes worse when you try to bend your head forward
- headaches that occur after a head injury, especially if they include nausea, vomiting, and lethargy
- recurring daily headaches that worsen over a period of time

- eye pain, blurred vision, or acute vision changes, such as blindness
- weakness, dizziness, difficulty speaking, and numbness that accompany a headache
- headaches accompanied by projectile vomiting
- severe pounding in the ear

Chronic Fatigue Syndrome

Chronic fatigue syndrome is a mysterious ailment characterized by severe, debilitating fatigue that can linger or periodically recur for several months or years. It usually begins abruptly with a flulike illness, often including sore throat, cough, low-grade fever, and sometimes swollen glands. About two-thirds of the victims are female, mainly white women in their 30s. Most have led active lives before becoming chronically ill.

A major mystery is just what causes it. Most experts believe there are a number of factors, none of which has yet been documented. Viruses, quirks in the immune system, and emotional factors are the current suspects.

The syndrome has gone by several names. In the mid-1980s, it was called "chronic mono" or chronic Epstein-Barr virus syndrome. But researchers now doubt that the Epstein-Barr virus has much to do with most cases of it. Some people know it by its media name, the "yuppie flu" (although people of any age or socioeconomic group can be affected). Whatever the name, it is almost certainly not a new illness. What's new about the ailment, now usually referred to as "CFS," is the large number of people who claim to be affected.

Symptoms and Diagnosis

No laboratory test can detect CFS. Indeed, physical exams and lab tests usually find no abnormalities. There's no effective treatment for it, and no way to predict its course. And a disparate mix of physical and mental symptoms invites debate over just what kind of illness it is.

People who have CFS—and many doctors who treat them—are convinced that it's a physical illness. They stress its sudden onset and flulike symptoms. Others point to the depression and anxiety common in CFS patients and contend that it's a form of emotional illness. Whether physical or emotional, CFS clearly disables. Chronic fatigue is usually accompanied by severe headaches, joint or muscle pain, general muscle weakness, and various psychological complaints—confusion, irritability, inability to concentrate, depression, sleep disturbances, and the like.

A Magnet for Quacks

Skeptical physicians, desperate patients, and a disease that's difficult to diagnose—all combine to make CFS ripe for quackery. Patients searching for cures eventually meet practitioners eager for income. The various treatments prescribed, ranging from homeopathic remedies to intravenous hydrogen peroxide, are useless at best and sometimes may be toxic.

If you have CFS or think you do, you have to walk a fine line when seeking medical care. You want a doctor who is sympathetic and well-informed about the illness. But you need to be wary about promises of cures, because there are none yet. Only one drug, acyclovir (an antiviral agent), has been rigorously tested in CFS patients, and it worked no better than a placebo. A few other drugs are now undergoing clinical trials or soon will be.

For now, the only other drugs that appear helpful against CFS symptoms are those used for treating fibromyalgia, a syndrome characterized by chronic muscle pain and fatigue. Several controlled studies have shown that low doses of tricyclic antidepressants were more effective than placebos in relieving symptoms in fibromyalgia patients. These antidepressants have not yet been rigorously studied in CFS patients, but experts say the drugs may be helpful.

Physicians also advise conservative measures for CFS: a balanced diet, adequate sleep, and avoidance of stressful situations. They recommend gradually increasing regular exercise but caution against overdoing it. Above all, most experts urge patience. Symptoms can wax and wane from day to day, but the general trend is toward stabilization with time. The illness tends to improve after the first year or two, and some people seem to make a complete recovery.

Joining a support group can help. For information about groups in your area, contact the National CFS Association, 919 Scott Avenue, Kansas City, Kansas 66105. Enclose $1 for postage and handling.

Dizziness and Vertigo

Occasional *dizziness,* the sensation of feeling light-headed for a few moments, is a common occurrence usually caused by physical and emotional strain. Working outdoors or playing strenuous sports in the hot sun without replenishing your fluids leaves you feeling dizzy. Drinking too much alcohol can create the sensation that the room is spinning. Jumping out of your chair or bed can create temporary dizziness because your blood pressure hasn't had enough time to adjust to the sudden change of position.

Dizziness may also occur as a symptom of influenza, a head injury, low blood sugar (hypoglycemia), irregular heartbeats, and severe allergic reactions. Some prescription and over-the-counter drugs may cause dizziness. Dizziness associated with a head injury merits immediate medical attention.

Vertigo is not synonymous with dizziness. Vertigo—defined as an illusion of movement—is a neurological disorder in which your body's automatic balance control system goes awry. It makes you feel unsteady—as if either you or your environment is constantly shifting. The disturbance in your equilibrium may occur because of a malfunction in the balance sensors deep inside your ear in the vestibular part of the auditory nerve.

Infection, head injury, and atherosclerosis in the blood vessels leading to the brain may produce vertigo as a symptom. An inflammation of the inner ear called *labyrinthitis* may cause nausea, vomiting, and vertigo. A disorder called *Ménière's disease* often has vertigo as a symptom, along with ringing in the ears, nausea, vomiting, and hearing loss.

Such vertigo-related disorders as *motion sickness* and *height vertigo* may bring symptoms such as sweating, nausea, vomiting, and weakness. *Positional vertigo* often occurs for no apparent reason after you change your physical position. Older adults occasionally experience positional vertigo after turning their heads a certain way, getting out of bed, or shifting their position too quickly.

If you have repeated episodes of vertigo, see your doctor. Diagnostic tests of your hearing and nerve function may be ordered. When the problem is due to bacterial infection, antibiotics may be prescribed, but vertigo that results from a viral infection is usually self-limiting and resolves on its own. If atherosclerosis is impeding blood flow to the brain, your doctor may prescribe anticoagulant drugs.

When the cause of vertigo remains elusive and attacks persist, antivertigo medications may be effective. These include prochlorperazine (Compazine), meclizine (Antivert), and scopalamine (Transderm-Scop), which is administered via patches applied to the skin.

Fainting

Fainting, also known as *syncope,* is a sudden—but brief—loss of consciousness. It occurs when blood flow to the brain is briefly reduced. Fear, anxiety, fatigue, emotional stress, hunger, and pain can cause fainting in otherwise healthy people. Standing in a hot and crowded room, seeing an accident, or hearing upsetting news can make you faint. If you've been sick in bed for several days and get up for the first time, you may faint because your blood pressure needs more time to adjust to your standing position.

Some symptoms that may occur just before you temporarily lose consciousness include a feeling of light-headedness, weakness, nausea, blurred vision, and breaking into a cold sweat. If you notice any of these symptoms, lie down at once—or sit with your head between your knees and breathe deeply.

Fainting may be associated with more serious conditions such as an abnormal heartbeat, heart disease, low blood sugar, diabetes, or anemia, so if you have repeated episodes of fainting, see your doctor. Fainting that occurs for no apparent reason or that accompanies a head injury or convulsion also requires medical attention.

If someone else faints, lay the fainting victim on the floor, with the person's feet raised a little higher than the rest of the body. Loosen any tight collars or constricting clothing. If consciousness doesn't return in a few moments, seek medical help immediately.

Neuralgia

Neuralgia is pain that runs along the course of a nerve. In some cases, the cause of neuralgia is clear. An attack of herpes zoster (shingles) causes a burning pain along the affected nerve of the back or face (see page 251).

Another form of neuralgia that affects older adults is called *trigeminal neuralgia*. It appears that blood vessels press on the trigeminal nerve and send bursts of pain across the lower part of the face. Such simple acts as eating, talking, and brushing your teeth may send off a volley of pain. If you have this kind of pain, see your doctor. To make a diagnosis, your physician must rule out sinus, ear, and tooth infections, but there are medications that help relieve this illness.

Causalgia is a pain syndrome that usually follows a small cut, a broken bone, or injury of a peripheral nerve just below the surface of the skin—usually in an arm or leg. Some time after the injury, the affected limb becomes extremely hot or cold, perspires, and changes color, followed by burning pain. In some cases, the skin may become so extremely sensitive that the touch of a bedsheet or a breeze can cause severe pain. Early diagnosis and treatment produce the best results. Local anesthetics may provide relief. Steroids may be effective when given during the early stages of causalgia. Doctors may also use drugs that block signals transmitted by the sympathetic nervous system and thus reduce the pain of causalgia.

Bell's Palsy

Bell's palsy is a paralysis of the muscles on one side of your face. Doctors can't explain why the nerve that controls the affected facial muscles suddenly becomes disturbed. It's possible that the nerve swells as a result of a viral disease, or reduced blood flow. A popular, although unproven, belief places the blame for Bell's palsy on a draft that gives you a chill.

In addition to the sudden paralysis of one side of your face, other symptoms of Bell's palsy include a flat appearance on the affected side. When you try to smile, your face may look distorted. Sometimes, one eye may remain open.

If you develop the symptoms of Bell's palsy, see your doctor. In making a diagnosis, your doctor must make sure that your sudden paralysis is due to Bell's palsy and not a stroke.

Treatment may include methylcellulose eye drops and an eye patch to help protect an exposed eye from infection. Prednisone (Deltasone) may be prescribed to reduce inflammation around the involved nerve. Your doctor may recommend that you gently massage your facial muscles for brief periods when muscle strength begins returning to your face.

Although Bell's palsy is frightening, most attacks are temporary and tend to clear up completely within several weeks. Though partial weakness may persist in the facial muscles, only in rare cases is there no recovery. If your doctor suspects that your case is severe, electrical tests of your facial muscles may be ordered. Surgery may be recommended to correct the problem.

Transient Ischemic Attacks

A *transient ischemic attack* (TIA) is a temporary decrease in the blood supply to part of the brain. When the blood flow is blocked, the affected areas of your brain can't function normally. TIAs may be caused by a blood clot or a fragment of atherosclerotic plaque that breaks away from an artery wall and temporarily jams blood flow.

During the minutes or hours that a TIA is in progress, you may have such symptoms as sudden visual changes or temporary blindness in one eye, muscle weakness, numbness in an arm or leg on one side of your body, slurred speech, and temporary loss of memory. These symptoms are similar to those of a stroke, but the main difference is that they are milder, last a relatively short time, and disappear spontaneously (see Chapter 6).

TIAs often recur and carry a strong likelihood that a full stroke may be imminent. If you experience TIA symptoms, visit your doctor as soon as possible. Advanced diagnostic imaging using computed tomography (CT) or magnetic resonance imaging (MRI) may help in making the diagnosis.

If an embolus, or traveling blood clot, is found your doctor may prescribe anticoagulant medications, which may include aspirin. Never attempt to treat yourself with aspirin for TIAs because the drug may have an adverse effect.

Treatment emphasizes stroke prevention. Your doctor will determine if you have certain risk factors that need to be controlled. These include high blood pressure, elevated blood cholesterol, uncontrolled diabetes, and cigarette smoking (see Chapter 1).

Carpal Tunnel Syndrome

Carpal tunnel syndrome is a neurological disorder in which the nerve running through a small bony passageway in your wrist, called the carpal tunnel, becomes pinched.

Compression of this nerve has been linked with repetitive motion, such as working on an assembly line, at a computer terminal, industrial piece work, and various jobs that require constant use of the hands and wrists. Some athletes and musicians may also have a high incidence of carpal tunnel syndrome.

Symptoms include numbness and tingling in the hand and fingers. The pain may suddenly shoot up your arm to your elbow, shoulder, or the back of your neck. Typically, the symptoms occur at night and may even rouse you from your sleep. Your hand may feel numb and floppy when you wake in the morning but come back to life after you use it. Simple tasks like writing, making a fist, and holding some objects may become difficult. Sometimes there may be symptoms without any nerve damage, while in other cases, muscles in the thumb and part of the palm may begin to waste away.

Diagnosis includes X rays and nerve conduction studies using electromyelography. Treatment may include rest, wearing a splint to immobilize the area, and injections of steroids or anti-inflammatory drugs to reduce the inflammation. If symptoms continue despite treatment, surgery may be recommended.

It is not certain whether carpal tunnel syndrome can be prevented. You may be able to reduce your risk by finding different ways to perform certain repetitive movements and by taking more frequent rest breaks.

Thoracic Outlet Syndrome

Thoracic outlet syndrome often produces pain and weakness in the arms, hands, and shoulders, especially in women. This disorder is caused by pressure on a network of nerves and blood vessels near the cervical ribs or collarbone. The pressure that causes the problem may come from repeatedly overextending your arms, muscle weakness in the shoulder, fatigue, having an extra cervical rib, or a tumor.

Symptoms include pain, numbness, and tingling in the arms, hands, shoulders, and neck. Your arms and hands may feel weak. If you have these symptoms, see your doctor. X rays and possibly diagnostic imaging will help confirm the diagnosis.

Treatment includes exercise and physical therapy. Aspirin or acetaminophen may help relieve the pain. In some cases, surgery may be recommended.

Peripheral Neuropathies of the Limbs

Damage in the sensory or motor (muscle) nerves outside the brain and spinal cord may produce symptoms of various nerve disorders collectively called *peripheral neuropathy*. Slowly and insidiously, the disorder damages the peripheral nerves that relay information about sensations and movement back to your brain. If left untreated, peripheral neuropathy can destroy the nerve endings in your limbs.

Diabetics often suffer from peripheral neuropathy as a complication of diabetes mellitus. Because a diabetic's tactile ability is reduced, a simple cut may turn into a serious infection because it goes unnoticed.

Possible causes of peripheral neuropathy, sometimes called neuritis, include viral infection, alcoholism, a deficiency in certain vitamins, reaction to certain prescription drugs, cancer, and exposure to toxic chemicals.

An early symptom of this disorder is constant tingling in the toes or fingers that spreads up through the rest of the limb. Numbness follows, usually beginning in the extremities and spreading up toward the trunk. The muscles in your hands and arms may gradually begin to feel weaker. Sometimes, your skin may feel very sensitive and painful around a single nerve.

See your doctor if you have these symptoms. Blood tests and nerve conduction studies (electromyelography) will be necessary to make a diagnosis.

Treatment varies depending on the cause of your neuropathy. If diabetes is the problem, your doctor will recommend a program of careful foot care to minimize the risk of injury, as well as other therapies. When a vitamin deficiency causes neuropathy, vitamin therapy may be administered. Some cases of neuropathy may respond to exercise and physical therapy.

In some cases, poor circulation in the feet and hands may cause numbness and tingling. When this is the case, your doctor may offer suggestions on promoting better circulation. These may include keeping your feet slightly elevated when you sit and not crossing your legs when sitting. Avoid wearing tight stockings. Occasionally, surgery may be necessary to improve blood flow.

Hiccups

An occasional attack of hiccups usually is not a problem, since most episodes disappear on their own or with any number of popular remedies. Some people say they prefer to drink a glass of water quickly, hold their breath, and count to 10; others breathe in and out of a paper bag to help dispel their hiccups. (The paper bag technique is dangerous if a plastic bag is used.)

When hiccups persist for several hours despite your home remedies, see your doctor. Your problem may be the result of an irritation of the vagus nerve, which runs from the brain into your gastrointestinal system. This nerve is responsible for much of the activity of your involuntary nervous system in the chest, abdomen, and intestines. Gastritis, peritonitis, lung disease, kidney disease, an inflammation of the outer lining of your heart, and cancer are among other conditions that may produce hiccups.

When the underlying condition that causes your prolonged hiccups is diagnosed and treated, the problem usually disappears.

Twitching

Rapid muscle movements of a small part of your body—usually the eyelid—are a phenomenon known as *twitching*. A benign condition called *fasciculation* sets a few muscle fibers into quivering. Tiredness or stress usually causes this involuntary movement. Some medications may also produce twitching. In most cases, the problem resolves on its own with rest.

Respiratory System

Your respiratory tract has a strong natural defense system to fight off infection, but viruses, bacteria, and allergens often manage to penetrate these barriers. When they do, you may experience a sore throat, cough, runny nose, sneezing, wheezing, or shortness of breath, some of the symptoms of colds, influenza, and other respiratory conditions that make you feel miserable. In most cases, these symptoms are self-limiting. But sometimes they can signify a more serious condition—a sore throat may really be strep throat; or a cough and shortness of breath may be bronchitis.

Colds

There are about 200 different viruses that cause what may be the most frequently occurring illness on this planet—the common cold. If you are infected with one of these viruses, you will likely develop an immunity to that particular strain of viral infection. This may be part of the reason that people tend to get fewer colds as they get older.

These microorganisms frequently enter your upper respiratory tract but usually don't have a chance at survival because your immune system mobilizes to defend the area. Naturally occurring mucus that coats the upper respiratory tract traps these particles. Fine hairlike cells lining the tract sweep out the viruses before they can latch on to the mucus membrane and cause an infection. But when a virus gains entry and infects a cell in the respiratory tract, the mucus membrane reacts by swelling and producing more mucus, which usually triggers the cough response.

The odd virus that gets through all these defenses incubates for one to five days, depending on the viral strain, before you notice any symptoms. The typical cold sufferer complains of nasal congestion, runny nose, sneezing, sore throat, and, occasionally, hoarseness and cough. Usually, these symptoms disappear within 7 to 10 days.

However, in some cases, complications may arise because of an underlying bacterial infection and lead to strep throat, bronchitis, sinusitis, or earache. If you have an extremely sore throat and notice white or yellow spots at the back of your throat, visit your doctor, who will do a culture for strep throat. This is especially important with children, in whom untreated strep throat often leads to rheumatic fever, with heart-threatening consequences. A deep, mucus-laden cough accompanied by shortness of breath and wheezing may be a sign of bronchitis, another respiratory ailment that should get prompt medical attention.

As with most viral infections, there is no cure for the common cold. Some remedies that may help reduce symptoms and provide some protection against secondary infections include getting rest, drinking plenty of fluids, keeping warm, and eating light meals.

Colds are transmitted from person to person, but we are not sure just how this happens. It may be that virus-laden droplets are released when a cold victim sneezes and then inhaled by those within range of the mist. Or perhaps it's all in the touch—touching the hands, face, or an object with a nonporous surface handled by a cold sufferer increases significantly the likelihood of transmission.

To help prevent a cold infection, wash your hands frequently when around a cold sufferer at home or at work. Your fingers can provide a direct route to your upper respiratory passages, so avoid touching your nose and eyes. Use tissues instead of handkerchiefs and dispose of them immediately.

Influenza

Although the viruses that cause *influenza* enter your body through the upper respiratory tract just as do cold viruses, the symptoms of influenza often cause greater discomfort and complications than those of the common cold.

Both major types of virus—influenza A and influenza B—produce new strains every few years; these new strains are named after the state or country in which they were first isolated. After a flu attack, your body may develop a temporary immunity to the strain with which you were infected, but remain susceptible to the newer strains.

Flu viruses are spread very much the way the cold virus is spread, by direct contact with infected people—by inhaling the mist from their sneezes or coughs or by shaking hands or touching a nonporous surface contaminated with microbes. Signs and symptoms may appear within one to three days after exposure to the flu virus.

The first signs of illness include fever that lasts two or three days, chills, headache, muscle pain, malaise, and loss of appetite. Joint pain may also occur. These symptoms are followed by continued feelings of lethargy and such respiratory complaints as coughing, nasal congestion, runny nose, and sore throat. Although most of these symptoms are gone within a week to 10 days, the cough and tiredness may persist for a few weeks longer.

In most cases, you can let the flu run its course without consulting a doctor. Antibiotics are not prescribed for influenza, because they are not effective against viruses. Treatment usually includes rest, drinking fluids (but not alcoholic beverages), cough suppressants, and a nonprescription pain reliever—aspirin, acetaminophen, or ibuprofen. However, it must be noted that aspirin should *never* be given to a child under 16 who has symptoms of the flu, chicken pox, or any other viral infections. Doing so may cause *Reye's syndrome,* which can be fatal. Rare cases of Reye's syndrome have been reported in adults.

The elderly, diabetics, heavy smokers, people with chronic lung disease, and children may have a higher risk of developing pneumonia if bacterial or viral infection spreads to the bronchial tubes or lower lungs.

If you are in this high-risk group, you may be advised by your doctor to get an annual flu vaccination at the beginning of the flu season in October. Each year, the vaccine's formula is updated so that it offers protection against the most current strains of influenza. Although vaccination is not guaranteed to protect you, it is considered about 80 percent effective.

The prescription drugs amantidine (Symadine) and rimantidine (Flumadine) are effective against the flu—but the protection is limited to type

A. Usually, amantidine is used to supplement the regular vaccine to prevent the flu, although it may be given alone as a treatment.

Bronchitis

Infection or irritation in the lining of the bronchial tubes—the large airways that lead into your lungs—may produce *bronchitis*. The viruses or bacteria occasionally settle in the bronchi and produce a deep cough accompanied by mucus. Other common symptoms include hoarseness, pain in the upper chest that may get worse whenever you cough, and fatigue.

An episode of *acute bronchitis* is usually self-limiting. Treatment with an over-the-counter cough suppressant, consuming plenty of fluids, and rest are recommended for simple cases. If you notice that the mucus you cough up turns from a clear or white color to green or yellow, it may indicate an underlying bacterial infection. For this kind of infection, your doctor may prescribe an antibiotic.

To help prevent acute bronchitis, take care of yourself when you get a cold by getting sufficient rest. Avoid polluted air. If you smoke, quit.

Chronic bronchitis is a persistent state of inflammation of the bronchial lining. Over time, this chronic infection eventually produces changes in the walls of the bronchial passages, including a narrowing of some small airways and congestion from increased mucus production.

Cigarette smoking is strongly connected with simple chronic bronchitis and with the asthmatic form of the disease. It increases the number of bouts of bronchitis and may make them last longer. *Emphysema,* a disease that gradually causes the lungs to lose their elasticity, may masquerade as bronchitis. People who encounter a lot of dust in their jobs, such as miners and grain handlers, tend to have a higher incidence of chronic bronchitis and emphysema.

Early symptoms of chronic bronchitis include a morning cough that contains mucus. As the condition progresses, the cough may persist all day and the volume of phlegm may increase. Wheezing and shortness of breath occur in the later stages. Infection with an upper respiratory virus may worsen the symptoms. Increased smoking and atmospheric irritants may also cause this chronic condition to flare up.

If you are a smoker, you will be advised to stop using cigarettes. Treatment includes antibiotics, medications called bronchodilators that help open the breathing passages, and often corticosteroids.

To help prevent chronic bronchitis from advancing into a disabling condition, avoid smoking and stay away from smoke-filled rooms.

Pneumonia

Pneumonia is a general term that doctors use to describe an inflammation of the lungs. Infection with bacteria, viruses, fungi, or microorganisms called mycoplasmas can cause pneumonia. The disease causes tiny air sacs in the lung called alveoli to become inflamed and fill up with fluid to the point that the normal exchange of air can't take place. The infection typically makes you cough and feel short of breath.

Doctors describe the different kinds of pneumonia based on the type and the extent of infection. The pneumonia may be patchy and affect part of one or both lungs, or it may be lobar, which means it has invaded an entire lobe or area of the lung. Infection of both lungs is called double pneumonia.

Healthy young adults occasionally encounter an infection with an atypical pneumonia commonly known as walking pneumonia. The mycoplasma organism causing this form of the disease spreads from person to person when an infected person sneezes or coughs.

Symptoms vary with the type of infection. Walking pneumonia can take a course so subtle that some sufferers may be misled into thinking they have a lingering cold. A mild fever is usually the first indication of an infection. A few days later, a severe cough erupts—often accompanied by a headache. The chest may feel sore or burning. In the majority of cases, this type of pneumonia is self-limiting. Your doctor may prescribe antibiotics.

The *Legionella* bacterium that causes Legionnaire's disease is responsible for another common form of pneumonia. It is spread through the environment—especially through air-conditioning and building ventilation systems. The symptoms of this type of pneumonia appear 2 to 10 days after infection. They may range from mild, flulike complaints to severe disturbances in major body systems. High fever, diarrhea, and impaired thinking are some of the clues that will make a doctor consider a diagnosis of Legionnaire's disease, which will then be confirmed by isolating the bacterium. Treatment is with antibiotics.

When the pneumococcus bacterium causes pneumonia, the symptoms usually occur within hours after infection. Chest pain and a cough that produces blood-stained mucus are typical. Other symptoms vary and may include fever, chills, nausea, and vomiting.

If you are over 65, have a chronic illness, or if your spleen has been removed, you have a higher risk of developing pneumonia. There is a vaccine that offers protection against the 23 strains of pneumococcal bacteria that are responsible for 90 percent of pneumonia infections. Estimates place the vaccine's effectiveness at 80 percent. In most cases, one dose of the vaccine confers immunity, although some people may need to be revaccinated every six years. Getting a yearly flu shot may offer additional protection.

To prevent a respiratory infection from escalating into pneumonia, call your doctor if over a few days' time the symptoms of a lingering cold get worse rather than better.

Asthma

Nearly 10 million Americans have *asthma,* a condition that creates bronchial spasms, increased mucus flow, and swelling of the tissue lining your airways.

An asthma attack can be a frightening experience because it suddenly produces the sensation of gasping for air without the ability to pull any oxygen into your lungs. Shortness of breath, wheezing, tightness in the chest, and coughing occur during an attack. A small number of people may have mild episodes that amount to nothing more than coughing. Others have attacks that may last up to a few hours.

When asthma begins during childhood and adolescence, it usually can be traced to a seasonal reaction to certain substances and a family history of allergies. Another form of asthma—one not linked to allergens—can develop in adults over 30. Among the triggering factors in adult-onset asthma are respiratory tract infections, especially those caused by viruses; airborne pollutants like fumes and odors; vigorous exercise; sensitivity to aspirin; and emotional stress.

If your doctor diagnoses asthma, effective treatment can be prescribed. Drugs called *bronchodilators* make it easier to breathe by relaxing the muscles around the airways and widening the passages so that air can enter and leave the lungs. Cromolyn sodium (Nasalcrom), a drug that is inhaled, can help prevent asthma attacks in some people. Other drugs that help relieve symptoms of an acute asthma attack include bronchodilators such as theophylline (Bronkolixir) and its derivatives, corticosteroids, and epinephrine (Adrenalin). These medications, which are usually reserved for emergency use, may be given in pill form, as inhalation therapy, or, if the attack is severe enough to require hospitalization, intravenously.

If you have asthma, you may be able to control it by avoiding substances to which you are allergic, taking your medication as prescribed, and following the management plan your doctor tailors for you. If you find that you are having an attack that doesn't resolve itself with your usual therapy regimen, seek medical attention. A severe asthmatic attack left untreated could result in *status asthmaticus,* a serious and often fatal form of asthma.

Lung Cancer

When you inhale cigarette smoke or certain pollutants in the environment, the chemicals you pull into your lungs may linger in the cells that line your breathing tubes. After enough exposure to these inhaled chemicals, the cells undergo changes and may begin to grow abnormally. Eventually, an area of abnormal growth, or a tumor, may slowly grow in the bronchial tubes and then invade the lungs.

There usually are no symptoms of lung cancer until the cancer reaches an advanced stage—often no signs appear until after 20 years of smoking cigarettes. When signs do occur, they may begin as a cough, persistent chest pain, and blood-stained phlegm. If the cancer is not detected until a late stage, cancer cells may have spread to other parts of the body.

When there is early detection and the tumor has not spread, surgery may be effective in some cases. Chemotherapy and radiation therapy are the only other treatments. The cure rate is low.

Screening tests such as X rays and checking samples of sputum for cancer cells are available. However, the routine use of these tests is not recommended for people without symptoms. The tests are expensive and they may not detect a tumor in its early stages. Also, there isn't enough evidence to show that these screenings can cut the number of deaths from lung cancer.

Lung cancer kills more men and women than any other form of cancer. Each year, about 150,000 new cases of lung cancer are diagnosed in the United States. About 85 percent of all cases of lung cancer have been attributed to cigarette smoking.

To help prevent lung cancer, don't smoke. Even if you've smoked for a number of years, you can begin to reverse your risk of lung cancer by quitting. Lung cancer is a largely preventable disease.

The Immune System and Allergies

Your immune system protects your body against infection and disease-causing organisms. But in one of every six Americans, the system over-reacts—not against germs, but against otherwise harmless substances in the environment. Allergies are so difficult a problem because the offending culprits that trigger the overreaction, called allergens, are commonplace: dust, pollen, mold, ragweed, pets, insect stings, food, certain medications, and even sunlight.

When your immune system is first introduced to an allergen, it may produce a protective substance, or antibody, called IgE for immuno-globulin E. The IgE then hooks onto mast cells in the skin, respiratory tract, and digestive system, and to basophil cells that travel in the bloodstream. When the antibody-armed mast or basophil cell next encounters the same allergen, it releases chemical substances—especially histamine—and you have an allergic reaction.

Knowing the difference between an allergy and a cold can make a great difference in terms of controlling your discomfort. In rare cases, one more exposure to an allergen that has caused problems in the past can trigger a reaction so severe that it may even be life-threatening.

The study and treatment of true allergy is a recognized medical specialty. If you develop allergies and your doctor suggests an allergist, be sure to check the specialist's qualifications and credentials.

Skin Allergies

Whether or not you react to airborne allergens, if you brush against a poison ivy plant, your skin will very likely react to the oil in the leaves, by swelling, itching, turning red, and forming fluid-filled blisters. Yet a reaction to poison ivy is only one form of *contact dermatitis*—an allergy triggered by touching certain plants, animals, or chemicals.

Any number of items you use regularly—the metal in some jewelry, particularly nickel, the substances in certain hair dyes and cosmetics, and the components of rubber used in some garments—can provoke allergic contact dermatitis. Oddly, you may have been able to wear or use these items for years with no problem, before you suddenly develop an allergy.

Atopic dermatitis. This type of eczema is often associated with an inherited tendency to develop allergies; episodes in which the skin becomes red, flaky, and extremely itchy occur periodically throughout childhood. Though this disease does not represent an allergic reaction to something that comes in contact with the skin, certain fabrics, soaps, and cleaning agents, and even such normally benign circumstances as a change in temperature or increased perspiration can be a source of irritation. Most often, this disease resolves itself spontaneously during the early teen years but does occasionally recur later in life.

Though this is a self-limiting disease, and certainly not a life-threatening one, it is one in which your doctor will particularly want to treat the symptom, the rash, usually with a topical steroid, to encourage quick healing and thereby avoid the infection often introduced by repeated scratching. If the rash is not promptly cleared up each time it occurs, the cycle of itching, scratching, infection, leading to more itching and scratching, can eventually traumatize the skin and leave it toughened.

Photosensitivity. An allergic reaction to certain wavelengths of ultraviolet light, photosensitivity often occurs in combination with other substances that you put on your skin or into your stomach. If you take certain medications or apply certain fragrances or sunscreens to your skin and go into the sunlight, you may develop a rash, redness, or swelling. This occurs because your body produces chemicals that ignite an immunologic reaction when your skin is exposed to light.

Urticaria, or hives.   Urticaria may erupt on your skin, sometimes in concert with respiratory, gastrointestinal, or cardiovascular symptoms. Foods, medications, insect stings, exposure to cold, a hot shower, and exposure to the contrast media used in some diagnostic tests can cause hives. Often, the cause remains unidentified. While a case of hives usually resolves within a matter of minutes or hours, sometimes the disorder may last longer.

A more serious but rare form of hives, called *angioedema,* is actually allergic swelling of deeper blood vessels in your body. It may involve your face, gastrointestinal tract, and respiratory tract. If the swelling progresses to the throat, it can block your airway and cause death by suffocation.

It usually takes some detective work to find the cause of your skin allergy. When you visit your doctor, be sure to mention anything that touched your skin or anything you consumed near the time your skin reaction appeared. Treatment includes identifying and avoiding the offending substance. A steroid cream may be prescribed to relieve the symptoms of a simple skin rash. In the case of light sensitivity, a properly prescribed sunblock may solve the problem. When hives tend to recur, your doctor may prescribe antihistamines, and in rare cases, epinephrine (Adrenalin).

Respiratory Allergies

The largest group of American allergy sufferers are easy to identify by their symptoms: watery eyes, a runny or stuffy nose, and fits of sneezing. Hay fever sufferers often experience itching in the eyes, mouth, and throat. Doctors call it *allergic rhinitis,* although it's best known as *hay fever.*

If you're bothered by seasonal hay fever, you know when trouble is in the air. Usually, the offending allergens are the pollens from trees in the spring, grasses in the late spring and summer, and ragweed and other weeds in late summer and early autumn. Mold spores are another common source of allergic rhinitis.

A sensitivity to any of these airborne allergens sets off an inflammation of your mucus membranes that can easily be mistaken for a cold. A key difference is the mucus discharge from your nose: a cold causes a thick discharge, while an allergy produces a clear nasal discharge. When hay fever symptoms don't quit regardless of the season, you may have perennial rhinitis.

Some people with mild allergy symptoms find relief by taking over-the-counter preparations, such as antihistamines or decongestants. Drowsiness is a frequent side effect with many of these products.

If your symptoms make you feel miserable, your doctor can take a history to help pinpoint the cause. When the answer isn't clear, a diagnostic test may be necessary. A simple skin test, such as the "scratch test," calls for placing a drop of allergen on your skin, scratching your skin with a needle, and observing your reaction.

Once the substance to which you are allergic has been identified, the first part of your treatment is avoidance of the allergen. For instance, if animal dander from a pet triggers your allergy, you may need to decide whether you'd be better off finding a new home for your furry friend. When mold spores irritate your nasal passages, inspect your home for signs of mold and mildew. If you can't avoid the problem, your doctor can prescribe medication to help control your symptoms.

Among the newer medications that have been effective in providing relief for many allergy sufferers with minimal side effects are: nonsedating antihistamines such as terfenadine (Seldane) and astemizole (Hismanal), which rarely cause drowsiness; cromolyn sodium nasal spray (Nasalcrom), and steroid nasal sprays, such as beclomethasone (Beconase) or flunisolide (Nasalide).

If it's impossible to avoid the allergen, and medications offer little relief, there are allergy shots, or immunotherapy. This kind of program consists of weekly or twice-a-week injections, usually for the first four to six months of treatment. After you gradually build a tolerance to the offending allergen, the allergist then tapers the schedule of shots to once a month. This is not a quick fix. In most cases, there is a noticeable improvement after a year or two, with the allergy shots usually continuing for about four years. Shots for ragweed pollen work for 85 percent of the people who take them.

Besides being time-consuming and expensive, this therapy doesn't work in all cases, and in rare cases may cause a serious reaction.

Asthma

The respiratory disorder *asthma* is often related to allergies. About half of the adults and 90 percent of children with asthma in this country have allergies. Those who develop the adult-onset form of asthma are likely to be devoid of allergies. Instead, their symptoms stem from such sources as respiratory infections, emotional stress, cigarette smoke, vigorous exercise, and cold weather. In either form of asthma, a multitude of inhaled substances can irritate the hypersensitive bronchial tissues and cause an asthma attack.

If you have asthma that is activated by allergies, avoid the offending substance. When avoidance isn't practical, your doctor may prescribe a bronchodilator spray or pill to help you to breathe more easily. The bronchodilator theophylline, or a steroid or cromolyn sodium spray may relieve your symptoms.

Some allergy sufferers who develop serious asthma attacks—especially from grasses and cats—may benefit from a program of allergy shots. But before undertaking such a regimen, your doctor must be able to document your allergy.

Food Allergies

Only a little more than 1 percent of American adults and about 5 percent of infants and children have a true *food allergy*. Truly allergic people must avoid the food to which they are allergic or else risk a serious immune response. The foods commonly associated with allergies include milk, egg whites, peanuts and other nuts, seafood, wheat (gluten sensitivity), and some fruits, such as berries. Additives, such as yellow food dyes and gum arabic, a food thickener, may also be responsible for some food allergies.

A *food intolerance* is a more common problem that is often erroneously thought to be a food allergy. Instead it is an adverse reaction to certain foods. Lactose intolerance is one of the best examples of this problem. Many people lack the enzyme lactase, which is necessary to digest the milk sugar, lactose. In this case, consuming milk, ice cream, and other dairy products may precipitate bloating, abdominal cramps, flatulence, and diarrhea.

An allergic reaction to food may vary from mild to severe. Typical skin symptoms include itching, redness, and hives. Gastrointestinal symptoms usually involve nausea, vomiting, cramps, and diarrhea shortly after eating the offending food. When there are respiratory symptoms, they may include wheezing, a runny nose, and difficulty breathing. A violent reaction may result in anaphylactic shock, a life-threatening situation.

The amount of food it takes to cause a serious reaction may be minuscule for highly sensitive people. Even with scrupulous avoidance of the forbidden food, if you have a documented food allergy you should be able to protect yourself in case of emergency. Special kits with preloaded epinephrine (Adrenalin) syringes are available by prescription when appropriate.

Drug Allergies

When you take a medication and notice that you develop symptoms such as hives, itching, wheezing, swelling, or a rash, you may have a *drug allergy*. If this happens, ignoring the reaction and continuing to take the medication can make you seriously ill or cause anaphylaxis (see page 246). Alert your doctor and explain what happened. Usually, a different medication can be prescribed.

While any number of medications cause allergic reactions in various people, the drug responsible for a large number of these is penicillin. Aspirin and other nonsteroidal anti-inflammatory drugs may also produce an allergic response—either to the substance itself or to the dye, usually tartrazine (yellow 5), added to the drug.

The contrast dyes injected into a vein used in some diagnostic X-ray tests will at times precipitate an allergic reaction—especially if you are sensitive to iodine. Local anesthetics used for dental work and minor surgery can also provoke a reaction.

If you have ever had an adverse reaction to a medication or diagnostic substance in the past, be sure to tell your doctor so that this information can be added to your medical chart. When your physician prescribes a new medication for you, don't rely solely on your doctor's remembering your allergy or prior reaction to certain drugs. Offer a reminder and be sure to mention whether you are taking any other medications.

Insect Sting Allergies

When an insect such as a honeybee, bumblebee, yellow jacket, hornet, wasp, or fire ant stings you, your immune system may respond immediately to the chemicals in the venom or the response may be delayed. Depending on how sensitive you are to the insect venom, you may experience a painful, but relatively mild local reaction limited to redness, itching, and irritation. But if you are allergic to the venom, the symptoms can involve other body systems besides your skin. Breathing may become difficult and you may feel tightness in your throat and chest. There may be nausea, vomiting, and abdominal pain. Hives may appear elsewhere on your skin. Anaphylactic shock may occur in a small number of people who are highly allergic.

Although millions of Americans have *insect sting allergies,* and large numbers of the population develop allergic reactions to these stings, the number of deaths from these reactions is estimated at 50 to 100 a year.

To treat an insect sting that produces a mild reaction, first inspect the wound. If a stinger is left behind, remove it immediately by gently flicking or scraping it out. Then apply ice to reduce swelling. Some popular remedies include applying a paste of baking soda and water to help relieve the pain. A paste made from a meat tenderizer that contains enzymes may also be helpful in neutralizing the venom. Calamine lotion may ease any itching. Aspirin or acetaminophen often helps reduce local inflammation.

A highly sensitive person who has suffered previous severe reactions to insect venom requires immediate medical attention. People who have strong reactions to insect stings should carry their own doctor-prescribed emergency kit, which consists of a tourniquet, one or two preset doses of epinephrine, and an antihistamine. Administering your own medication is no substitute for medical care, only a way of protecting yourself until you can reach a doctor.

Allergy shots have been shown to offer virtually complete protection against the severe systemic effects of insect stings to people who are highly sensitive.

To help prevent insect stings, be cautious when you venture outdoors. Avoid wearing bright colors and bold patterns because bees and other members of the Hymenoptera clan may mistake you for a flower and alight on your skin. Wear long-sleeved, long-legged garments, as well as shoes and socks. Don't wear any fragrances or scented cosmetics. If a stinging insect approaches you, don't panic or try to shoo it away. Just stand still or make a slow, quiet exit.

Anaphylaxis

Anaphylaxis, an abnormal response to certain foods, medications, or insect venom, is the most severe and dramatic allergic reaction that can occur. Typically, it comes without warning and may be life-threatening if left untreated.

In an anaphylactic reaction, your immune system overreacts so violently to the offending substance that it can throw your system into shock. It begins with hives on the skin, swelling in the throat, and spasms in the tissue of your airways that result in wheezing. Nausea and vomiting may follow. Blood pressure may drop so low that you lose consciousness. Swelling in the throat may be so severe that it can lead to death by asphyxiation.

Only emergency treatment with epinephrine and antihistamine can stop the reaction. If you have a known allergy to a food, a medication, or to insect venom, carry a doctor-prescribed emergency kit with a preloaded epinephrine syringe and an antihistamine.

Penicillin, insect venom, seafood, and nuts are the substances most likely to cause anaphylaxis. Allergy shots are an effective way to become desensitized to insect sting allergies. In the case of food or drug allergies, avoidance is the only way to prevent a reaction.

The contrast dyes used in some diagnostic X-ray tests may provoke a severe allergic reaction in susceptible people. This type of response is called an *anaphylactoid reaction.* Although it produces the same symptoms and outcome of anaphylactic shock, an anaphylactoid reaction is immunologically different.

Some runners and others who exercise strenuously may develop a form of "food-dependent, exercise-induced anaphylaxis." Typically, symptoms of anaphylaxis appear when they eat and then exercise. If you have ever had such a reaction, see your doctor. You may be ordered to carry an emergency kit with epinephrine when you exercise. By fasting for two to four hours before your exercise period, you may be able to prevent such a reaction.

The Skin

Your skin is a highly protective barrier, but its function also makes it vulnerable to disorders, discolorations, disease, and damage. Occasionally, you may develop a rash, itching, an irritation, or a growth that is annoying, painful, or unsightly. Sometimes, these flare-ups clear up on their own, but when they persist and become severe, or look suspicious, seek medical attention. More than 500,000 new cases of skin cancer are diagnosed each year. With early detection and treatment, much skin cancer can be cured.

Acne

Acne, a common affliction of adolescence, occasionally persists through the 20s and even into the 30s. Overactive oil glands, bacteria on the skin, and other factors—such as cosmetics and oily skin creams—may all contribute to the common form of acne. There's no evidence that diet (including chocolate) has a role in acne.

Blackheads and pimples may fill with pus and become infected if you tamper with them. Over-the-counter preparations that contain benzoyl peroxide may help clear up mild or moderate cases of acne. If you have a severe case of acne, consult a dermatologist, who can prescribe an appropriate treatment to help control the condition.

Acne treatment may include topical or oral antibiotic therapy, injection of corticosteroids into acne cysts, cryotherapy, or opening and draining of large pustules. A vitamin-A derivative, widely known as tretinoin (Retin-A), may also be prescribed to help clear up acne (see page 160).

Pregnant women are advised to avoid using tretinoin, as it may have adverse effects on fetal development.

Acne Rosacea

Some adults may develop a form of acne called *acne rosacea* that begins around the mid-30s. This chronic disorder causes inflammation of the skin on the nose and cheeks and dilation of the blood vessels in this area. Facial skin may tend to flush and blush when you drink alcoholic beverages or eat foods that are hot and spicy. Caffeine may aggravate the condition. Acne rosacea is not a serious condition, but it can affect the way you feel about your appearance. There is an antibiotic therapy that can control acne rosacea. Discuss the benefits and risks of this drug therapy with your physician.

Eczema and Dermatitis

When your skin becomes irritated and inflamed, doctors may describe the condition as *dermatitis*—a problem that can be triggered by a number of causes. *Eczema* is a term used to group several types of dermatitis. Some of these skin reactions stem from contact with external irritants, such as the chemicals in soaps or cleaning agents. Other reactions may be set off by internal triggers—namely, allergies.

Different types of eczema tend to produce the same reaction, including redness, swelling, and itching in the early stages of irritation. Later on, oozing blisters erupt in the affected area. Eventually, a crust forms and the area heals. If the reaction continually recurs, the irritated skin gets thicker and may turn darker. If some forms of dermatitis are left untreated, the condition may spread.

Contact dermatitis results from contact with an irritating substance that touches your skin. The reaction you suffer may be one of two kinds: irritant or allergic. If an external agent that contains an acid, alkali, solvent, or a detergent causes your reaction, you have the irritant form of contact dermatitis. The allergic variation results from touching certain plants (poison ivy, oak, and sumac), metals, preservatives, cosmetics, and some medications.

Once the offending irritant is identified, you can prevent irritation by avoiding the substance. Treatment of mild contact dermatitis includes topical steroids and antihistamines.

Hand eczema occurs among people whose work requires regular exposure of their hands to the irritants in soaps, detergents, solvents, and water. To help protect your hands, wear thin cotton gloves under rubber gloves.

Seborrheic dermatitis is marked by redness and flaking of the skin around the glands that produce oil in parts of the face, around the ears, and on the scalp. In more severe cases, other parts of the body may be affected, including the armpits, groin, and other areas where the skin creases. *Dandruff,* another form of this condition, makes the scalp scaly, but without inflammation.

To control seborrheic dermatitis of the scalp, use a shampoo that contains tar, sulfur, salicylic acid, selenium sulfide, or zinc pyrithione. If these shampoos don't help, your doctor may prescribe topical corticosteroids for application to the affected areas. When the face is affected, hydrocortisone cream may be prescribed to help control the inflammation. Check with your doctor before applying any type of medicated cream or ointment to your skin.

Atopic dermatitis often begins in childhood, then disappears, only to return during the adult years. This condition, which is inherited, produces sensitivity to several ordinary substances. The main symptoms are itching, redness, and thickening of the affected skin on the face, neck, upper chest, insides of the elbows, and behind the knees. Treatment includes choosing fabrics that don't irritate the skin, applying skin emollients, and using topical steroids as prescribed.

A nervous habit of repeated rubbing and scratching of the skin may cause a thickening of the skin. This condition, called *lichen simplex chronicus,* results in itchy patches of dermatitis on the neck, lower legs, groin, and other easy-to-reach areas. Steroid injections into the affected area may help to stop the itching.

Circular patches of scaly, thickened, itchy skin may appear during the winter months. A dry indoor environment, irritation from soap, and frequent bathing may aggravate this condition, known as *nummular dermatitis.* Treatment may include topical steroids, a lotion that contains coal tar, and ultraviolet light treatments.

Infections

It's normal to have many kinds of microorganisms on areas of your skin and not even be aware of these tiny skin dwellers. They are harmless on the surface of the skin, but if your skin breaks and they enter, you may develop an infection. When the conditions are right for them, other kinds of infection may also occur—fungal and viral.

Bacterial infections. These include boils, impetigo, folliculitis, and cellulitis. Hair follicles on the face, thighs, or buttocks may become infected with bacteria and produce redness and swelling, called *folliculitis*. A pimple may develop in the area. If the infection runs deep into the hair shaft, the inflammation progresses into a *boil* filled with pus. To help prevent these infections, keep your skin clean. If you tend to develop folliculitis, use an antiseptic soap that contains chlorhexidine. When the infection is extensive, antibiotics may be prescribed.

Impetigo, another superficial infection, usually begins with a patch of blisters around the mouth, nose, or other skin areas. When the blisters break, they release fluid. Eventually, a crust forms over the area. Infants and children are more likely to develop impetigo than adults. You may be able to treat mild impetigo by gently cleansing the area to remove the crusts and applying an antibiotic ointment. If the infection is extensive, consult a physician. Impetigo is contagious and is more easily communicated among children than among adults. Treatment is with oral antibiotics or antibacterial ointments.

Cellulitis most often affects children and the elderly. Bacteria enter the skin through a cut or sore—usually on the face, arm, or leg—and cause redness, swelling, and tenderness. The area feels warm to the touch. Red streaks may appear in the infected area, suggesting *erysipelas,* a form of cellulitis, indicating that the infection is spreading rapidly. Fever, chills, and a feeling of tiredness are common. A severe infection left untreated can be fatal. As with any infection involving a fever, consult a physician. Antibiotics can be prescribed to clear up the infection.

Fungal infections.   Common fungal infections include athlete's foot, jock itch, nail fungus, and candida, or yeast infection.

When your feet remain moist from water or perspiration, the area between the toes becomes vulnerable to *athlete's foot.* Foot odor is not a sign of athlete's foot; in some cases, sweaty feet may cause foot odor without infection. When the fungus that causes athlete's foot thrives, it causes itching, scaling, and cracked skin.

Moisture in the groin can produce *jock itch*—an annoyance that can affect women as well as men. Tight clothing, obesity, or an allergic reaction to chemicals in clothing help moisture and certain fungi trigger jock itch. This infection produces an itchy rash and often tiny blisters.

To prevent athlete's foot and jock itch, keep the feet and groin area dry. You can help keep your feet dry by lightly dusting them with powder, and by wearing absorbent socks. To help prevent jock itch, wear loose-fitting clothing and underwear. You may find over-the-counter powders and ointments helpful for mild irritation. These antifungal preparations generally have miconazole, tolnaftate, or undecylenic acid as active ingredients.

Candida albicans is a yeast organism that normally inhabits the mouth, intestinal tract, and vagina. Infection, disease, and other conditions may cause these fungi to multiply and infect the skin or mucus membranes. Candida of the mouth, called thrush, appears as white patches on the tongue. A vaginal infection caused by candida produces a white or yellow discharge. Your doctor will take cultures and stain the secretions to diagnose candida. Treatment of this local infection is with prescription antifungals, such as amphotericin B (Fungizone) or ketoconazole (Nizoral).

Candidiasis hypersensitivity is currently touted as the cause of a large number of diseases by practitioners who may call themselves clinical ecologists. Beware of anyone who claims that a wide range of your health problems are "yeast-connected."

Viral infections.   Viral skin infections that occur most commonly are warts, herpes simplex, and herpes zoster, or shingles.

The papilloma virus causes various kinds of *warts* on different parts of the body. So-called common warts occur on the hands, plantar warts appear on the sole of the foot, and filliform warts, or small, narrow growths, may sprout on the eyelids or elsewhere around the face. Venereal warts (condyloma) occur in the genital area (see Chapter 4).

Warts can be dome-shaped and rough or flat and smooth. They can appear at any age, last for years, and then disappear without treatment. Doctors aren't certain why some people get warts and others don't. Skin that is irritated or damaged may be more susceptible to the wart virus. An over-the-counter preparation may be helpful in removing hand warts. Consult a doctor if you have warts on your feet, face, or genitals. Several kinds of treatment are available to remove warts.

Some types of skin cancer may be mistaken for a wart—especially squamous cell carcinoma and melanoma. Many people presume that any type of growth on their skin is a wart or a mole. If you notice a suspicious-looking growth, consult a doctor, especially when it has suddenly changed in size, color, or shape (see page 254).

The *herpes* viruses are responsible for a variety of infections. Herpes simplex type I causes infections above the waist—often around the face. Herpes simplex type II infects the genital area. Although some people contract the virus without experiencing any symptoms, most develop the characteristic painful, fluid-filled blisters. Before the blisters form, tingling or itching often occurs.

When the blisters pop open, the liquid that oozes from the area is highly contagious. Within a few days, scabs form and the healing process begins. Because the herpes virus remains in the nervous system in a dormant state, infection may recur at the site of the original eruption. Repeat infections may be triggered by stress, the ultraviolet light from the sun, menstruation, physical trauma, or fever.

Acyclovir (Zovirax) may be prescribed in ointment form, but the oral form is more effective and works to prevent recurrent infections. To help prevent infection with herpes simplex type I, avoid kissing or sharing eating utensils with someone who has open blisters around the face, lips, or nose. Avoid open blister contact with any of the body's mucus membranes. If you're in direct contact with someone who is actively infected, wash your hands before you touch your eyes or mucus membranes. To help prevent the spread of genital herpes, avoid intimate sexual contact with a person who has an active infection.

Herpes zoster, or shingles, mostly affects people over 50. If you had chicken pox as a child or adolescent, you are at a higher risk for shingles, since the virus that causes chicken pox (varicella-zoster virus) remains dormant in certain nerve cells. For unknown reasons, it travels back to the skin during later adulthood to produce herpes zoster.

You may notice chills, fever, and tiredness at first, but the main early symptoms are burning pain and tingling, as well as increased sensitivity of certain areas of your skin. A rash then breaks out, followed by blisters that may persist for one to two weeks before scabs form and the skin heals. In some people, the pain from shingles may last for months after the skin has healed.

Depending on which nerves are involved, herpes zoster may occur on the front and back of the trunk, or an extremity, or on the face—but only on one side of the body. Analgesics may help relieve the pain of shingles. If you have a severe case of shingles your physician may prescribe acyclovir, corticosteroids, or a combination of both. Most people who suffer an attack of herpes zoster never develop another one.

Psoriasis

About 4 million Americans have *psoriasis,* a disease in which the skin overproduces new cells, causing thickness and scales in the affected areas.

The cause of psoriasis remains unknown, though it is known that the disorder tends to run in families. It may be linked to a faulty control mechanism that steps up the process of skin production even when no new skin is needed.

Psoriasis is not an infectious disease. Some cases are so mild that no treatment is necessary. In other cases, sufferers need to consult a dermatologist to get a treatment plan and medication that will help keep the disorder under control. For reasons that aren't known, a small number of people with psoriasis are vulnerable to arthritis—often in the small bones of the hands and feet.

Young adults are the most likely group of people to develop psoriasis, although it does occasionally begin later in life. The symptoms include reddened patches, or plaques, of scaly skin usually on the scalp, elbows, knees, and lower back. The groin, genital area, and fingernails may also be involved.

The course of psoriasis is unpredictable. The plaques may suddenly disappear, only to recur at a future time. At other times, the skin may not respond well to any treatment.

Treatment varies according to the severity and extent of the psoriasis. Moisturizing creams and lotions help improve the appearance of the skin and reduce itching. Your doctor may prescribe a topical medication containing cortisone, tar, or anthralin. The topical tars may be used in combination with ultraviolet light from the B spectrum or ultraviolet light from the A spectrum administered in combination with a drug called psoralen, a treatment known by the acronym PUVA, for psoralens plus ultraviolet A. The light therapy is carefully given while the patient stands in a booth wearing protective eye gear. For severe cases, certain cancer chemotherapy drugs, such as methotrexate (Folex), or a newer form of vitamin-A derivative known as etretinate (Tegison), may be recommended.

Nail Disorders

Because your nails are a part of the outer layer of your skin, they take a lot of abuse. Hangnails and small cuts may result in infection. Frequent exposure to water may cause brittleness. Reactions to the chemicals in some products may cause splitting or breakage of your nails.

Fungal infections may also occur—especially in the toenails. An infected toenail may become thick and dull-looking, but the problem is harmless and usually painless. If the appearance of the nail prompts you to seek treatment, an antifungal drug such as griseofulvin (Fulvicin, Grisactin) or ketoconazole (Nizoral) may be prescribed. These drugs must be taken orally, and in most cases, for up to a year or more. Because the toenails grow at a much slower rate than fingernails, it takes longer for the fungus to work its way out of the nail plate. These medications are fairly expensive, so you may decide to live with the unsightly condition. In severe cases, a doctor can remove the toenail under local anesthesia.

Ingrown toenails result from cutting the nail in too much. If the problem doesn't resolve by itself and the pain persists, see your physician.

Ridges, white spots, splitting, and bumps may occur on normal, healthy nails for no good reason. But some serious disorders can produce changes in the fingernails. Psoriasis often produces small pits on the nails. Chronic liver disease may cause a white area near the bed of the nail. In chronic lung disease, the nails often turn thick and yellow. Clubbing of the nails—actually an enlargement of the fingertips accompanied by curving of the fingernails—is often a symptom of lung or congenital heart disease.

Vitiligo

When the skin cells that control the color of your skin stop working, new skin grows in with the color missing. This disease, called *vitiligo,* is a cosmetic problem with an unknown cause. Most of the people who get vitiligo are otherwise healthy. In some cases, the disease is associated with disorders of the endocrine system, including thyroid disease and diabetes mellitus.

More than a third of all cases run in families. Vitiligo can be especially troubling to dark-skinned people as white patches appear on knees, elbows, hands, and around body openings of the face and genital area. PUVA therapy, which uses drugs called psoralens and ultraviolet A light, may stimulate the skin's pigment-producing cells to recolor the area. Many PUVA treatments are necessary to restore skin color. Repeat visits for therapy are time-consuming, expensive, and in the end may not be fully effective.

Moles

Moles are benign growths made up of pigment-producing cells that can appear anywhere on your skin. They come in various sizes and shapes, and are usually some shade of brown. Doctors often refer to a mole as a nevus, for the type of cell from which it originates. Most moles develop by the time you reach 20, although some may appear later—especially during pregnancy.

Moles often darken, become elevated, and change in size over the years. Sometimes they fade into the skin and seem to disappear, or they rise up from the skin and fall off on their own. A mole can enlarge and hairs may begin to grow out of it. These changes are normal.

If you have a type of mole called a *dysplastic nevus,* you need to watch this growth for changes in size, shape, color, or itching. This could be an early warning sign of skin cancer, or melanoma.

Dysplastic nevi often run in families. Unlike the common circular or oval-shaped moles, these have an irregular border, variations in color, an asymmetrical shape, and are wider than the eraser on a pencil. If you have this type of mole or notice a new growth or a sore that doesn't heal, consult a doctor. Regular monitoring and a biopsy of the area, if it is considered necessary, can help determine whether removal is indicated.

Skin Cancer

Prolonged exposure to the ultraviolet light of the sun is the main cause of *skin cancer*. Suntanned skin may be seen as a sign of health by many people but it may also be a forerunner of skin cancer. Thirty percent of adults and 50 percent of adolescents are aware of the risks of severe sun exposure but continue to pursue a tan, according to a survey by the American Academy of Dermatology.

Basal cell carcinoma is the most common form of skin cancer. It usually begins with a small, shiny nodule, or collection of cells with a raised surface. It slowly enlarges and in a few months, blood vessels may be noticeable on the surface of this skin-colored lump. A crust may form over the area, or it may bleed. Without treatment, the area continues to bleed, crust over, seems to heal, and starts to bleed again. Sun-exposed parts of the body are most affected, including the face, neck, arms, and hands.

Squamous cell carcinoma growths may begin as a reddish lump that later looks like a wart or, in some cases, an ulcerated area of skin. These growths tend to be more aggressive than basal cell carcinoma, and if left untreated, the cancer cells can spread to other parts of the body.

Although *malignant melanoma* is the least common form of skin cancer, it is the most serious. If the melanoma is caught before it penetrates into the second layer of skin there is an excellent chance of a cure. Examine your skin regularly to look for any changes in moles or any new growths.

To confirm the diagnosis, your doctor will take a skin biopsy to check for cancerous cells. Depending on the location and the extent of the skin cancer, there are different types of treatment. The growth may be scraped away, frozen with liquid nitrogen, or excised. Topical chemotherapy cream may also be prescribed to destroy cancerous or precancerous cells.

To help protect yourself from skin cancer, use a sunscreen with a sun-protection factor of at least 15, wear protective clothing and a hat, and stay out of the sun—especially the midday sun when the ultraviolet rays are strongest. If you go swimming or your work or exercise causes perspiration, reapply the sunscreen. Avoid tanning parlors and sun lamps.

If you notice a suspicious-looking growth on your skin, seek medical attention immediately.

Eyes

Our eyes are among the few organs of the body that must function without the protection of the skin. Considering the complex job they do, and how vulnerable they are when doing it, it is remarkable how few problems they cause us. At times, you can chalk up your irritated eyes to a day's work. Most often getting some rest or avoiding offending substances will relieve the problem. But if your eyes suddenly become blurry, painful, produce a discharge, or if you notice other changes in your vision, you should consult a doctor at once.

Eyestrain

Focusing your eyes on the same area for too long at close range can bring on *eyestrain*. Fatigue makes reading difficult and you may experience a headache. Contrary to popular opinion, eyestrain doesn't come from working your eyes too much. It occurs when you force the six small muscles around each eye to stay in the same position for too long.

To help prevent eyestrain, periodically exercise your eye muscles by looking away from your work for a few moments and focusing on objects at varying distances. At regular intervals, rotate your eyes a few times clockwise and then counterclockwise. Make sure the lighting is good and position yourself and your work area so that there is no glare. If you frequently suffer eyestrain, consult an ophthalmologist or optometrist.

You may need a pair of reading glasses, or a different prescription, if you already wear glasses.

Floaters and Flashes

Small specks that float into your field of vision when you are looking at something with a plain background—for instance, a plain white sheet of paper—are called *floaters*. These tiny clumps of debris are cast off from that gelatinous transparent fluid called the vitreous body that fills up the inner part of your eyeball. When these floaters cross in front of the light-sensitive retina at the back of your eye, a speck or fine line appears.

Virtually all of us experience floaters from time to time, especially as we grow older. They are usually more of an annoyance than a serious concern. If floaters drift into your field of vision, move your eyes around; the fluid in your eyes helps to move the speck out of the way.

If you are nearsighted or have had cataract surgery, you may have a larger number of floaters. But when a group of floaters develops suddenly, consult a medical eye doctor at once. It may signify a torn retina—a serious condition that can develop into a detached retina (see Chapter 6).

Streaks of flashing light may also appear across your field of vision. The shrinking vitreous gel pulling against the retina is responsible for many of these *flashes,* which commonly occur as we age. But the flashes may be linked to the sudden development of floaters—and may be a warning sign of a detached retina. If you experience a sudden onset of spots and flashes, consult an ophthalmologist immediately.

Foreign Bodies

Foreign bodies that lodge on the conjunctiva—the mucus membrane that covers the outer surface of the eye—or on top of the transparent outer covering of the eye called the cornea, are among the most common problems that affect the eyes. In many cases, a piece of soft dirt or a stray eyelash causes discomfort but then washes out of the eye on its own. But when dirt, metal, or any other substance cuts into the cornea or becomes embedded, infection may occur if the foreign body isn't removed promptly.

If the foreign body doesn't come out when you rinse the affected eye with clear water, consult a doctor at once. Ideally, you should see an ophthalmologist who will use special equipment to locate and remove the foreign body. Antibiotic ointment may be prescribed. An eye patch may need to be worn for a few days until the area heals.

Eyelid Infections

The skin on the edge of your eyelids contains tiny glands and hair follicles, which can become infected. One such condition is *blepharitis,* an infection of the lid margins, which produces redness, itching, burning, swelling, and scaling. In severe cases, eyelashes fall out and small ulcers appear on the eyelid. Some milder cases may be linked to allergies or to dandruff associated with seborrheic dermatitis, but the severe form of blepharitis is a result of bacterial infection. Milder forms of blepharitis often respond to regular washing of the scalp to control dandruff and the gentle application of warm compresses to the eyelids. When blepharitis recurs—or suddenly flares up—consult a physician. Prescription ointments can help relieve your symptoms.

A *sty*—or boil-like swelling in a hair follicle—may develop along the eyelid edge when bacteria enter the area. This swollen area becomes red, painful, and filled with pus. The sty usually bursts on its own. Or you can gently apply hot compresses to the eyelid to help draw out the infection. When the pus is released, it relieves the pain. Carefully wash the area after clearing away the pus. Never squeeze the pimple because it can cause the infection to spread. If the sty persists or doesn't respond to hot compresses, consult a physician. An antibiotic ointment may be prescribed.

Sties may recur, especially if they involve the tiny glands along the eyelid. Sometimes they are associated with blepharitis. Neither blepharitis nor sties is contagious.

Conjunctivitis

The transparent mucus membrane that covers the front of your eyes and lines your eyelids is called the conjunctiva. When a bacterial or viral infection, certain allergens, or irritating substances slip into this thin protective coating, the resulting problem is called *conjunctivitis.*

Because conjunctivitis gives the eyes a characteristic bloodshot appearance it is also known as pinkeye. Other symptoms include itching, burning, and a discharge from the affected or infected eye. The discharge crusts over at night, causing the eyelids to stick together. (A wakening child may panic when he finds he cannot open his eyes.)

When infectious conjunctivitis caused by a virus is mild, it usually is self-limiting and clears up on its own. The bacterial form, which usually produces a heavy discharge and swollen lids, responds well to antibiotics. In either case, applying a warm compress to the crusty eyelids in the morning helps to dissolve the crust and open the eyes. Viral and bacterial conjunctivitis are caused by person-to-person contact and are highly contagious.

Allergic conjunctivitis may occur as an adverse reaction to pollen, cosmetics, air pollution, and chemicals. Itching, redness, and heavy tearing are the major symptoms of allergic conjunctivitis—which is not contagious. Your physician may prescribe corticosteroid drops, but these are not meant to be taken on a long-term basis. You can best relieve your symptoms by identifying and avoiding the substance that irritates your eyes.

To prevent the spread of infectious conjunctivitis, don't share a towel with anyone else. Never share eye medications or eye makeup with another person, and try to avoid touching your eyes. Don't use over-the-counter eye solutions for bloodshot eyes. These preparations may appear to relieve the symptoms of conjunctivitis at first but they do not cure infections, which may continue to worsen even while the symptoms are somewhat relieved.

Corneal Ulcers and Infections

When a foreign body strikes or scratches your cornea—the transparent covering at the front of the eye—this outermost part of your eye is highly vulnerable to infection. Irritation from a contact lens or wood or metal shavings is among the many causes of open sores on the cornea.

If this open sore, or ulcer, isn't treated immediately, scar tissue can form on the cornea. Left untreated, the ulcer can perforate the cornea, produce a severe loss of vision, and may result in permanent damage to eyesight. Symptoms include pain, redness, swelling, and reduced vision.

Bacterial and fungal infections may enter the ulcerated area and set up housekeeping. But the most likely invader is a virus—especially herpes simplex, which may produce a small white-colored patch that you often can see yourself.

If you suspect that you have a corneal ulcer or infection, consult an ophthalmologist, who will use a special dye to stain the area and confirm the diagnosis. Depending on the type of infection, your doctor may prescribe drops or ointment. In the event of serious injury to the eye, a corneal transplant may be necessary.

To help prevent corneal injuries, wear protective eyegear when working around particles that potentially could blow into your eyes.

If you have a tendency to develop cold sores around your mouth, never touch your eyes after touching your mouth, because the herpes infection can easily spread to your eyes.

Subconjunctival Hemorrhage

A *subconjunctival hemorrhage* is a fancy name for a red patch on the white of your eye. It may occur as the result of a minor injury, or from sneezing, coughing, straining, or anything that increases the blood pressure in your head and neck veins. These red patches usually require no treatment and resolve on their own in several days. If the red patch causes pain, occurs after recent eye surgery, or otherwise bothers you, consult an ophthalmologist.

Ears

Your ears allow you to maintain your sense of balance as well as your hearing. Tiny hairs and glands in the outer part of your ear produce wax that protects your auditory canal from bacteria, insects, and dirt. A variety of common ear complaints are often caused by water, accumulated wax, injury from cleaning the ear, changes in pressure, and infection. A hearing disturbance resulting from one of these problems is called conductive hearing loss—because conduction of sound waves from the outside air to the fluid inside your ear is blocked. Occasionally, an upper respiratory infection works its way into the ear channels and causes pain, a feeling of fullness, and impaired hearing.

Earwax

One of the most common causes of impaired hearing is impacted wax in the canal of the outer ear. Each person produces a different amount of earwax. Some people rarely have an accumulation of too much wax, while others build up enough earwax to require regular visits to a doctor for professional removal. The symptoms include a feeling of fullness in the ear, slight hearing loss, ringing in the ear, and, occasionally, pain. Your doctor can remove the wax with a special instrument or by irrigating the ear. Using a cotton-tipped swab, hairpin, or a fingernail to try to remove impacted wax may cause damage to the eardrum.

External Otitis

An infection of the outer ear canal is called *external otitis,* but is popularly known as *swimmer's ear.* Water or other irritants can produce a single boil or widespread infection in the ear canal. Symptoms include itching, pain, discharge, swelling, and, at times, temporary loss of hearing. Young adults are most likely to develop external ear infections. The condition needs treatment by a physician. Untreated it can result in damage to the structures of the inner ear. Treatment includes cleaning and draining the infected area, and the prescription of topical antibiotic or steroid ointments. To help prevent future infections, wear ear plugs when swimming or bathing. A shower cap may also help keep water out of your ears.

Aerotitis

Flying can cause sudden changes in atmospheric pressure that may block your ears. The condition, called *aerotitis,* can be painful and may last for hours or days. What happens is that the pressure in your middle ear—which is normally the same as the pressure of the outside atmosphere—for one reason or another fails to adjust to match the new pressure on the outer side of your eardrums. To help reduce the risk of blocked ears, chew gum, suck on candy, or yawn frequently during takeoff and landing.

You might also try a decongestant spray or drops in each nostril shortly before takeoff and landing. If you prefer an oral decongestant, take it 30 minutes to an hour before boarding. If you suffer from allergies, you may be able to avoid pressure discomfort by taking an antihistamine before takeoff.

If you have a cold or an acute upper respiratory infection, try to avoid flying. If your sinuses are infected too, air pressure changes from flying can aggravate the condition and cause a complication known as *barometric sinusitis.* People with colds who can't avoid air travel are at less risk in a larger, well-pressurized plane, as opposed to smaller commuter aircraft.

Otitis Media

The term *otitis media* refers to an infection of the middle ear. Both viruses and bacteria can cause middle ear infections, sometimes as secondary infections during a cold, influenza, or measles. Although children tend to suffer more middle ear infections, adults may develop otitis media too.

The symptoms of *acute otitis media* include a feeling of fullness in the ear and a severe earache. You may not be able to hear from the affected ear. When a bacterium is responsible for otitis media, pus that forms in the area may cause the eardrum to burst. If the infection is caused by a virus, it often clears up by itself without affecting the eardrum, unless a bacterial infection follows.

If you have a severe earache, see your doctor. Antibiotics may be prescribed to stop a bacterial infection. If otitis media is left untreated, it can spread to another part of the ear and cause permanent hearing loss.

Chronic otitis media may occur after a bout of acute otitis media, trauma, or an upper respiratory infection. This recurring infection, which may not even be noticeable, is thought to be the result of an earlier ear infection that never completely healed. Typically, there is a slight discharge of pus and some degree of hearing loss. This infection usually results in a permanent tear in the eardrum. If you notice a discharge from your ear, see a doctor. Antibiotics may be prescribed to clear up the infection. The doctor will also examine your ears to determine whether the infection has spread into the mastoid bones behind the ear.

Tinnitus

Like virtually everyone, you've probably experienced noise in the ears at times. Ringing, buzzing, roaring, or blowing sounds not generated by any outside source are the hallmarks of a condition called *tinnitus*.

In some cases, tinnitus may follow exposure to a loud noise but often it's difficult to pinpoint a definite cause. It may also occur when there is impacted earwax, an ear infection, or a progressive hearing disorder of the middle ear called *otosclerosis*.

Tinnitus may also be due to *Ménière's disease,* a condition that causes dizziness (also called *vertigo*), a feeling of pressure in the ear, and variation in the ability to hear.

Certain drugs have been linked with noise in the ears. Among these are aspirin or aspirin-containing drugs, caffeine, alcohol, nicotine, quinidine, indomethacin (Indometh, Indocin), carbamazepine (Epitol, Tegretol), propranolol (Inderal), levodopa (Dopar, Larodopa), and aminophylline. If you develop noise in your ears after you begin taking a drug, tell your doctor. Your prescription can be changed or modified until the ringing disappears.

If you notice a mild ringing in your ears that doesn't soon resolve on its own, consult an otolaryngologist, a specialist in ears, nose, and throat. Tinnitus may be an early sign of a correctable hearing disorder.

Mouth and Tongue

The soft tissue inside the oral cavity is vulnerable to injury. You may bite your tongue or constantly irritate it with a raggedy-edged tooth, jab the inside of your mouth with a toothbrush, or burn your mouth with piping hot food. A virus may cause a mouth ulcer, or a fungus may set the stage for oral thrush. Mouth tumors are rare in people under 40, but the incidence rises in people 60 and older. If you notice a lump, sore, or strange color change that doesn't clear up on its own in a short time, see your doctor. It may be an early warning sign of a more serious condition.

Mouth Infections

Canker sores (apthous ulcers) commonly occur on the inside of the mouth, gums, and tongue but not on the lips. A break in the mucus lining of your mouth or a viral infection can lead to a mouth ulcer or a group of them. The cause still remains unclear, although it appears that canker sores run in families. Young adults seem to develop more canker sores, but eventually have fewer attacks as time goes by. Usually, the sores heal within 5 to 10 days—even without treatment. To help reduce the pain, you may find an over-the-counter topical anesthetic or mild mouth rinse helpful. If you have a problem with recurring canker sores, see your doctor. In some cases, steroids may be prescribed.

Cold sores, or blisters on the lips, are an oral form of the herpes simplex virus type I. Occasionally, the inner lining of the mouth may have blisters, too. Symptoms often include fever, tiredness, and occasionally, swollen lymph glands a few days before the sores appear. In some cases, there may be no symptoms, although the virus lingers on in your nerve cells in a dormant state. When the virus reactivates at a later time, you may feel tingling and itching prior to the eruption of a cold sore.

When the characteristic blisters form, burst, and begin to heal, the area may be extremely painful, making it hard to eat. If you have an active cold sore, never touch your eyes after touching your mouth. Exposure to sunlight, stress, and having a cold or fever all have been linked to new attacks of cold sores. If you have a tendency to develop severe or frequent cold sores, you may be able to help control recurring attacks by using the antiviral drug acyclovir (Zovirax). This drug is available by prescription.

Thrush, or a *Candida albicans* infection of the mouth, is a series of sore, white patches on the tongue and mucus lining of the mouth. Symptoms include a feeling of dryness in the mouth and raised white or yellow patches, which may be raw when the patch is removed. If you have thrush, see your doctor. A topical antifungal drug may be prescribed to clear up the infection.

Thrush is likely to reappear even after treatment if the underlying cause for the susceptibility to new infection isn't addressed. Some of these are: the use of certain antibiotics, diabetes mellitus, dry mouth caused by reduced saliva production, medications or infections that suppress the immune system, and poor hygiene in denture wearers.

Dry Mouth

Dry mouth—or *xerostomia*—occurs when you can't produce enough saliva, which you need to keep your teeth and mouth healthy. Saliva not only helps digest your food but is also important because it protects the oral environment against bacteria and fungi. In some cases, dry mouth may be annoying but not a serious problem. For instance, if you snore or breathe through your mouth while you sleep, you may have a dry mouth upon awaking—and a temporary mouth odor that usually disappears after rinsing your mouth with water or brushing your teeth. Anxiety may produce dry mouth and temporary mouth odor as well.

A reversible cause of dry mouth is the regular use of certain medications. You may be able to alleviate the problem by sucking on sugarless candies or drinking more fluids.

Other causes of dry mouth include cigarette smoking, infection or obstruction of the salivary glands, radiation treatment for head and neck cancer, and Sjögren's syndrome, an autoimmune disease that dries up moisture-secreting glands in the body, including those in the eyes and mouth, and produces joint pain.

Sometimes the cause of dry mouth is unknown. If you suffer from dry mouth, drink plenty of fluids throughout the day. It is particularly important that you practice good oral hygiene by brushing and flossing your teeth daily; a chronic lack of saliva may endanger your teeth and gums and lead to infections. If you have a serious problem with dry mouth, let your dentist know about it.

Leukoplakia

A condition called *leukoplakia* can produce white patches on the inside lining of your mouth. While anyone may develop leukoplakia, it is more likely to occur if you constantly use tobacco, have dentures that don't fit well, eat hot and spicy foods, or have poor oral hygiene. If the problem is due to any of these conditions, it often can be corrected. Still, there is a risk that the thickened patch may indicate a more serious condition—especially if it has red markings.

In a small percentage of cases, changes in the cells may indicate a precancerous stage of growth. Symptoms often are hardly noticeable. The patchy area may give you slight discomfort and become tougher than the surrounding tissue. There may be no pain. If you notice such patches, see your doctor or dentist. A biopsy can determine if there are any changes in the cells.

Oral Cancer

The association between tobacco and alcohol use and mouth cancer is clear. Unfortunately, by the time many of these cancers are diagnosed, malignant cells have spread to other parts of the body. Most oral cancers appear on the tongue. Malignant growths also may occur on the floor of the mouth, the soft palate, and other areas that you can't see yourself when you look in a mirror.

Some tumors that grow in the mouth are benign and may cause bleeding but no significant pain. One of the first symptoms of a malignant tumor is a sore that is painful and doesn't heal. If you notice any kind of lump or patchy area of irritation that persists without healing after a reasonable time, see your doctor or dentist at once. If oral cancer is caught in its early stages, simple surgery often can contain it.

Regular dental examinations are an important strategy in detecting early oral cancer. Dentists are believed to give the most thorough and effective examination of the mouth and therefore most likely to detect oral cancer in its early stages.

Approximately 50 percent of the deaths from oral cancer have been associated with smoking, but another large percentage has been linked to the use of smokeless tobacco products, such as snuff and chewing tobacco. A growing number of male teenagers and young adults are using smokeless tobacco regularly and may be increasing their risk of oral cancer.

Tongue Infections

Your tongue normally looks pink, plush in texture, and has a certain number of creases, or fissures. If you develop oral thrush or are a heavy tobacco user, you may develop discolorations on your tongue. Such discolorations are often little cause for concern. Gently brushing your tongue with your toothbrush when you brush your teeth may help. If the discoloration doesn't soon disappear, see your doctor. You may have an underlying condition that needs to be treated.

You may notice an inflammation of the tongue called *glossitis*. This fairly common condition may include redness and pain, or burning without any signs of inflammation. You may notice that the texture of your tongue feels oddly smooth or has whitish spots. Or it may begin to look hairy. These symptoms may be caused by injury, aging, poor nutrition, reaction to a drug, or disease.

Because there are so many possible causes, an essential part of diagnosis is your medical history—including a consideration of any drugs you take. Once the underlying cause is identified, treatment can begin and the tongue inflammation should subside.

Temporomandibular Joint (TMJ) Syndrome

The jaw muscles you use to chew your food work as a team with the temporomandibular joint in your jawbone. When the area becomes painful and chronically sore, the discomfort may point to a disorder commonly known as *TMJ syndrome*. Besides pain, other symptoms of TMJ include clicking or popping noises when you chew, difficulty in opening your jaw fully, and perhaps headaches. Clenching the teeth during times of stress or grinding your teeth while you sleep may help precipitate TMJ. Other possible causes include an abnormal bite and rheumatoid arthritis.

TMJ appears to be linked to stress. If you develop persistent pain in your jaw muscles, see your dentist or doctor. Often, wearing a mouth guard during sleep helps to prevent grinding the teeth. Some dentists may be able to recommend simple exercises to help alleviate the pain. Most TMJ sufferers can find effective relief by taking simple analgesics. To help relieve TMJ pain, as well as for your general health, try to determine what is causing stress and tension in your life and then make an effort to eliminate it.

8

Using the Health Care System

Mack Lipkin, Jr., M.D.,
and Joan H. Marks, M.S.

As we proceed into the 1990s, we can expect much change and uncertainty in the health care delivery system in the United States. The annual tab for health care soared to $620 billion in 1989, and by 1995 this figure is expected to double. The price tag is enormous, and those who are footing the bill—the government and employers as well as patients—are increasingly asking if they're getting the best value for their money.

As costs soar, public satisfaction remains low. A national survey taken in 1989 showed that Americans think the U.S. health care system needs "fundamental change or complete rebuilding." Whether the drastic change of a national health insurance program or universal coverage could ever materialize in the United States remains to be seen.

It's impossible to predict what our health care system will look like in the future. Health care expenditures now average about $2,500 per person a year, the highest of any country. At the same time, a glaring inequity surfaces: about 18 percent of the population is without a source of health care financing. The need for health and medical services can only increase in the future, especially as our population ages and the AIDS epidemic creates new demands on the delivery system.

Some health care analysts predict that as employers and government struggle to reduce their share of costs, the burden of payment will fall on consumers, who will have to pay higher premiums or deductibles. Others predict that by the end of the decade, consumers will be forced to pay out-of-pocket costs for all health care except catastrophic illness, which would be covered by insurance.

Your ability to access the health care system in times of need and the quality of care you receive may depend on how well you understand the services you are purchasing. You may have to make a few tradeoffs, you may have to be vocal in asserting your rights, but for certain, you must know how the system works to be able to use it. You need a sound strategy for protecting your health, your assets, and your peace of mind. This strategy includes choosing a health care plan and a primary doctor, selecting a hospital if serious illness strikes, having an awareness of your rights as a patient, and educating yourself to avoid medical quackery.

Choosing a Health Care Plan

Even the most sophisticated medical consumer may pale at the bewildering array of health insurance plans now available for purchase. Competition among insurers is intense and the products they offer are increasingly complex.

Depending on your family size and state of health, your insurance needs change during young adulthood, middle age, and as you near retirement. Before you decide on a plan, make sure that it is one that fits your needs. A few of your considerations might include: will you be allowed to choose your own doctor and how important is this choice to you? If you must be hospitalized, must you go to the hospital of the plan's choice? Does the plan cover pregnancy and well-baby care? How long a waiting period is there before your benefits begin?

While a written explanation or materials may come with your health insurance policy, very often the language is too general and too full of jargon. Phrases such as "preexisting condition," "not medically necessary," and "reasonable and customary charges" are written into many policies. Make sure you know in advance how these phrases will affect what the company will pay. Find out what categories of treatment are excluded. Ask the health insurance plan's representative to explain terms you don't understand.

The long-accustomed ability to receive virtually any type of test or treatment up to the limits of your policy—currently described as *unmanaged care*—is now only one option in coverage plans. Now, many more Americans are in one form or another of *managed care,* offered through health maintenance organizations, preferred providers, or groups of doctors who offer their services at discount. As well, many people who still use doctors who charge on a fee-for-service basis are in plans that will pay for hospitalization in nonemergency situations only if prior clearance was obtained.

When you consider your options in choosing a health care coverage plan, there are four points to keep in mind: *cost, freedom of choice, comprehensiveness,* and *quality.* Here is a guide to the types of plans now available and some criteria for making an informed choice.

Fee-for-Service Plans

In the traditional *fee-for-service* insurance plan, you visit your doctor or hospital, have your examination, test, or procedure, get a bill for the services performed, and pay it. In return for paying a premium that you or your employer pays, your health insurance company reimburses you a certain percentage (usually 70 to 90 percent) either of the actual cost of service performed or of that which a schedule within the policy has established as "usual, reasonable, and customary." If your policy has such a schedule and your doctor or hospital charges more for a procedure than the schedule calls for, you are responsible for paying the difference. This is in addition to the remaining percentage of the covered amount your plan does not pay.

Under the fee-for-service arrangement, a doctor can take a defensive approach and offer all-inclusive testing and treatment with little concern for cost because the insurance plan covers the expenses. Such a carte blanche approach to health care with no budgetary constraints is considered by many health care analysts to be one of the main causes of inflated costs in the health care sector.

This form of insurance doesn't cover routine checkups or immunizations, thus reducing the incentive to perform preventive care.

The *advantage* of fee-for-service coverage includes the ability to choose your own doctor, whether it is the family physician you have grown to like and trust, or a top specialist anywhere in the country who can treat you for a disorder you may develop. The plan should also cover you if you are away from home and need a doctor's care. If your doctor finds that a test, procedure, or treatment is necessary, you should have easy access to the care you need, since there is no incentive to skimp on services.

Among the *drawbacks* to a fee-for-service plan are having to pay for routine medical care (including periodic health checkups and preventive screening), paying deductibles, and making copayments. You may have to shell out a certain amount of out-of-pocket costs (perhaps $2,500 to $3,000) until you reach a fixed maximum each year. Once these requirements are met, some plans kick in with full coverage.

Managed Fee-for-Service

Managed fee-for-service plans are basically the same as traditional coverage, with some additions to the rules of the game. The difference is known as *utilization review,* a process that determines in advance whether a certain procedure or hospital entry is justified, and how long your stay should be. In the event of an emergency, you do not need prior approval to receive treatment.

Under utilization review, your doctor must present the diagnosis and proposed treatment plan that calls for hospitalization to a cost management review program hired by your employer or insurer. The review team, or cost-management company, uses its own physicians, nurses, and computer software to determine whether the proposed treatment is appropriate and necessary, and if the price is right.

If utilization review turns down the proposed treatment, you must look to your physician to become your advocate and defend your need for surgery or the procedure in question. The current concept behind utilization review is cost control as opposed to improving the quality of care. However, it is also designed to track a small number of physicians who may perform one procedure but submit a bill for reimbursement in a higher-priced category.

Health Maintenance Organizations

Prepaid health insurance, which offers comprehensive medical care for a fixed overall annual fee that you pay in advance, is a major alternative to traditional coverage. The most common prepaid plan is the *health maintenance organization,* or HMO, which covers members for medical, surgical, and hospital care, as well as emergency, maternity, prescription, and preventive services.

In an HMO, there usually is no deductible and the member need only make a small "nuisance" payment (about $5) for each visit to the doctor. The monthly or quarterly premiums for HMOs have been less than for standard insurance, with savings estimated to be 15 to 25 percent when costs for both types of insurance are compared.

But HMOs have not been immune to the same high costs that keep forcing up the price of medical care. In recent years, many HMOs have increased their charges to members or have cut back on services. The result has been disenchantment among some of the 30 million Americans who have enrolled in the plans since their introduction in the mid-1970s.

HMOs have managed to be less expensive than fee-for-service insurance by using less hospitalization and more utilization review of all services, including lab tests, referrals to specialists, inpatient surgery, and high-technology diagnostic tests. In an HMO, the primary care physician acts as a "gatekeeper," who coordinates the member's care. The gatekeeper's job is to make decisions about the use of the HMO's resources in order to eliminate any unnecessary tests, care, or use of the system.

The fee each member pays is derived from an estimate of what the HMO expects its expenditures to be for the year. The figure is based on the number of members, expenses in the previous year, and an estimate of inflation. Since it is done on a per capita (literally, "by the head") system, it is called *capitation*. If the HMO's costs are higher than the prepaid amount, the organization loses and operates at a deficit. To make a profit, the HMO must keep costs below the total of prepayments.

In some HMOs, the physician who makes too many referrals to specialists and orders too many tests stands to lose income. As a result, there is concern over whether such financial incentives affect the decisions a doctor makes. A major question has been: do HMO physicians skimp on patient care in favor of keeping their organization profitable? In reputable HMOs, the answer is no.

Studies on quality of care and member satisfaction in HMOs by independent analysts indicate that care is comparable to that delivered under fee-for-service coverage. One of the main incentives to reduce costs in HMOs is to lower the number of days in the hospital. To achieve a reduction in hospitalization, HMOs provide more ambulatory care and perform less surgery. HMO doctors order as much as 50 percent fewer medical services, such as electrocardiograms and chest X rays, than physicians in traditional settings.

Types of HMOs.   Many employers now offer HMO plans to their employees. At some companies, HMO enrollment is optional; at others, it is mandatory. Cost-conscious employers are painfully aware of the many inefficiencies in the present health care system and now offer several types of HMO coverage. There are four types of HMO: staff, group, network, and independent practice association.

• *Staff HMO.* Here the HMO delivers health care services directly through its own salaried staff of primary care physicians, specialists, nurses, pharmacists, radiologists, and ancillary staff. Staff and clinical services are located under one roof, including doctors' offices, laboratories, X-ray facilities, and pharmacies.

• *Group HMO.* In this arrangement, an HMO contracts with an independent group practice of doctors to provide health care services to its members.

• *Network HMO.* When two or more large group practices contract with an HMO to provide care to members, the system is called a network HMO.

• *Independent practice association (IPA).* In an IPA, doctors in independent practice sign contracts with HMOs to offer medical care to members in their own private offices so that members of a plan that uses IPAs have a larger number of doctors from which they can choose a personal physician. Each participating doctor is paid in advance an agreed-upon amount for that patient's care. An IPA doctor is also likely to provide care for fee-for-service patients.

Preferred Provider Organization

A *preferred provider organization (PPO)* is yet another alternative to conventional insurance plans. Among the organizations or associations offering this kind of coverage are large insurance companies, health care companies, hospitals, and large physician groups. Unlike HMOs, there is no formal organization and there is no capitation. A growing number of employers have been striking deals with PPOs to offer prepaid or discount prices for their employees' medical care.

People who use the PPO system often have no deductible and usually no out-of-pocket costs other than a small fee for an office visit. Routine physical examinations and well-baby care are covered. The main disadvantage is that if you seek care from a physician or a hospital not under contract with the PPO, you're penalized in the form of higher fees.

Other People, Other Needs

People who are self-employed or whose employers don't offer health insurance usually can purchase coverage through a professional organization, union, or trade association. If you are in this category, you pay the entire premium on the policy. But obtaining coverage through your association is still a better buy than independently buying an individual policy.

Depending on the size of the organization with which you are affiliated, you may receive as a member a menu of plans from which to make a choice. In some cases, an HMO may be among the listings.

Disability coverage may also be available through your organization. A disability plan is important for self-employed people because it provides a monthly income if you become disabled for several months and cannot do your work. The National Insurance Consumer Organization recommends that you buy disability coverage that pays benefits until age 65. If you have a sufficient cash reserve to cover your expenses for two or more months, select a 60-, 90-, or 180-day waiting period for your diasability benefits to keep your premiums at a lower price.

A worker who has been laid off or fired from the job is eligible to continue group health insurance coverage for up to 18 months after the termination. In order to keep the coverage, the former employee pays the full premium. The law that made this continuation of coverage possible is called COBRA, the acronym for Consolidated Omnibus Budget Reconciliation Act of 1985.

Under COBRA, employers with more than 20 employees are required to offer discharged workers, their dependents, and spouses of employees becoming eligible for Medicare the opportunity to continue their coverage. At the end of the 18-month period, you may be eligible to convert your coverage to an individual policy, a type of coverage that is always more expensive than similar coverage offered to groups.

Retirees and Medicare

If you're retired or age 65 and about to retire, you're eligible for Medicare, the federal government's health insurance program for older Americans. But there are some gaps in Medicare, and it is important to know which gaps may require backup coverage. For Medicare Part A, which pays for hospital and related services, these gaps include an annual hospital deductible ($592 in 1990), and coinsurance payments for hospital stays that last longer than 60 days. For those requiring care in a skilled nursing care facility, there is a coinsurance payment for the 21st through 100th days of care, after which Medicare no longer pays any part of the bill. For Medicare Part B, which covers doctors' fees, outpatient services, laboratory fees, and ambulance services, there are separate gaps. Among these gaps are the $75 annual deductible and any excess charges by a physician over the amount that Medicare allows for a particular service performed. Under Part B, a 20 percent copayment is required. For more information, contact your local Social Security office or call the Medicare Hotline: 1-800-638-6833.

Consumers Union studied and rated supplemental policies being sold to cover the gaps left by Medicare and found significant differences in quality and price. Some policies are comprehensive and cover most of the gaps while others don't provide the benefits that retired people need. More than half of all the supplemental insurance sold was purchased through Blue Cross and Blue Shield organizations and the American Association of Retired Persons (AARP). However, the 1989 CU study found that, overall, the policies these two organizations were selling were "relatively mediocre."

Many employers continue coverage for their workers past retirement and fill these gaps, so you may not need any additional coverage. However, as a result of soaring health care costs, some companies have begun to set limits on how much they will contribute to retirees' health plans. This includes an end to picking up the remaining expenses after Medicare pays its portion of coverage. In other instances, the company pays benefits based on years employed, so if you've worked for the firm for 30 years, they'll pick up more of the costs than if you're only a 10-year employee.

If you decide to buy a Medicare-supplement policy, Consumers Union advises that you keep these points in mind:

• Buy just one policy.

• If you qualify for Medicaid, you don't need a policy because Medicaid will pay your bills.

• If your income is low but you don't qualify for Medicaid, join an HMO instead of buying a Medigap policy.

• Avoid buying any policies that cover only certain major diseases, or that say they'll pay a flat rate per day in the hospital.

• If you're older or in poor health, seek out an insurance company that won't examine every aspect of your health and that charges every policyholder the same rate.

• If you're healthy and just turned 65, look for a company that carefully scrutinizes the health of prospective policyholders and charges low premiums.

• If you have a Medicare-supplement policy and it doesn't cover excess charges, ask your insurance carrier if it sells a plan with this coverage. It's possible that if you upgrade your policy, the company may waive the "preexisting condition" clause on your new policy.

• Shop around and compare policies. Ask the agent for each policy's outline of coverage and then compare policies from different companies.

Long-term-care Insurance

As the nation's elderly population grows, especially the segment of "old-old," who are over 85, so grows fear of nursing home costs by retirees, their families, and older middle-aged adults. To allay their fears, many are purchasing long-term-care insurance to protect themselves against the financial devastation that usually results from a lengthy stay in a nursing home.

Buying a long-term-care policy might be a good idea for some people, but not for others. If you're over age 60, buying a good long-term-care policy may be a reasonable choice. People under age 60 shouldn't buy one unless the policy has a mechanism for keeping benefits current with inflation in the cost of a nursing-home stay. If you have fairly modest income and assets, don't buy long-term-care coverage because you would soon qualify for Medicaid benefits if you require nursing home care.

Depending on your age and your health, the annual premium may range from around $610 for a 55-year-old to over $3,100 and higher for a 75-year-old. More than 100 insurance companies sell long-term-care policies, some of which offer good coverage and others of which are severely limited in many aspects.

If you are shopping for a long-term-care policy, consider these guidelines before you buy:

• Does the policy have a rider that offers inflation protection? This feature will annually adjust the benefit for inflation. Without it, a daily benefit of $50 could be meager in 10 years as inflation continues to climb.

• What is the daily nursing home benefit? A 1988 Consumers Union study recommended $80 a day. This figure is adjusted by region.

• The waiting period before benefits can begin ranges from 20 to 100 days. Look for a 20-day elimination period.

• How long do the benefits last? For all nursing-home stays, there should be an unlimited number of days.

• Does the policy cover skilled, intermediate, and custodial care? Your insurance should pay benefits for all of these. Most people in nursing homes need custodial care (assistance with basic activities such as getting out of bed, bathing, eating, and walking). Often, residents may also need intermediate care that requires a nurse to give injections or to change bandages. A good policy will cover custodial care.

• Does the payment of benefits hinge upon a prior hospital stay of at least three days before entering a nursing home? Most elderly patients with Alzheimer's disease or arthritis are unlikely to need hospitalization but may need custodial care.

• Are benefits paid for home care? Is a previous hospital or nursing-home stay required to qualify for benefits?

• Does the policy contain a clause that covers "organically based brain disease"? That's one form of insurance industry jargon for Alzheimer's disease. Some policies may be vague in this area.

• Is the policy "guaranteed renewable" for life? If it says "conditionally renewable," then while the insurer may not cancel one policyholder because that policyholder has become a bad risk, it can cancel the coverage at its discretion.

• Is there a waiver of premium? When an insured person has been in a nursing home for a period of time—usually about three months—the insurer will waive the premium.

• What is the A.M. Best & Company rating of the insurer? This company rates the financial stability of insurance companies in its "Best's Insurance Reports," which may be available at your public library. Or ask an insurance agent to provide you with this information. While an A or A+ rating is recommended, a lower rating doesn't necessarily mean the insurer is in failing financial health.

The Poor, the Near-Poor, and Poor Risks

Since the 1980s, continuous cutbacks in the federal government's health insurance program for the poor have left more people who need health care without access to the system. Certain categories of poor and disadvantaged people qualify for the Medicaid program, including the aged, blind, disabled, medically needy, and families with dependent children.

In 1989, a family of four with an annual income of about $11,000 was eligible for Medicaid, although this figure may have been higher or lower depending on the state. Another qualified Medicaid recipient is a person over 65 whose total assets are less than $1,800. Each state decides which people are medically needy and which services it will cover for Medicaid recipients.

People whose income is low, but not low enough to meet the Medicaid standard, are often considered the near-poor. They cannot afford to pay health insurance premiums or medical bills, but they aren't poor enough to use government-sponsored programs.

Of the 31 million Americans without health insurance, an estimated 18 million work but are self-employed or have employers who don't offer health benefits. Surprisingly, about 5 million of the uninsured are members of households where the annual income exceeds $40,000.

When people have disabilities or major illnesses, they may be refused health insurance or be asked to pay huge premiums because commercial carriers consider them poor risks. People with AIDS may encounter difficulty from some insurers when applying for a health or disability policy. A growing number of insurance companies now require testing for AIDS, but they must obtain a signed consent from each policy applicant before that applicant's blood can be tested for AIDS.

Those who have had insurance for a period of years and are diagnosed as having AIDS should have no problem with their health coverage. However, many of the drugs used in AIDS therapy are considered experimental and as such may not be covered under a typical insurance policy. Some insurers may limit the dollar amount of coverage for AIDS care.

How to Choose and Use a Doctor

People who feel healthy don't usually think of doctors. But for anyone who doesn't already have a personal physician, the best time to shop for a doctor is when you're healthy. You feel more savvy, confident, energetic, and in control of your health when you're well—generally the opposite of how you feel when you're sick and don't know where to turn.

Although the myth persists that all doctors are alike in knowledge or competence, it's not true. Aside from such basic differences as training, area of specialization, and number of years in practice, there are other considerations that separate the caring, concerned, and competent physician from the mediocre or incompetent doctor. The first of these is an aptitude for the specific work the doctor is doing, followed by availability, accessibility, affordability, and attitude.

Before you can select a doctor, you need to know which kind you want—a primary care physician or a specialist?

A *primary care physician* is trained to be the doctor you see first—the one who takes care of most of your medical problems and encourages you to prevent illness. This doctor should serve as your advocate in the health care system and determine when a problem is serious enough to refer you to a specialist. Primary care physicians have training in internal medicine, pediatrics, and family medicine. Women who consult a gynecologist for an annual checkup should not consider that examination a substitute for a periodic visit to a primary care physician.

An *internist,* or doctor who practices internal medicine, may also serve as a primary care physician. Some internists may also be qualified as subspecialists in one of several fields, including cardiology, endocrinology, gastroenterology, hematology, infectious diseases, oncology, nephrology, pulmonary diseases, and rheumatology.

A *specialist*'s training focuses on specific organ systems, with an emphasis on disease treatment and hospital care. A specialist cares for serious or puzzling disorders of these organ systems that may be too rare or complicated for your primary care physician to treat. Unless you have a chronic problem, or your problem recurs, you can expect to have a short-term relationship with a specialist.

Because it is the commonplace that occurs most commonly, a primary care physician or internist is your best choice for a doctor with whom you look to develop a continuing relationship. If you experience uncommon symptoms, this personal physician—who knows you, your medical history, and your health profile—will be able to recognize if these symptoms indicate that you need more specialized care, providing advice and direction for you, or simply confirmation, as you make the difficult decisions about choosing or continuing specialized care.

The next step is to get recommendations and referrals from which you can narrow your choice. There are many sources for the names of doctors. These include friends, neighbors, coworkers, relatives, local medical societies, and referral services operated by local hospitals. If you live near a university medical school, you can call the department of primary care or internal medicine and ask the office manager for the names of doctors with private practices. People enrolled in HMOs can ask other patients which doctors they prefer.

Although friends, neighbors, and other personal acquaintances may readily offer the name of their doctor, carefully weigh their recommendations. Be sure to ask them why they like their doctors. Your friend may either be a truly satisfied customer, or someone who focuses on the doctor's personality with little thought about medical competence.

Whether a doctor is a man or woman, older or younger, has a warm or serious personality is all a matter of personal preference. Whether or not the doctor is competent and dedicated can be a matter of your continued good health.

Checking Up

Once you've compiled a list of names, call the medical licensing board in your state and ask if any of the doctors on your list have ever been subject to disciplinary action for professional misconduct. By checking with the state licensing board, you may be able to eliminate a doctor with a poor reputation. Unfortunately, states vary in the degree to which they discipline errant doctors. Some are very strict in enforcing medical professional standards and weeding out doctors who are incompetent or impaired, while others may be more lax.

When you have your list of possibilities, here are some of the main points to cover as you complete your search:

• To make a *credentials check,* find out whether the doctor went to medical school in the United States or Canada, completed a residency, and performed a fellowship, and if the physician is board-certified. If so, be sure to find out which board provided the certification. You can get this information from the doctor's office or HMO office or, better yet, you may prefer to look it up in your local library.

Ask the librarian for the *Directory of Medical Specialists.* This directory will list various information, including whether the physician is board-certified, board-eligible, or recertified. One shortcoming of this directory is that some excellent physicians who are board-certified choose not to be listed or decline to give biographies that list their training. Much of the information that is supplied is not verified by the publishers of the directory.

A board-certified physician is one who has successfully passed the examinations given by the specialty board in a certain area of expertise, such as primary care, orthopedics, or gynecology. A board-eligible doctor has completed the necessary training in the specialty but for some reason may not have taken or perhaps failed the board examinations. Some doctors remain board-eligible their entire medical careers because the current system allows it. If a doctor is represented as a specialist but has not become board-certified in that specialty, you have a right to know why not.

When a doctor has obtained recertification, it indicates that the physician has passed yet another test by demonstrating that he or she has stayed current with the latest medical developments by attending approved continuing education courses and participating in certain other professional activities. Some specialties require periodic recertification, while in others it is voluntary.

• Find out where the doctor has *hospital admitting privileges*. Each hospital must carefully examine the credentials of all physicians who practice there. Many major hospitals require high-level training and demonstrated competence before they will grant staff privileges to doctors.

• How does the doctor *stay current* with the constant advances in the field of medicine? Many physicians regularly take continuing medical education courses or teach at a university hospital or medical school to ensure that they don't isolate themselves from new knowledge and newly developed techniques.

• Can you *afford* this doctor? Ask what is the charge for the first visit, for regular and follow-up visits, and for other services. Get all of this information before making a visit. If you don't feel comfortable with the fee schedule, look for another doctor.

• Do you feel comfortable dealing with the *office staff*? Can you get the information you need? Are your requests and inquiries handled promptly and pleasantly?

• *Access* to the doctor's office is another practical consideration. Is it easy to travel to? Will getting there entail a long bus ride, an expensive taxi ride, or a large bill for parking? A long ride may not seem much of a problem when you're well but may be a real burden when you're ill.

• *Who covers for the doctor* on days off and during vacations? Is the covering physician as qualified in terms of skills and board certification?

• How does the doctor handle *emergencies*? As a regular patient, can you call any time of day or night if you have a true emergency?

• What is the doctor's *attitude* on prevention and health maintenance? To what degree is health education available?

Book an office visit with the doctor you have selected. Bring up your health concerns and your questions during your visit and then decide if you'd like to work with this doctor on maintaining your health. Unfortunately, many doctors insist that a first visit with them involve an extensive, and expensive, generalized examination. Ask the person making the appointment what a first visit will cost you.

The First Visit

During your first or return visit to your doctor, the two of you need to set some ground rules. These include mutually agreed-upon ideas about when you should be in contact. Although you won't be able to cover every theoretical situation in which you should or shouldn't call, at least you'll have a mutual understanding.

If you have a particular health concern, ask your doctor under what circumstances you should call and when you should take care of yourself. If you can treat yourself, what does the doctor recommend?

The doctor should make sure that a patient leaves the office with a clear understanding of the diagnosis and the treatment. If a physician lapses into professional jargon when talking to you, ask for a definition of anything you don't understand.

When medication is prescribed, the physician should explain its use. This includes: when and how to take it, possible side effects, the cost, when you can expect to see an improvement in your condition, and what happens if you stop taking the medication prematurely or abruptly.

A doctor must be willing to answer questions. If a doctor declines to give you information about your diagnosis, proposed treatment, prognosis, and alternative treatments, discuss your concern with the doctor. If the physician still isn't willing to talk, find another doctor. People who live in small towns or rely on a particular specialist may have to try to train that physician about the value of openness and communication. If that still doesn't work, voice your complaint to your local medical society.

If You Need a Specialist

For some serious, complicated, or life-threatening problems, your primary care physician may refer you to a specialist. But your doctor should not refer you to a specialist every time you report a minor complaint in an area of medicine for which there is a specialty. When you are told to consult a medical or surgical specialist, be sure you understand the reason you are being sent to another doctor.

Medicine and surgery both have their own major specialties. There are 16 types of major surgical specialists, including general surgeons. The areas of medical specialization are even more vast. Finding the right specialist may help save your life.

Your choice of a specialist must be highly selective. A surgeon should have considerable technical skill in the specific area you need and perform this type of surgery often. A medical specialist should have finely tuned investigational skills, backed by knowledge and clinical judgment, in order to unravel any puzzling medical mysteries.

Choosing a surgical or medical specialist may begin with your primary care physician. If your personal physician recommends a specialist, and you have confidence in your own doctor, you may want to go with the recommendation that is made. If you have questions or concerns, discuss them with your primary care physician. If you still have concerns about the specialist who was recommended, do some research on your own. To be absolutely sure, follow these guidelines:

Ask your personal physician for the names of two or three medical specialists or surgeons. Find out why these names were recommended—because of reputation, friendship, or because they have a known track record?

Ask for a recommendation at the nearest university medical school. Call the director's office or department division of the specialty you need and ask for the names of top doctors in the area in your geographical location, in the region, and in the nation. Find out which specialist the director would personally want to see for the problem you have.

Check the specialist's training and credentials. The reference section of your public library should have a copy of the *Directory of Medical Specialists,* which lists physicians' credentials. The American College of Surgeons will give you the names of member surgeons who practice in your area. To request information, contact The American College of Surgeons, 55 East Erie Street, Chicago, Illinois 60611. Telephone: (312) 664-4050.

If you have been told you are facing surgery, the following are particularly important.

Find out how often a surgeon performs the operation you are considering. Then ask for the surgeon's personal track record. A surgeon who frequently does certain procedures may have plenty of experience. However, you want experience that has produced good results. At your first appointment, ask for the surgeon's success rate and rate of complications on the type of surgery you are discussing. A highly skilled surgeon will be proud of a good record and readily offer this information. If a surgeon balks at your request, look for another doctor.

It is important to learn the surgeon's hospital affiliation. A well-regarded surgeon will have admitting privileges at major medical centers and good community hospitals. Although there may be a number of hospitals in a certain city, they may not all excel in certain types of surgery. Whereas a community hospital may be a good choice for simple surgery, a major teaching hospital affiliated with a medical college is usually a better setting for a more complicated procedure.

Ask if the surgeon you are consulting will actually perform the operation. If your surgery will be performed at a teaching hospital, is there a chance that a surgical resident—a surgeon in training—will perform the procedure under the supervision of the attending surgeon? You have the right to know in advance if the surgeon you have chosen will do all or part of the operation. If you don't approve of what your surgeon tells you, don't be afraid to assert yourself. Insist on getting the surgeon you are paying for.

Discuss the surgeon's fee and whether this price includes postoperative follow-up visits. Ask the doctor if advance payment is required of if the amount your insurance plan pays is an acceptable form of payment. If your insurance covers only a portion of the cost, and you have limited financial resources, discuss your concern with the surgeon. You may find a sympathetic physician who is willing to adjust the fee or accept your share over time. A doctor's fee doesn't always correlate with the quality of the services provided.

Aside from getting the answers to these questions, you must decide whether surgery is really the only or the best form of treatment for your illness. Here are some questions to consider:

• Before you consult the surgeon, ask your primary care physician if there are any possible alternative treatments other than surgery. If so, ask for information and then do some research on your own. Check the *Readers Guide to Periodical Literature* at your local library. Look for health-related newspapers, magazines, and journals.

• When you see the surgeon ask what the proposed procedure will entail. Find out exactly what will be done and the risk of complications. Inquire as to whether the surgery requires hospitalization or if it can be done on an outpatient basis. If the former, how many days in the hospital will be necessary? Find out how long it will be before you're fully functioning again. Ask the surgeon to explain why the operation will help you. Tell the surgeon your expectations of the end result. Are they in line with the expected benefits for this kind of surgery? Ask if the condition is likely to recur.

A Second Opinion

Faced with a prospect of surgery, you may want a second opinion but feel uncomfortable discussing the subject with your doctor. On the other hand, you don't want to disrupt the relationship you have with your physician, but at the same time, you feel a second opinion would give you some peace of mind.

If you have been told you need immediate emergency surgery, there's no time to quibble over a second opinion. But there are situations, other than surgery, when it's appropriate for a patient to seek another point of view. These include: when you have pain that recurs despite extended treatment, when you have a disabling illness, and when your physician says that nothing more can be done for you. However, the most important reason to seek another opinion is when elective surgery has been recommended.

Several insurance companies and employers now require their policyholders to obtain a second opinion before undergoing elective surgery. Under some plans, getting a second opinion is optional. Among the most common elective surgical procedures are:

hysterectomy	back surgery
gallbladder removal	(lumbar laminectomy)
(cholecystectomy)	knee surgery (arthroscopy)
coronary artery bypass	hernia repair
angioplasty	cataract removal
prostate section	removal of the tonsils
(prostatectomy)	(tonsillectomy)

Under a second-surgical-opinion program, you consult a second physician to obtain more information in deciding whether surgery is the right choice for you. Your insurance company will usually pay for the second opinion, even if it is optional under its policy. Medicare and most state Medicaid programs will pay for the cost of a second opinion.

If the surgeon to whom you've been recommended suggests scheduling surgery, and you'd like to have a second opinion, here's how you can get one:

• Ask your own doctor or the surgeon for the name of another surgeon qualified in the same specialty. Ask if the name you are given is an associate or friend of either of the first two. Don't seek a second opinion from a physician who is associated with a doctor who has already provided an opinion.

• Contact your local medical society, major area hospitals, or a medical school to get the names of surgeons in the area you need. Also, a hospital's patient representative department may be able to steer you toward the right office to call for information.

• Call the federal government's Second Surgical Opinion Hotline for the name of a medical organization in your area that may be able to give you referrals. The toll-free number is (800) 638-6833. When calling from Maryland, dial (800) 492-6603. You will be referred to another phone number in your own state.

Once you've decided upon a physician to provide a second opinion and scheduled an appointment, contact your doctor's office and ask to have your X rays and the results of any tests sent to the consultant's office.

When you seek a second opinion from another surgical physician, bring the same concerns and questions that you took to the first surgeon.

Ask the second-opinion doctor for his or her own diagnosis of your problem. If it differs from the diagnosis offered by the first physician you saw, then ask what could have accounted for the difference. Ask how your treatment might differ following one recommendation or the other.

If the physician agrees with the first opinion, ask for an explanation of the problem, the risks and hoped-for benefits of the proposed surgery, length of recovery, and what to expect in costs. You might also ask about possible alternative treatments and how you'd fare if you delayed the surgery. Getting a second opinion allows you to confirm not only that the surgery is indicated but as well that you have been given an accurate picture of your illness.

If the second doctor agrees that surgery is the best choice, your records will be returned to your first doctor. If you decide to have the recommended operation, the first doctor will perform the surgery, if that is your choice.

When the second doctor disagrees with the opinion of your first doctor, you may want to discuss it with your primary care physician. Or, you may even prefer to seek a third opinion to help you make your decision.

Getting a second opinion does not always provide clear-cut answers, but it should make you feel better informed about the possible choices you have. Surgery is never something to be taken lightly.

Studies have pointed to variations in the types of surgery performed in different cities and parts of the country. Regional patterns have been found to emerge, which appear to be based on the common values and preferences that doctors in a particular city or region have come to share. Researchers comparing these variations identified certain patterns of surgery peculiar to certain regions. For instance, the number of hysterectomies is higher in some cities, while the number of prostatectomies and tonsillectomies is greater in others.

When Hospitalization Is Necessary

Hospitals need to keep their rooms filled to stay profitable. As the national hospital occupancy rate hovers around 60 percent, many hospitals are losing money and some have been forced to close. To fill their beds, several hospitals have launched mass marketing campaigns with the goal of stimulating demand for their services. The amenities they now boast include concierge service, gourmet meals on china, and designer decor in VIP suites. These are not substitutes for an excellent medical, nursing, and laboratory staff.

The promise of state-of-the-art treatments and the accompanying hospitality may be appealing, but think carefully before you decide to enter a hospital: it may be dangerous to your health. Among the potential dangers are complications from postoperative infection, hospital-acquired infection, and adverse reaction to medication and blood transfusions.

Estimates vary, but it is thought that many hospital admissions may be unnecessary. When your doctor says that hospitalization is necessary, you or your health insurance company may want to ask some questions.

Your insurer's focus will be on whether the proposed treatment is medically necessary, and if it is being done in the hospital for appropriate reasons. As a patient, one of your concerns may be whether alternative treatments could be used and whether they could be administered outside the hospital.

Because a hospital stay is expensive and does add its own health risks, ambulatory care units have emerged as an alternative for several surgical procedures that once were almost always done in a hospital. The growing trend toward ambulatory care is expected to increase in the 1990s and beyond. Some ambulatory surgical units may be located in or near a hospital, while others may be in different parts of the community.

In addition, freestanding emergency care centers have sprung up in many communities. These urgent care centers offer quick treatment to patients who otherwise might go to a hospital emergency room for care. Among their advantages are convenience and accessibility, as well as a lower cost than a hospital emergency room. They are open from 12 to 24 hours a day, you don't need an appointment, and waiting time is usually no more than 20 minutes.

However, these units offer quick fixes only. The staff may not take a complete medical history. You may find some urgent care centers lacking in continuity of care, rigorous quality control, or top doctors. Most states don't require licensing of urgent care centers because they are viewed as extensions of doctors' offices.

It's a good idea to visit some urgent care centers in your area before you need them and check on the type and the quality of services available. Talk to the staff and ask about the doctors' credentials and qualifications. The American College of Emergency Physicians has recommended that these centers be operated under the direction of a doctor who is board-certified in emergency medicine.

Which Hospital?

In the past, virtually all hospitals were not-for-profit institutions. Increasingly, large profit-making chains that specialize in health care services have entered the medical marketplace and spurred competition for patients and income. Both not-for-profit and for-profit hospitals run facilities that offer short-term care (30 days or less) as well as long-term care for patients who may have chronic disabilities, severe acute illness, or who need extensive rehabilitation.

There are many types of short-term-care hospitals, including specialty hospitals exclusively for the treatment of illness relating to one body system, such as the eyes or the musculoskeletal system.

The other major types of hospitals are usually classified as teaching, community, or public institutions.

A *teaching hospital* may be affiliated with a medical school, a voluntary not-for-profit hospital, or a public hospital. "Teaching" refers to the staffing pattern, not to the level of care. In a teaching hospital, medical interns, residents, and fellows handle much of the medical care—under the supervision of an attending physician, who is often board-certified in one or more specialties. (A resident is a licensed doctor who has completed a medical internship and is pursuing further postgraduate training in a specialty area, including such fields as internal medicine and family practice, as well as the more unusual specialties.)

Because some larger teaching hospitals may offer highly specialized treatment, they are known as tertiary care centers. They treat people with the rarer illnesses as well as those with common maladies. Because most teaching hospitals are located in major cities, and because many are public hospitals as well, they provide primary care to poor inner-city residents who rely on the hospitals' clinics or emergency rooms for treatment.

Many teaching hospitals are recognized for excellence in certain specialties and for having the latest and the best technology. Certain doctors who are ranked tops in their field by their medical colleagues may have their practices affiliated with a teaching hospital. If you want to be treated by a particular doctor who is associated with a teaching hospital, and the doctor recommends hospitalization, you most likely will have to enter a teaching hospital.

When you enter a teaching hospital, you benefit from frequent contact with the medical staff and double checking of proposed treatments. Several doctors may examine you and follow your case. This system, in which doctors are looking over each other's shoulders, helps guarantee your safety and allows for new insights into your care if your health problem is unusual.

As a private patient of an attending physician who has admitting privileges at a teaching hospital, your daily care may be managed by residents, although your private doctor remains responsible for all final decisions. If you don't have an attending physician, you still will be admitted to the hospital. In this case, your care is placed under the supervision of an attending physician with admitting privileges. Still, most of your care will be delivered by residents.

Your stay may end up being more expensive because doctors in training at teaching hospitals tend to order more tests than other physicians. If you decide you want to receive a particular treatment at a teaching hospital, and your insurance company requires advance clearance, you'll need a doctor who is willing to argue your case.

It's important to learn the names, specialties, and telephone or beeper numbers of any residents who stop by your bedside and say they'll be taking part in your care. Never allow yourself to be treated by anonymous people. Feel free to ask these residents questions and to assert yourself when necessary during your stay in a teaching hospital.

Residents and interns, known as house staff, work on schedules that may include a rotation to a different unit during the course of your care. If residents rotate while you are a patient in a teaching hospital, you'll need to adjust to the new medical team.

A *public hospital,* or city hospital, is supported by public funds derived from the federal, state, or local government. Although public hospitals offering short-term care account for more than 20 percent of the hospitals serving communities of various sizes, they are most likely to be found in large cities. Public hospitals also provide long-term care for patients with psychiatric illness or certain chronic conditions.

Public hospitals include military hospitals, the hospitals and facilities operated by the Veterans Administration, as well as hospitals for American Indians and merchant seamen. Municipal hospitals, such as Bellevue in New York, Cook County Hospital in Chicago, and New Orleans Charity Hospital, are public hospitals. Most of the larger public hospitals are affiliated with medical schools, and so in effect are also teaching hospitals.

Because public hospitals are the only source of health care to the poor, there is a public perception that they deliver substandard care. It's true that some public hospitals are understaffed, overcrowded, and located in aging buildings in declining inner-city areas. However, because they are teaching hospitals, they have top doctors and residents on their medical staff.

Several public hospitals offer superior care for special medical needs, including microsurgery to reattach severed limbs, burn treatment, organ transplants, cardiac care, trauma treatment, and specialized care for high-risk pregnant mothers or very sick, premature newborn infants.

When people who cannot afford health care need medical treatment, they are usually admitted or transferred to a public hospital or a teaching hospital. Although public hospitals are reimbursed at least in part by Medicaid or Medicare for many patients, a large amount of the treatment they provide is without compensation. To survive, the hospital must depend on government support.

A *community hospital* may be best known as a general hospital in many towns. The number of beds may range from 50 to 500. Community hospitals are often designed to provide care for common medical and surgical needs. Many have a medical and cardiac intensive care unit (ICU).

In the past, most community hospitals were strictly voluntary not-for-profit institutions, or else were owned by a small group of doctors. Since the mid-1960s, when the federal government launched the Medicare and Medicaid programs which offered reimbursement for health care, investor-backed corporations entered the hospital industry with an eye on profits. Today, scores of these for-profit hospital chains or multihospital systems operate more than 1,000 hospitals around the country. Additionally, they run hundreds of HMOs and so-called convenience-care clinics, thousands of nursing homes, and other health care operations.

Investor-owned community hospitals are usually located in affluent suburbs or in growing upscale communities. In some cases, a for-profit hospital may be the only health care facility in town. Many health care analysts note that in deciding whether or not to admit you, for-profit hospitals first examine your wallet and then your illness. If you don't have private insurance or the funds to cover the care you need, you'll either be asked to apply for a loan or find yourself transferred to the nearest public hospital.

An inpatient at a for-profit community hospital may pay about the same costs for a given treatment as a patient at a voluntary not-for-profit hospital, but it is more likely that charges will be higher at a for-profit hospital. The quality of care is considered to be equal in both types of hospital. While the for-profit hospitals may be able to boast of more amenities for patients, many voluntary hospitals also offer a range of special suites and services.

Assuring Quality Care

When a hospital meets quality standards, it receives accreditation from the *Joint Commission on Accreditation of Healthcare Organizations* (JCAHO). About 5,400 of the nation's hospitals have JCAHO accreditation. Each year, about 2 percent of these hospitals fail to earn full accreditation.

JCAHO reviewers visit participating hospitals every three years and scrutinize various aspects of the institution. If a hospital fails to meet JCAHO standards, it risks being placed on conditional status until the shortcomings are corrected. A highly rated hospital may prominently display its formal JCAHO accreditation for patients and visitors to see.

In July 1989, the Joint Commission began a new policy under which it now will disclose the names of hospitals that are only conditionally accredited or not accredited. To check on a hospital's status, ask a hospital representative or contact the Joint Commission on Accreditation of Healthcare Organizations directly. They are at 875 North Michigan Avenue, Chicago, Illinois 60611. Telephone: (312) 642-6061.

Accreditation is an important assurance that a hospital meets certain standards. If the JCAHO revokes a hospital's rating or puts it on a six-month term of probation with a conditional accreditation, find out why.

Many insurers require JCAHO accreditation before they will pay any bills for certain categories of hospital care.

The state health department also may be a source of information about hospitals. To learn whether other patients have filed complaints against the hospital you are considering, call the state health department and ask for this information. This office also should be able to provide you with the up-to-date JCAHO accreditation status of a hospital.

To avoid outside censure, hospitals strive to assure quality care to their patients by various internal mechanisms. A hospital may have a quality assurance department or committee as well as a risk management department to reduce the incidence of potential problems that could lead to lawsuits.

Monitoring Physicians

From the standpoint of government regulators and consumers, the demand for accountability and guaranteed quality care would appear to be a simple request. But creating an effective and acceptable method of evaluating the competence of physicians, dentists, and other health care professionals has long been elusive. Traditionally, doctors have been successful in resisting monitoring by any outside group—including their own peers.

Though estimates as to exact number vary, it's believed that at least a small percentage of the country's doctors are unfit for practice. These are physicians who have a history of incompetence, professional misconduct, impairment from alcohol or drug abuse, or mental illness. No matter how great the risk to patients, it's a frustrating and difficult struggle to put an incompetent physician out of business.

Doctors assert that they are the best qualified to police the medical profession, but in reality, like most professionals, they are reluctant or unwilling to turn in their own colleagues. Unfortunately, bad medical practice often is not brought to public attention until someone outside the field speaks up or notices that an unfit doctor has left a trail of injury or even death.

Until recently, there was no system to learn the identity of these physicians. In 1989, a major force in the drive to weed out delinquent doctors was put into action: the *National Practitioner Data Bank*.

The data bank was created by an act of Congress in 1986 to track incompetent medical practitioners and to encourage peer review in the health care profession. Using a national computer system, the data bank essentially serves as a clearinghouse of data on how physicians perform. The data bank collects information on professional disciplinary actions by state medical boards, the courts, hospitals, peer review groups, and medical societies. Professional liability insurance companies must report any malpractice payments to the data bank or face a fine. A physician's dismissal from a hospital staff or license suspension in one state will now show up if the doctor attempts to set up practice in another state.

Hospitals are required by law to use the data bank as a major source of information on all licensed health care professionals. For instance, when a physician applies to a hospital for an appointment to its medical staff or seeks renewal of privileges every two years, the hospital must consult the data bank. Failure to use the data bank can result in hefty fines.

The public will not have access to the data bank. Those who will be able to obtain information include medical professionals who would like to check their own records, state licensing boards, health care groups and hospitals who need the information to screen job applicants, the Department of Defense, and the Drug Enforcement Agency. Plaintiff attorneys involved in litigation against a hospital or one of its doctors also will have access to the data bank under certain situations. One such situation would be if it can be proven that the hospital didn't query the data bank before hiring a doctor or renewing his or her privileges. The only other situation in which an attorney would have access is if the information is going to be used in relation to the case in question.

The law that created the data bank doesn't spell out what a hospital must do with the data it compiles on its practicing physicians and prospective employees. When problem physicians are identified, it is expected that they will be reeducated and their patient care monitored. If necessary, the hospitals will move to suspend or revoke their licenses.

Peer Review

Each state is required by law to have a physicians' Peer Review Organization (PRO) to monitor the quality of care that doctors deliver to patients receiving Medicare. The PRO is an independent group that uses doctors from each specialty area to review physicians in their own field of practice. Among the areas that come under the PRO's scrutiny are patient care that is given in doctors' offices and the documentation of that care in the medical chart.

If the PRO finds that a physician has compiled a number of violations, it may recommend that the doctor take remedial education, or continuing medical education courses. In some cases, the PRO may assign a doctor with quality-of-care problems to work under a senior physician who is willing to serve as an interim mentor.

Doctors who have been assigned to remedial education and don't comply may be subject to disciplinary action. However, many state PROs report that physicians who have been asked to take some remedial study are more than willing to undergo the training and keep their licenses.

Patient Representatives

Traditionally, patient advocacy was a role assumed by doctors, nurses, and social workers. Since the early 1970s, the delivery of health care has become more sophisticated, more specialized, and more fragmented. As a hospital patient, you have needs, but they often may fall through the cracks. When you are sick and in an intimidating hospital environment, you may be too frightened or too ill to ask questions or to speak up if you have a problem.

Negotiating today's complex, high-technology medical centers may now be a little smoother in many hospitals because of the advent of a relatively new health care specialist—the *patient advocate*, also called a *patient representative* or ombudsman.

Patient representatives are not to be confused with the hospitality hostesses or stewards that may be a part of the promotional amenities a hospital offers. Nor are they volunteers who bring you magazines and snacks, or public relations staffers who want to make the hospital look good. Patient representatives are specially trained to help you negotiate the hospital system if you encounter a problem that you feel is compromising your care.

Complaints about care, poor communication with doctors and nurses, inconvenience, second opinions, and grievances that could lead to costly lawsuits are among the issues that patient representatives confront every day. Because patient representatives are familiar with all levels of the hospital's power base, they know which department head or administrator can help to resolve your problem. By working as mediators between the patient and the institution, patient representatives have defused many situations before they became major problems.

But even when a hospital has a patient representative program in place, there may be some limitations. Ask which office the patient representative reports to—the business office or the vice president for administration? When high-level administrators are responsible for the program, the program is likely to be stronger. Find out the size of the patient representative department. If there is only one advocate for a 500-bed hospital, that patient representative will be very busy and may not have the time to be very effective on your behalf.

A true patient representative, though employed by the hospital, is diligent and responsive in meeting your needs as a patient—even when the end result works out in your favor instead of the hospital's. In this era of competition for patients among health care institutions, astute hospital administrators want each patient to leave their hospital healthy and satisfied.

To get information about a hospital's patient representative department, you can call the hospital before your admission and get information about location, hours, extension, and the name of the advocate. Some hospitals may include this information in a preadmission packet that is mailed to your home. Others may give you this information at the time of admission, or leave a card at your bedside with the name and number of the representative.

Patients' Rights

Today, most people—including doctors—accept that patients have rights. These basic rights to consideration and respect were earned as a result of growing consumer frustration with the changing health care system over the last few decades.

In a show of support for patients, the American Hospital Association created a 12-point document that acknowledges a patient's rights and privileges. This document, known officially as the *Patient's Bill of Rights,* was released in 1973. Some states follow the AHA's original guidelines exactly as written by the association. Other states, such as New York, have added more rights that become a part of the state's public health code.

If you want to take an active part in your care, it can help to be familiar with these rights. Many states require hospitals and nursing homes to give each patient a complete list of these rights upon admission. The AHA and the Joint Commission on Accreditation of Healthcare Organizations support you in your pursuit of these rights.

The main points that the bill addresses are such rights as:

- knowing the name and function of any health care professional who is treating you (see point 2)
- informed consent, or your right to have all necessary information before the start of any operation, procedure, or treatment (point 3 covers these concerns)
- your right to refuse treatment (point 4)
- the right to personal privacy and the privacy of medical programs, and the right to confidentiality of your medical records (points 5 and 6)
- the right to know if you will be offered any experimental treatment (point 9). Based on this information, you have the right to refuse treatment, without prejudice to continued medical treatment.

(See Appendix for a full listing of the Patient's Bill of Rights.)

Ideally, a family member or someone close to you should serve as your personal representative or ombudsman during your hospital stay. If you are very weak or ill, having a personal advocate can help keep the lines of communication open between you and your health care team. If you have communication problems with the medical staff when you are a patient, and you have no one close to count on, ask the patient representative department for assistance.

Patients who feel they are poorly treated while in the hospital can complain. If a hospital sends you a patient survey questionnaire after your discharge, use this form to say you weren't pleased during your stay. Similarly, if things went well, let the hospital administration know.

If you have a serious complaint, write to your state health department's Office of Consumer Affairs. Send a copy to the JCAHO. If your grievance involves a doctor, contact the state board of medical examiners or the state Office of Professional Misconduct.

The state health department investigates every complaint it receives. When the investigation is complete, the department will let you know whether it considers your complaint valid. One of your alternatives in our litigious society is to consult an attorney. If you decide to take legal action, remember that new laws in some states have set a $10,000 penalty for nuisance claims.

If you make a formal complaint, stick to the facts and be concise when you discuss your problem. Although you may be angry for good reason, it's to your benefit to give a factual account of the incident or person involved, not an emotional one.

Informed Consent

By law, no one has the right to do anything to your body without your consent. But under the legal principle of *informed consent,* consent based on insufficient or inaccurate information holds no validity. That means your doctor must spend some time discussing your options with you. For a doctor to recite only statistics or to hand you a fact sheet to read does not meet the minimum requirements of informed consent.

Some physicians find informed consent bothersome and consider a consent form with your signature as proof that they have obtained your informed consent. They are in error about this, for your signature alone is not a substitute for a process that must take place.

In a healthy doctor-patient relationship, informed consent is not just a legal issue, but an opportunity to further expand the dialogue between patient and physician. Here is your chance to get a complete lowdown on your medical condition and treatment options—in plain English. Don't sign anything if you need time to understand and absorb the pros and cons of a proposed treatment and to reflect on what you've learned.

If you are contemplating a treatment or procedure, always be aware of this right to make an informed consent. This includes the right to know:

• What is your current medical condition, or diagnosis?

• What will the proposed procedure or treatment entail? What is its purpose? What is the expected outcome?

• Who is the doctor that will perform the procedure? Except under extenuating circumstances it should be done by the same physician who is obtaining the consent. That the doctor who will be performing the procedure is too busy to bother with informed consent procedures is not a properly extenuating circumstance.

• What other alternatives are there to this treatment?

• What are the benefits of each alternative treatment?

• What are the risks of each alternative treatment? How serious are these risks?

• What would be the likely outcome if you had no treatment at all?

A Few Exceptions

If there is an *emergency* and you need immediate treatment to save your life, a doctor may treat you without obtaining informed consent. When a person is unconscious, it is implied that a reasonable person would want to be treated. But if an injured person regains full consciousness and refuses treatment, the doctors would have to be guided by the request for refusal. It must first be determined whether the patient is competent to make a decision about treatment. A patient who is confused or delirious is not considered competent to accept or refuse treatment.

When a doctor determines that disclosing the alternative treatments and risks would harm a patient more than the proposed treatment, this exception is called *therapeutic privilege*. This privilege is rarely used. A savvy doctor would provide the necessary information to the patient's family or personal representative before using therapeutic privilege.

Another exception to informed consent is the patient who doesn't want any information. Such a *waiver* of the right to be informed is acceptable, if the patient doesn't really want to know. If you really don't want to hear the details about risks you needn't be forced to endure hearing about them. In this case, your doctor may ask you to sign a waiver form.

Medical Research

Major medical centers around the country regularly conduct experiments that measure a new drug's effectiveness against another medication, or against an inactive substitute, or placebo. If you are being treated for a certain condition—and in some cases, if you are healthy—a doctor may ask you to participate in a clinical trial of a new therapy. Although these trials enable medical researchers to gain new knowledge that benefits society, you have no obligation to participate.

Few people embark on a research protocol without some fear and misgivings. A common feeling is: why should I be a guinea pig? For a person with an illness that has not responded to approved drugs or therapies, treatment with an experimental drug may represent a last desperate search for a chance at better health. For others, the promise of payment for participation may be a factor. Most who participate simply wish to be helpful and contribute to new knowledge.

Informed consent is crucial to anyone considering becoming a human research subject. If you decide to join a clinical trial, be sure you fully understand the nature of the research. You are entitled to a clear explanation of the drugs being used and the possible side effects, benefits, and risks. You never should allow yourself to feel pressured into entering an experiment.

Never sign a consent form that you don't fully understand without asking for a full explanation. Improperly omitted material may include a full description of the risks, the fact that it is experimental, and the right of participants to withdraw at any time.

The federal government's Office for Protection from Research Risks lists general requirements for informed consent in its code of federal regulations. Among these are:

• If you decide to participate in a research protocol, you must receive information that describes the purpose of the experiment, how long it will last, and which aspects are experimental.

• The researcher must tell you what kind of risks or discomfort you may experience, as well as the benefits you may expect. Similarly, the physician must explain any alternative treatments or procedures that may be beneficial to you.

• The doctor running the experiment must explain whether your medical records will remain confidential during this treatment. If others will see this information, ask who will have access and why.

• If the risk to you is more than minimal, the physician owes you an explanation as to whether any compensation and any medical treatment is available if you are injured. You need to know what the compensation and medical treatment will consist of and where you can get further information.

• The physician must explain who you can contact for answers to questions about the research and your rights as a participant. This should include the name of a person to contact if you suffer an injury related to the research.

• The doctor must clearly tell you that your decision to participate is voluntary. If you refuse to participate your treatment will not suffer as a result. You may drop out of the clinical trial at any time.

Your Medical Records

Keeping a copy of your own medical records is a good idea. If you move or your doctor retires, you'll have everything you need to give a copy to your new doctor. But more important than convenience is the simple fact that it's one of your fundamental rights to see your records at your request. Information about your health belongs to you.

Some doctors may discourage you from keeping a current copy of your medical record. But it's your right to have access to your records in a doctor's office or hospital in 23 states and the District of Columbia, according to a recent survey. Depending on where you live, if you request a copy of your file, your doctor's office or hospital may have a legal obligation to provide you with a photocopy. Usually, there is a fee for making photocopies. If you live in a state that does not require that you be given a copy of your records upon your request, write or call your state department of health, and your representative in each house of your state legislature, demanding a change in the law or regulation. There are people in the medical profession who believe, and so report to these lawmakers and regulators, that only a small number of patients really want to see their medical records. It's up to you to let them know how you feel about the issue.

Even if you live in a state where you have a right to your records, expect resistance here. You may have to be both persistent and patient before getting them. If you ask your doctor or hospital for your records and get no response, make a written request. If you receive no answer within a reasonable time you may have to call your state department of health to find out if you have a right to these records in your state. If you do, write to your doctor or hospital again telling them of what you have learned. Even where you are entitled to these records by law, in the end you may have to engage an attorney to obtain them.

Even if you are not especially interested in reading your file, a periodic review of your medical records can ensure that they are accurate and complete. If an error creeps into your file, it can cause you problems. There have been cases in which erroneous information has resulted in rejection by insurers, employers, and potential spouses, as well as misguiding future doctors who treat you.

Every time you apply for health, disability, or life insurance, you must sign a waiver that allows the insurer to obtain your complete medical history, giving many people access to your medical records. Insurance companies, employers who handle their employees' insurance, utilization review groups, government agencies, and consumer reporting groups all have a look at your medical history, and transmit all or part of it to other data banks.

Insurance companies rely on two large computerized data banks for information on applicants. They check to see if you are on file at the Medical Information Bureau, a trade group of insurance companies whose members exchange information on people who apply for insurance. They also may use Equifax, a consumer reporting agency, which collects authorized-release records from doctors and hospitals.

In a typical file are a person's weight, blood pressure, electrocardiogram results, and any illnesses or chronic conditions. Life-style habits, such as smoking or drinking alcohol, are included. A person's driving record may be included. Hobbies also may be listed—especially risky ones, like hang gliding.

Under the Fair Credit Reporting Act, these computerized file keepers have an obligation to collect and maintain accurate information on each person. You have the right to see a copy of your file and to make corrections if there are errors.

To get a copy of your record from the Medical Information Bureau, write to the bureau at P.O. Box 105, Essex Station, Boston, Massachusetts 02112. Telephone: (617) 426-3660. It releases only nonmedical information to consumers. For medical information, you must designate a medical professional to whom the bureau can disclose your medical file.

To request a copy of your investigative report from Equifax, check your area telephone directory for an Equifax listing and call the company. If no office is located nearby, you may want to write to the director of consumer affairs, Equifax Services, P.O. Box 4081, Atlanta, Georgia 30302.

If you find a mistake in your file, notify the bureau. It will conduct an investigation, and if it determines that you are right, your file will be corrected. If you aren't satisfied with the response, you can write a letter of dispute, which will become a part of your file.

The Right to Die

If you are 18 or older, consider this question: if a serious accident or illness left you in an irreversible coma with no chance of recovery, would you want to be tethered to a respirator or stomach feeding tube to stay alive indefinitely?

Dying is complicated these days. As medical technology saves more lives, it also prolongs the lives of people who permanently lose consciousness and cannot speak for themselves.

If you've ever thought about this issue, you can take steps to let your family or friends know what you'd want them to do if you were in such a medical situation. To buy some peace of mind for yourself and your loved ones, preparing an advance directive, such as a living will or a health care proxy, should be high on your list of priorities.

Living Wills

A living will is a document that tells your family and your doctor how you want them to proceed in regard to life-prolonging medical treatment or equipment when your condition is hopeless and your chance of regaining a meaningful life is nil.

Doctors, lawyers, a presidential commission on ethics, and the American Medical Association have endorsed living wills. Forty states and the District of Columbia have laws that recognize living wills. One recent opinion survey for the AMA indicated that 73 percent of the American public agrees that artificial life support should be withdrawn from hopelessly ill or comatose patients if the patient or the family requests it. Yet only about 9 percent of Americans have written a living will.

You can draft a living will without an attorney. The Society for the Right to Die will send you a living will declaration and guidelines for its proper use in your state. In states where there is no living will law on the books, the society will send you a document and information that will cover you under the current laws in your state.

This nonprofit organization doesn't charge for the living will forms. It is recommended that you send a stamped, self-addressed envelope along with your request. If you can afford a donation, the money is used to help cover the costs of materials and printing.

To get your living will, write to the Society for the Right to Die, 250 West 57th Street, New York, New York 10107. Or call the society at (212) 246-6973.

Every state has a *durable power of attorney* statute, in which you can delegate power to a family member or trusted friend to act on your behalf if you should become terminally ill or incompetent. But the existence of the statute doesn't necessarily apply to health care decisions in all states. Different laws apply in each state.

When you fill out your forms, be clear in writing your instructions. You can state that you wouldn't want your life prolonged by a mechanical ventilator or artificial feeding. You can also say that you would like medication to reduce your pain.

A living will is not an absolute guarantee that your family will avoid legal tangles regarding your care. It is more of a guide for your family or designated personal representative and communicates to your doctor and the courts, if they become involved, how you would likely make the decision for yourself if you could. Decisions over whether life should be prolonged are heart wrenching and rarely clear-cut. In many institutions, if you have a signed, recently dated living will, this document strengthens the chances that your wishes will be honored.

Two adults who are not relatives must witness your signature on a living will. You may even want to have the document notarized. When you have completed your living will, discuss it with your family and close friends so that they are familiar with your wishes. Give a signed copy to the person who you would like to act as your personal representative or proxy if medical decisions must be made.

Bring a signed copy to your doctor and discuss the contents of the living will. Tell your doctor you would like to have a copy of the living will placed in your medical file. If your doctor disagrees with the idea or content of your living will, you need to find a new doctor who will respect your request.

If you require hospitalization or must enter a nursing home, see that a signed copy of your living will becomes a part of your medical chart. You may want to request that the facility give you a written confirmation that it has a copy of your living will and that it will honor your requests.

After giving a signed copy of the living will to your personal representative, your doctor, and your attorney, if you have one, keep a copy with your own important personal papers. The copy should be located in an easy-to-access place so that if your living will is needed, it will be easy to find.

If you decide to make a living will, you can change it any time you like. It's a good idea to make an occasional review of your living will to make sure it exactly reflects your choices. If you make changes of any kind, initial them and date them, just as you would with any legal document. Be certain that the date is current—this will help establish that the will reflects your current thinking. Be certain to make these same changes and put your initials on additional copies on file with your doctor and your personal representative.

To Resuscitate or Not?

When you enter a hospital, it is presumed that you would want to be resuscitated, or revived, if your heart and lungs suddenly stopped working—an emergency state called cardiopulmonary arrest. In the past, doctors made decisions over whether or not to resuscitate gravely and terminally ill patients. As patients assume a greater responsibility in their own care and decision making, many may choose to make these decisions for themselves. If you don't want cardiopulmonary resuscitation, you can request a *DNR,* or Do Not Resuscitate order.

The JCAHO now requires hospitals and other health care organizations to have formal written policies on DNR standards. The policies must spell out how DNR decisions are to be reached, the role of health care professionals in these decisions, and how to protect the patient. In some states, patients now receive information about DNR upon admission to the hospital.

A DNR order is not the same as a living will. It is a separate order that is a part of each state's public health law. DNR provisions change from state to state.

A DNR order must be documented in your medical chart by a physician when you or your designated representative gives it. Similarly, if you change your mind and decide you want resuscitation, the physician is required by law to note this immediately in your chart. You should discuss life support and DNR orders with your primary care physician at the earliest opportunity.

Appendix

THE PATIENT'S BILL OF RIGHTS
(as established by the American Hospital Association)

The hospital shall establish written policies regarding the rights of patients upon admission for treatment as an inpatient, outpatient, or emergency room patient, and shall develop procedures implementing such policies. These rights, policies, and procedures shall afford patients the right to

1. receive emergency medical care, as indicated by the patient's medical condition, upon arrival at a hospital for the purpose of obtaining emergency medical treatment;

2. considerate and respectful care;

3. obtain the name of the physician assigned the responsibility for coordinating his/her care and the right to consult with his/her private physician and/or a specialist for the type of care being rendered, provided such physician has been accorded hospital staff privileges;

4. the name and function of any person providing treatment to the patient;

5. obtain from his/her physician complete current information concerning his/her diagnosis, treatment and prognosis in terms the patient can be reasonably expected to understand. When it is not medically

advisable to give such information to the patient, the information shall be made available to an appropriate person on the patient's behalf;

6. receive from his/her physician information necessary to give informed consent prior to the start of any nonemergency procedure or treatment or both. An informed consent shall include, as a minimum, the specific procedure or treatment or both, the reasonably foreseeable risks involved, and alternatives for care or treatment, if any, as a reasonable medical practitioner under similar circumstances would disclose;

7. refuse treatment to the extent permitted by law and to be informed of the medical consequences of his/her action;

8. privacy to the extent consistent with providing medical care to the patient. This shall not preclude discreet discussion of a patient's case or examination of a patient by appropriate health care personnel;

9. privacy and confidentiality of all records pertaining to the patient's treatment, except as otherwise provided by law or third-party contract;

10. a response by the hospital, in a reasonable manner, to the patient's request for services customarily rendered by the hospital consistent with the patient's treatment;

11. be informed by his/her physician or designee or the physician of the patient's continuing health care requirements following discharge, and that before transferring a patient to another facility the hospital first informs the patient of the need for and alternatives to such a transfer;

12. the identity, upon request, of other health care and educational institutions that the hospital has authorized to participate in the patient's treatment;

13. refuse to participate in research and that human experimentation affecting care or treatment shall be performed only with the patient's informed effective consent;

14. examine and receive an explanation of his/her bill, regardless of source of payment;

15. know the hospital rules and regulations that apply to his/her conduct as a patient;

16. treatment without discrimination as to race, color, religion, sex, national origin or source of payment, except for fiscal capability thereof;

17. designate any private accommodation to which admitted as a nonsmoking area. In the event that private accommodations are not available, a patient shall have a right to be admitted to accommodations which have been designated by the governing authority as a nonsmoking area. It shall be the duty of the governing authority of the hospital to afford priority to the rights of nonsmokers in all semiprivate, ward, and pediatric common patient areas;

18. voice grievances and recommend changes in policies and services

to the facility's staff, the governing authority and the state department of health without fear of reprisal; and

19. express complaints about the care and services provided and to have the hospital investigate such complaints. The hospital is responsible for providing the patient or the patient's designee with a written response if requested by the patient indicating the findings of the investigation. The hospital is also responsible for notifying the patient or the patient's designee that if the patient is not satisfied by the hospital response, the patient may complain to the state department of health's Office of Systems Management.

A copy of the provisions of this section shall be made available to each patient or patient's representatives upon admission for treatment as an inpatient, outpatient and/or emergency room patient and posted in conspicuous places within the hospital.

References

Altman, L. K. "The Evidence Mounts on Passive Smoking." *The New York Times,* May 29, 1990.

Amara, R. "Health Care Tomorrow." *Hospital Topics,* Vol. 67, No. 1 (January/February 1989).

American Cancer Society. *Cancer Facts and Figures.* 1990.

American College of Sports Medicine. Position Stand. "The Recommended Quantity and Quality of Exercise for Developing and Maintaining Cardiorespiratory and Muscular Fitness in Healthy Adults." *Medicine and Science in Sports and Exercise,* April 1990.

American Dental Association. "Keeping a Healthy Mouth. Tips for Older Adults." 1989.

———. "Periodontal Disease." 1984.

American Heart Association. *1990 Heart and Stroke Facts.* 1990.

American Medical Association. *The American Medical Association Family Medical Guide.* Edited by J. R. M. Kunz and A. J. Finkel. New York: Random House, 1987.

———. *The American Medical Association Guide to Heart Care.* Consumers Union Edition. Mount Vernon, N.Y.: Consumers Union, 1986.

American Psychiatric Association. *Diagnostic and Statistical Manual of Mental Disorders.* Third Edition. Revised. Washington, D.C.: American Psychiatric Association, 1987.

"Are You a Good Insurance Risk?" *Consumer Reports,* June 1986, pp. 401–402.

Arthritis Foundation. *Understanding Arthritis.* Mount Vernon, N.Y.: Consumers Union, 1984.

"Aspirin—An Rx to Prevent Heart Attacks?" *Consumer Reports,* October 1988, pp. 616–618.

Bailey, J. "Built to Last." *Health,* October 1989.

"Baldness—Is There Hope?" *Consumer Reports,* September 1988, pp. 543–547.

Barrett, S., and Cornacchia, H. J. *Consumer Health.* Fourth Edition. St. Louis: C. V. Mosby, 1989.

Barrett-Connor, E. "Postmenopausal Estrogen Replacement and Breast Cancer." Editorial. *The New England Journal of Medicine,* Vol. 321, No. 5 (August 3, 1989), pp. 319–320.

Bedell, S. E., and Delbanco, T. L. "Choices About Cardiopulmonary Resuscitation in the Hospital." *The New England Journal of Medicine,* Vol. 310, No. 17 (April 26, 1984), pp. 1089–1093.

Belloc, N. B., and Breslow, L. "Relationship of Physical Health Status and Health Practices." *Preventive Medicine,* 1 (1972), pp. 409–421.

"Beyond Medicare." *Consumer Reports,* June 1989, pp. 375–391.

Birren, J., and Schaie, K. W., editors. *Handbook of the Psychology of Aging.* New York: Van Nostrand Reinhold, 1985.

Blair, S. N., et al. "Physical Fitness and All-Cause Mortality." *Journal of the American Medical Association,* Vol. 262, No. 17 (November 3, 1989), pp. 2395–2401.

Blakeslee, S. "The Return of the Mind." *American Health,* March 1989.

Blum, K., Noble, E. P., et al. "Allelic Association of Human Dopamine D2 Receptor Gene in Alcoholism." *Journal of the American Medical Association,* Vol. 263, No. 15 (April 18, 1990), pp. 2055–2060.

Bonner, J., and Harris, W. *Healthy Aging.* Claremont, Calif.: Hunter House, 1988.

The Boston Women's Health Collective. *The New Our Bodies, Ourselves.* New York: Simon and Schuster, 1984.

Bouchard, C., et al. "The Response to Long-term Overfeeding in Identical Twins." *The New England Journal of Medicine,* Vol. 322, No. 21 (May 24, 1990), pp. 1477–1482.

Brownell, K. D. "The Psychology and Physiology of Obesity: Implications on Screening and Treatment." *Journal of the American Dietetic Association,* April 1984.

Burros, M. "Decoding a Nutrition Label." *The New York Times,* July 12, 1989.

Calderone, M. S., and Johnson, E. W. *The Family Book About Sexuality.* New York: Harper & Row, 1989.

"Can You Rely on Condoms?" *Consumer Reports,* March 1989, pp. 135–141.

"Chronic Fatigue Syndrome." *Consumer Reports,* October 1990, pp. 671–675.

Columbia University College of Physicians and Surgeons. *Complete Home Medical Guide.* Medical Editors: D. F. Tapley, R. J. Weiss, and T. Q. Morris. New York: Crown, 1985.

"A Consumer's Guide to Food Labels." *FDA Consumer,* September 1988, HHS Publication #FDA 88-2083.

Council on Scientific Affairs, American Medical Association. "Mammographic Screening in Asymptomatic Women Aged 40 Years and Older." *Journal of the American Medical Association,* Vol. 261, No. 17 (May 5, 1989), pp. 2535–2542.

Dandoy, S. "Preventive Medicine." *Journal of the American Medical Association,* Vol. 263, No. 19 (May 16, 1990), pp. 2674–2675.

Davis, R. M. "Uniting Physicians Against Smoking: The Need for a Coordinated National Strategy." Editorial. *Journal of the American Medical Association,* Vol. 259, No. 19 (May 20, 1988), pp. 2900–2901.

Derogatis, L. R., and Wise, T. N. *Anxiety and Depressive Disorders in the Medical Patient.* Washington, D.C.: American Psychiatric Press, 1989.

Doress, P. B., Siegel, D. L., and the Midlife and Older Women Book Project. *Ourselves, Growing Older.* New York: Touchstone, 1987.

Dranov, P. "How Do You Know If It's PMS?" *American Health,* December 1989, pp. 54–58.

Eckert, E. D., and Mitchell, J. E. "An Overview of the Treatment of Anorexia Nervosa." *Psychiatric Medicine,* Vol. 7, No. 4 (1989), pp. 293–313.

Edlin, G., and Golanty, E. *Health & Wellness.* Third Edition. Boston: Jones and Bartlett, 1988.

Emanuel, L. L, and Emanuel, E. J. "The Medical Directive. A New Comprehensive Advance Care Document." *Journal of the American Medical Association,* Vol. 261, No. 22 (June 9, 1989), pp. 3288–3293.

"Fascinating Facts." *Berkeley Wellness Letter,* April 1990, p. 1.

"Fast Food: A Survival Guide to Greasy Kid Stuff." *Consumer Reports,* June 1988, pp. 355–361.

Fielding, J. E., and Phenow, K. J. "Health Effects of Involuntary Smoking." *The New England Journal of Medicine,* Vol. 319, No. 22 (December 1, 1988), pp. 1452–1460.

Finch, C., and Schneider, E. L., editors. *Handbook of the Biology of Aging.* New York: Van Nostrand Reinhold, 1985.

"Finding Help to Quit Cigarettes." *Harvard Medical School Health Letter,* November 1987, pp. 6–8.

Fineberg, H. V. "The Social Dimensions of AIDS." *Scientific American,* October 1988, pp. 121–134.

Fiore, M., et al. "Methods Used to Quit Smoking in the United States. Do Cessation Programs Help?" *Journal of the American Medical Association,* Vol. 263, No. 20 (May 23/30 1990), pp. 2760–2765.

Flieger, K. "Why Do We Age?" *FDA Consumer,* October 1988, pp. 20–25.

Folkenberg, J. "Hair Apparent? For Some, a New Solution to Baldness." *FDA Consumer,* December 1988/January 1989, pp. 8–11.

Ford, D. E., and Kamerow, D. B. "Epidemiologic Study of Sleep Disturbances and Psychiatric Disorders. An Opportunity for Prevention?" *Journal of the American Medical Association,* Vol. 262, No. 11 (September 15, 1989), pp. 1479–1484.

"Forget About Cholesterol?" *Consumer Reports,* March 1990, pp. 152–159.

Gabel, J., et al. "Employer-Sponsored Health Insurance in America." *Health Affairs,* Vol. 8, No. 2 (Summer 1989), pp. 116–128.

Gawin, F. H. "Cocaine Abuse and Addiction." *Journal of Family Practice,* Vol. 29, No. 2 (1989), pp. 193–197.

Glynn, T. J. "Methods of Smoking Cessation—Finally, Some Answers." Editorial. *Journal of the American Medical Association,* Vol. 263, No. 20 (May 23/30, 1990), pp. 2795–2796.

Goldbloom, R. B., and Lawrence, R. S., editors. *Preventing Disease: Beyond the Rhetoric.* New York: Springer-Verlag, 1990.

Goleman, D. "When to Challenge the Therapist and Why." *The New York Times Good Health Magazine,* October 9, 1988.

Hall, R.C.W. and Beresford, T. P. "Bulimia Nervosa: Diagnostic Criteria, Clinical Features and Discrete Clinical Sub-Syndromes." "Anorexia Nervosa: Diagnostic, Prognostic and Clinical Features." *Psychiatric Medicine,* Vol. 7, No. 3 (1989), pp. 13–23; 3–9.

Halperin, J. L., and Levine, R. *Bypass.* New York: Times Books, 1985.

Harrison, W., Endicott, J., and Nee, J. "Treatment of Premenstrual Dysphoria with Alprazolam." *Archives of General Psychiatry,* No. 47 (March 1990), pp. 270–275.

Hein, K., DiGeronimo, T. F., and the Editors of Consumer Reports Books. *AIDS: Trading Fears for Facts.* Mount Vernon, N.Y.: Consumers Union, 1989.

Henderson, D. "Early Detection the Key to Success Against Testicular Cancer." *FDA Consumer,* December 1988/January 1989, pp. 16–19.

Henig, R. M. *How a Woman Ages.* New York: Ballantine, 1985.

Higgins, L. C. "Chronic Pain." *Medical World News,* August 28, 1989, pp. 43–48.

Hillman, A. L., et al. "How Do Financial Incentives Affect Physicians' Clinical Decisions and the Financial Performance of Health Maintenance Organizations?" *The New England Journal of Medicine,* Vol. 321, No. 2 (July 13, 1989), pp. 86–92.

Hogan, N. S. *Humanizing Health Care.* Oradell, N.J.: Medical Economics, 1980.

Horne, J. A. "Sleep Loss and Divergent Thinking." *Sleep,* Vol. 11, No. 6 (1988), pp. 528–536.

Horowitz, L. C. *Taking Charge of Your Medical Fate.* New York: Random House, 1987.

"How Good Is Retin-A?" *Consumer Reports,* February 1989, pp. 112–113.

Hunt, M. "Navigating the Therapy Maze." *The New York Times Sunday Magazine,* August 30, 1987.

Jenike, M. A. "Obsessive-Compulsive and Related Disorders." *The New England Journal of Medicine,* Vol. 321, No. 8 (August 24, 1989), pp. 539–541.

Joint National Committee on the Detection, Evaluation and Treatment of High Blood Pressure. *The 1988 Report of the Joint National Committee on the Detection, Evaluation and Treatment of High Blood Pressure.* NIH Publication No. 88-1088.

Jonas, S., editor. *Health Care Delivery in the United States.* Third Edition. New York: Springer, 1986.

Kaplan, H. S. *Disorders of Sexual Desire.* New York: Simon and Schuster, 1979.

Karasek, R., and Theorell, T. *Healthy Work.* New York: Basic Books, 1990.

Keeler, E., et al. "The External Costs of a Sedentary Life-style." *American Journal of Public Health,* Vol. 79, No. 8 (August 1989), pp. 975–980.

Kenney, R. A. *Physiology of Aging.* Second Edition. Chicago: Year Book Medical Publishers, 1989.

Kolata, G. "Eye Protection Urged After New Study Links Cataracts to Sun Rays." *The New York Times,* December 1, 1988.

Kottke, T. E., et al. "Attributes of Successful Smoking Cessation Interventions in Medical Practice. A Meta-analysis of 39 Controlled Trials." *Journal of the American Medical Association,* Vol. 259, No. 19 (May 20, 1988), pp. 2883–2889.

Kramon, G. "Psychiatric Care: Orphan of Insurance Coverage." *The New York Times,* February 9, 1989.

Krane, R. J., et al. "Impotence." *The New England Journal of Medicine,* Vol. 321, No. 24 (December 14, 1989), pp. 1648–1656.

Kwiterovich, P. *Beyond Cholesterol.* Baltimore: Johns Hopkins University Press, 1989.

Lamberg, L. *The American Medical Association Guide to Better Sleep.* New York: Random House, 1984.

Langsley, D. G., and Signer, M. M., editors. *Hospital Privileges and Specialty Medicine.* American Board of Medical Specialties in collaboration with the American Hospital Association, Evanston, Ill., 1986.

Larson, E. B. "Alzheimer's Disease in the Community." *Journal of the American Medical Association,* Vol. 262, No. 18 (November 10, 1989), pp. 2591–2592.

Larson, E. B., and Bruce, R. "Exercise and Aging." Editorial. *Annals of Internal Medicine,* Vol. 105, No. 5 (November 1986), pp. 783–785.

Lawrence, R. S., Mickalide, A. D., et al. "Report of the U.S. Preventive Services Task Force." *Journal of the American Medical Association,* Vol. 263, No. 3 (January 19, 1990), pp. 436–437.

Levine, R. J. Letter to the Editor. *IRB.* The Hastings Center, Vol. 4, No. 1 (January 1982).

Love, S. *Dr. Susan Love's Breast Book.* Reading, Mass.: Addison-Wesley Publishing Co., 1990.

Manson, J. E., et al. "A Prospective Study of Obesity and Risk of Coronary Heart Disease in Women." *The New England Journal of Medicine,* Vol. 322, No. 13 (March 29, 1990), pp. 882–889.

"Marijuana: What We Know." *Berkeley Wellness Letter,* March 1990, pp. 2–3.

Massachusetts Medical Society Committee on Nutrition. "Fast Food Fare. Consumer Guidelines." *The New England Journal of Medicine,* Vol. 321, No. 11 (September 14, 1989), pp. 752–756.

Masters, W. H., Johnson, V., and Kolodny, R. C. *Sex and Human Loving.* Boston: Little, Brown, 1988.

Mastroianni, Jr., L., Donaldson, P. J., and Kane, T. T. "Development of Contraceptives—Obstacles and Opportunities." *The New England Journal of Medicine,* Vol. 322, No. 7 (February 15, 1990), pp. 482–484.

Matthews, T. J., and Bolognesi, D. P. "AIDS Vaccines." *Scientific American,* October 1988, pp. 120–127.

Mechanic, D. "Consumer Choice Among Health Insurance Options." *Health Affairs,* Vol. 8, No. 1 (Spring 1989), pp. 138–157.

"Medical Research Shows Link Between Fish, Health." *Community Nutrition Institute Nutrition Week,* March 6, 1986, p. 6.

Mehta, J. L., et al. "Aspirin in Myocardial Ischemia: Why, When, and How Much?" *Clinical Cardiology,* Vol. 12 (April 1989), pp. 179–184.

Meyer, J. K., Schmidt, Jr., C. W., and Wise, T. N., editors. *Clinical Management of Sexual Disorders.* Washington, D.C.: American Psychiatric Press, 1989.

Milgram, G. G. *The Facts About Drinking.* Mount Vernon, N.Y.: Consumers Union, 1990.

Miller, A., et al. "Can You Afford to Get Sick?" *Newsweek,* January 30, 1989, pp. 44–52.

Monsen, E. R. "What's New in the 1989 RDAs?" *Journal of the American Dietetic Association,* December 1989, pp. 1748–1752.

Nachtigall, L., and Heilman, J. R. *Estrogen.* Los Angeles: The Body Press, 1986.

National Cholesterol Education Program. *Report of the Expert Panel on Detection, Evaluation, and Treatment of High Blood Cholesterol in Adults.* Public Health Service, National Institutes of Health. NIH Publication No. 89-2925, 1989.

National Commission on Sleep Disorders. *Formation/Correspondence/ Backgrounder.* From the office of William C. Dement, M.D., Director, Sleep Disorders Clinic. Stanford University, Palo Alto, Calif., May 1990.

National Institutes of Health. *Consensus Development Conference Statement: Treatment of Early Stage Breast Cancer.* June 18–21, 1990.

National Institute of Mental Health. *A Consumer's Guide to Mental Health Services.* DHHS Publication No. (ADM) 87-214.

National Insurance Consumer Organization. *The Buyer's Guide to Insurance.* Alexandria, Va.: National Insurance Consumer Organization, 1989.

National Research Council, Committee on Diet and Health. *Diet and Health.* Washington, D.C.: National Academy Press, 1989.

Norton, C. "Absolutely Not Confidential." *In Health,* March/April 1989, pp. 52–59.

Office for Protection from Research Risks, Department of Health and Human Services. *OPRR Reports. Protection of Human Subjects.* Code of Federal Regulations. 45 CFR 46. Revised March 8, 1983.

Office of Economic Affairs. American Psychiatric Association. *Status Report on Developments in the Health Care Industry and the Impact on Psychiatry.* Washington, D.C.: American Psychiatric Association, May 1989.

Olsen, E. "Exercise, More or Less." *In Health,* January/February 1988.

Peck, W. A., and Avioli, L. V. *Osteoporosis—The Silent Thief.* Glenview, Ill.: AARP/Scott Foresman, 1988.

Pesmen, C. *How a Man Ages.* New York: Ballantine, 1984.

Public Health Service. *Healthy People. The Surgeon General's Report on Health Promotion and Disease Prevention. 1979.* DHEW (PHS) Publication No. 79-55071.

Raloff, J. "Revised RDAs Add a Few Good Nutrients." *Science News,* October 28, 1989, p. 277.

Rapaport, E. "Thrombolytic Agents in Acute Myocardial Infarction." Editorial. *The New England Journal of Medicine,* Vol. 320, No. 13 (March 30, 1989), pp. 861–863.

Ravich, R. "Patient Advocacy." In *Advocacy in Health Care,* edited by J. H. Marks. Clifton, N.J.: Humana Press, 1985.

Reade, J. M., and Ratzan, R. M. "Access to Information—Physicians' Credentials and Where You Can't Find Them." *The New England Journal of Medicine,* Vol. 321, No. 7 (August 17, 1989), pp. 466–468.

Redfield, R. R., and Burke, D. S. "HIV Infection: The Clinical Picture." *Scientific American,* October 1988, pp. 90–98.

Regestein, Q., and Ritchie, D. *Sleep Problems and Solutions.* Mount Vernon, N.Y.: Consumers Union, 1990.

Reisberg, B., editor. *Alzheimer's Disease.* New York: The Free Press/ Macmillan, 1983.

Reynolds III, C. F. "The Implications of Sleep Disturbance Epidemiology." Editorial. *Journal of the American Medical Association,* Vol. 262, No. 11 (September 15, 1989), p. 1514.

Riggs, B. L. "A New Option for Treating Osteoporosis." Editorial. *The New England Journal of Medicine,* Vol. 323, No. 2 (July 12, 1990), pp. 124–125.

Riggs, B. L., and Melton III, L. J. "Involutional Osteoporosis." *The New England Journal of Medicine,* Vol. 314, No. 26 (June 26, 1986), pp. 1676–1684.

Robertson, J. A. "Taking Consent Seriously: IRB [Institutional Review Board] Intervention in the Consent Process." *IRB* (The Hastings Center), Vol. 2, No. 5 (May 1982), pp. 1–5.

Rowe, J. W., and Kahn, R. L. "Human Aging: Usual and Successful." *Science,* Vol. 237 (July 10, 1987), pp. 143–149.

Rubinstein, E., and Federman, D. D., editors. *Scientific American Medicine.* New York: Scientific American, 1988, 1989.

Rudman, D., et al. "Effects of Human Growth Hormone in Men Over 60 Years Old." *The New England Journal of Medicine,* Vol. 323, No. 1 (July 5, 1990), pp. 1–6.

Rydman, E. J. *Finding the Right Counselor for You.* Dallas: Taylor, 1989.

Scallet, L. J. "Paying for Public Mental Health Care: Crucial Questions." *Health Affairs,* Vol. 9. No. 1 (Spring 1990), pp. 117–124.

Schnall, P. L., et al. "The Relationship Between 'Job Strain,' Workplace Diastolic Blood Pressure and Left Ventricular Mass Index." *Journal of the American Medical Association,* Vol. 263, No. 14 (April 11, 1990), pp. 1929–1935.

Schneider, I. *Patient Power: How to Have a Say During Your Hospital Stay.* White Hall, Va.: Betterway, 1986.

"Second-hand Smoke." American Lung Association, 1988.

Segal, M. "Should You Take Aspirin to Help Prevent a Heart Attack?" *FDA Consumer,* June 1988, pp. 19–21.

Segal, S. "Mifepristone (RU 486)." Editorial. *The New England Journal of Medicine,* Vol. 322, No. 10 (March 8, 1990), pp. 691–693.

Shlian, J. N., and Shlian, D. M. *Self-help Handbook of Symptoms and Treatments.* Chicago: Contemporary Books, 1986.

Sims, E. A. H. "Destiny Rides Again as Twins Overeat." Editorial. *The New England Journal of Medicine,* Vol. 322, No. 21 (May 24, 1990), pp. 1522–1524.

Smith, W. *The Doctor Book.* Los Angeles: Price, Stern, Sloan, 1987.

Sobel, D. "Social Phobia." *The New York Times Sunday Magazine,* January 1, 1989, pp. 24–25.

Starr, P. *The Social Transformation of American Medicine.* New York: Basic Books, 1982.

Stockton, W. "Can Exercise Alter the Aging Process?" *The New York Times,* November 28, 1988.

Stoline, A., and Weiner, J. *The New Medical Marketplace. A Physician's Guide to the Health Care Revolution.* Baltimore: Johns Hopkins University Press, 1988.

"The Stress-Resistant Person." *Harvard Medical School Health Letter,* Vol. 14, No. 4 (February 1989), pp. 5–7.

Stunkard, A. J., et al. "The Body-Mass Index of Twins Who Have Been Reared Apart." *The New England Journal of Medicine,* Vol. 322, No. 21 (May 24, 1990), pp. 1483–1487.

Sweet, C. A. "Rethinking Eating Out." *FDA Consumer,* November 1989, pp. 8–13.

Thomas, L. "On Magic in Medicine." *The New England Journal of Medicine,* Vol. 299, No. 9 (August 31, 1978), pp. 461–463.

Thomason, J. L., et al. "Pelvic Inflammatory Disease." *Clinical Microbiology Newsletter,* Vol. 8, No. 24 (December 15, 1986), pp. 181–184.

Thygerson, A. L. *Fitness and Health.* Boston: Jones and Bartlett, 1989.

Tomb, D. A. *Psychiatry for the House Officer.* Second Edition. Baltimore: Williams & Wilkins, 1984.

Ulene, A. *Safe Sex in a Dangerous World.* New York: Vintage, 1987.

U.S. Centers for Disease Control. "Estimates of HIV Prevalence and Projected AIDS Cases: Summary of a Workshop, Oct. 31–Nov. 1, 1989." *Morbidity and Mortality Weekly Report,* February 23, 1990.

U.S. Centers for Disease Control. "1989 Sexually Transmitted Diseases Treatment Guidelines." *Morbidity and Mortality Weekly Report,* September 1, 1989.

U.S. Department of Health and Human Services. *Surgeon General's Report on Nutrition and Health.* DHHS (PHS) Publication No. 88-50210, 1988.

U.S. General Accounting Office. *Mental Health: Prevention of Mental Disorders and Research on Stress-Related Disorders.* GAO/HRD-89-97, September 1989.

U.S. Preventive Services Task Force. *Guide to Clinical Preventive Services.* Baltimore: Williams & Wilkins, 1989.

Van Cauter, E., and Turek, F. W. "Strategies for Resetting the Human Circadian Clock." *The New England Journal of Medicine,* Vol. 322, No. 18 (May 3, 1990), pp. 1306–1308.

Vance, M. L. "Growth Hormone for the Elderly." Editorial. *The New England Journal of Medicine,* Vol. 323, No. 1 (July 5, 1990), pp. 52–54.

"The Vitamin Pushers." *Consumer Reports,* March 1986, pp. 170–175.

Walzer, R. A. *Healthy Skin.* Mount Vernon, N.Y.: Consumer Reports Books, 1989.

Watts, N. B., et al. "Intermittent Cyclical Etidronate Treatment of Post-menopausal Osteoporosis." *The New England Journal of Medicine,* Vol. 323, No. 2 (July 12, 1990), pp. 73–79.

Weiss, R. "Wrestling with Wrinkles." *Science News,* September 24, 1988.

Whitbourne, S. K. *The Aging Body.* New York: Springer-Verlag, 1985.

"Who Can Afford a Nursing Home?" *Consumer Reports,* May 1988, pp. 300–311.

Williams, Jr., R. B. "An Untrusting Heart." *The Sciences,* September/October 1984, pp. 31–36.

Williams, R. B. "The Role of the Brain in Physical Disease." Editorial. *Journal of the American Medical Association,* Vol. 263, No. 14 (April 11, 1990), pp. 1971–1972.

Williams, S. R. *Essentials of Nutrition and Diet Therapy.* Fourth Edition. St. Louis: C. V. Mosby, 1986.

Wise, T. N. "The Complaint of Pain." *Primary Care,* Vol. 2, No. 1 (March 1975), pp. 1–8.

———. "Sexual Dysfunction in the Mentally Ill." *Psychosomatics,* Vol. 24, No. 9 (September 1983), pp. 787–805.

Woods, N. F. *Human Sexuality in Health and Illness.* Second Edition. St. Louis: C. V. Mosby, 1979.

Wyngaarden, J. B., and Smith, Jr., L. H., Editors. *Cecil Textbook of Medicine.* Philadelphia: W. B. Saunders, 1988.

Zuercher, A. "A Look at the Latest AIDS Projections for the United States." *Health Affairs,* Vol. 9, No. 2 (Summer 1990), pp. 163–170.

Index